AF247601

PHARMACOLOGY OF STEROID CONTRACEPTIVE DRUGS

MONOGRAPHS OF
THE MARIO NEGRI INSTITUTE FOR
PHARMACOLOGICAL RESEARCH, MILAN

SERIES EDITOR: SILVIO GARATTINI

Amphetamines and Related Compounds
Edited by E. Costa and S. Garattini

Basic and Therapeutic Aspects of Perinatal Pharmacology
Edited by P. L. Morselli, S. Garattini, and F. Sereni

The Benzodiazepines
Edited by S. Garattini, E. Mussini, and L. O. Randall

Chemotherapy of Cancer Dissemination and Metastasis
Edited by S. Garattini and G. Franchi

Drug Interactions
Edited by P. L. Morselli, S. Garattini, and S. N. Cohen

Insolubilized Enzymes
Edited by M. Salmona, C. Saronio, and S. Garattini

Isolated Liver Perfusion and Its Applications
Edited by I. Bartošek, A. Guaitani, and L. L. Miller

Mass Spectrometry in Biochemistry and Medicine
Edited by A. Frigerio and N. Castagnoli, Jr.

Pharmacology of Steroid Contraceptive Drugs
Edited by S. Garattini and H. W. Berendes

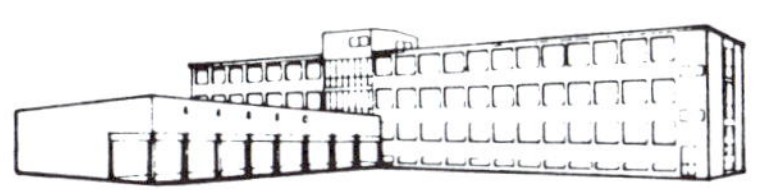

MONOGRAPHS OF
THE MARIO NEGRI INSTITUTE FOR
PHARMACOLOGICAL RESEARCH, MILAN

Pharmacology of Steroid Contraceptive Drugs

Editors

S. Garattini, M.D.
*Director, Mario Negri Institute
for Pharmacological Research
Milan, Italy*

H. W. Berendes, M.D., M.H.S.
*Chief, Contraceptive Evaluation
Branch
Center for Population Research
National Institute of Child
Health and Human Development
National Institutes of Health
Bethesda, Maryland 20014*

RAVEN PRESS ■ NEW YORK

Raven Press, 1140 Avenue of the Americas, New York, New York 10036

Made in the United States of America

Library of Congress Cataloging in Publication Data

Main entry under title:

Pharmacology of steroid contraceptive drugs.

(Monographs of the Mario Negri Institute for
Pharmacological Research)
    Includes bibliographical references and index.
    1.   Oral contraceptives—Physiological effect.
2.   Oral contraceptives—Side effects.
I.   Garattini, Silvio.   II.   Berendes, H. W.
III.   Series: Instituto di ricerche farmacologiche
Mario Negri. Monographs. [DNLM: 1.   Contra-
ceptives, Oral—Pharmacodynamics. QV177 P536]
RG137.5.P5   615'.766   77–6100
ISBN 0–89004–187–3

Preface

Numerous meetings have been organized and many books published in attempts to clarify the mechanism of action of steroid contraceptive drugs. In contrast, relatively little effort has gone into studying their side effects. Particularly felt is the lack of animal models of real use in predicting adverse reactions in women.

It is widely believed that steroid contraceptive combinations are all the same, but, as is shown in this book, there is evidence that the various progestogens do in actual fact differ in their pharmacological properties.

In part, as the result of a program of the National Institute of Child Health and Human Development at the NIH studying the pharmacological effects of steroid contraceptive drugs—in which the Mario Negri Institute has the privilege of taking part—we have attempted to ascertain a variety of current opinions concerning the side effects of these agents. This volume reviews the kinetics and metabolism of steroid contraceptive drugs, effects on the central nervous system, carcinogenesis and immunology, cardiovascular effects, and drug interactions.

We sincerely hope that this volume will be of interest and utility not only to specialists in this field, but also to physicians and health workers whose difficult task it is to assess in individual cases or in the population as a whole, the complex balance between risks and benefits of this treatment; this decision is always delicate, and it is our duty to ensure that it is based on thoughtful appraisal of factual information rather than on emotional reactions.

Silvio Garattini

Contents

Contributors

H. Adlercreutz
Department of Clinical Chemistry
University of Helsinki
Helsinki, Finland

John J. Albers
University of Washington School of Medicine
Department of Medicine
Seattle, Washington 98195

S. Algeri
Istituto di Ricerche Farmacologiche
"Mario Negri"
20157 Milan, Italy

Norma K. Alkjaersig
Department of Internal Medicine
Washington University School of Medicine
St. Louis, Missouri 63110

A. Anaclerio
Istituto di Ricerche Farmacologiche
"Mario Negri"
20157 Milan, Italy

Deborah M. Applebaum
University of Washington School of Medicine
Seattle, Washington 98195
and
Northwest Lipid Research Center
Seattle, Washington 98104

C. Barale
Istituto di Ricerche Farmacologiche
"Mario Negri"
20157 Milan, Italy

C. Wayne Bardin
The Milton S. Hershey Medical Center
The Pennsylvania State University
Hershey, Pennsylvania 17033

Etienne-Emile Baulieu
Unité de Recherches sur le Métabolisme
Moléculaire et la Physio-Pathologie des
Stéroides de l'Institut National de la
Santé et de la Recherche Médicale
Département de Chimie Biologique
Faculté de Médecine Paris-Sud
94270 Bicêtre, France

S. Beier
Department of Endocrine Pharmacology
Schering AG Berlin/Bergkamen
1000 Berlin 65, West Germany

Heinz W. Berendes
Contraceptive Evaluation Branch
Center for Population Research
National Institute of Child Health and
Human Development
National Institutes of Health
Bethesda, Maryland 20014

R. von Berswordt-Wallrabe
Department of Endocrine Pharmacology
Schering AG Berlin/Bergkamen
1000 Berlin 65, West Germany

A. Bizzi
Istituto di Ricerche Farmacologiche
"Mario Negri"
20157 Milan, Italy

Hermann-Maximilian Bolt
Institute of Toxicology
University of Tübingen
D–7400 Tübingen, West Germany

Mechthild Bolt
Institute of Toxicology
University of Tübingen
D–7400 Tübingen, West Germany

M. Bonati
*Istituto di Ricerche Farmacologiche
"Mario Negri"
20157 Milan, Italy*

W. E. Braselton
*Departments of Endocrinology and Obstetrics and Gynecology
Medical College of Georgia
Augusta, Georgia 30902*

A. Breckenridge
*Department of Pharmacology and Therapeutics
University of Liverpool
Liverpool L69 3BX, England*

Heinz Breuer
*Institut für Klinische Biochemie
Universität Bonn
D 5300 Bonn-Venusberg, West Germany*

Terry R. Brown
*Departments of Pharmacology and Medicine
The Milton S. Hershey Medical Center
The Pennsylvania State University
Hershey, Pennsylvania 17033*

John D. Brunzell
*University of Washington School of Medicine
Department of Medicine
Seattle, Washington 98195
and
Veterans Administration Hospital
Division of Metabolism
Seattle, Washington 98108*

Leslie P. Bullock
*The Milton S. Hershey Medical Center
The Pennsylvania State University
Hershey, Pennsylvania 17033*

Robert Burstein
*Department of Obstetrics and Gynecology
Washington University School of Medicine
and
Jewish Hospital
St. Louis, Missouri 63110*

L. Cantoni
*Istituto di Ricerche Farmacologiche
"Mario Negri"
20157 Milan, Italy*

P. W. Concannon
*Department of Animal Science
Cornell University
Ithaca, New York 14853*

S. Beach Conger
*South of Market Health Center
San Francisco, California 94122*

M. Curcio
*Istituto di Ricerche Farmacologiche
"Mario Negri"
20157 Milan, Itlay*

W. Elger
*Department of Endocrine Pharmacology
Schering AG Berlin/Bergkamen
1000 Berlin 65, West Germany*

J. O. Ellegood
*Departments of Endocrinology and Obstetrics and Gynecology
Medical College of Georgia
Augusta, Georgia 30902*

S. El Mahgoub
*Department of Gynecology
Ain Shams University
Cairo, United Arab Republic*

Jack Fishman
*Institute for Steroid Research
Montefiore Hospital and Medical Center
Bronx, New York 10467
and
Department of Biochemistry
Albert Einstein College of Medicine
Bronx, New York 10461*

Anthony P. Fletcher
*Department of Internal Medicine
Washington University School of Medicine
St. Louis, Missouri 63110*

Edward H. Fowler
University of Rochester Cancer Center
Division of Laboratory Animal Medicine
and
Department of Pathology
University of Rochester School of Medicine
and Dentistry
Rochester, NY 14642

Claude Gagne
University of Washington School of Medicine
Division of Metabolism, Endocrinology, and Gerontology
Seattle, Washington 98195

S. Garattini
Istituto di Ricerche Farmacologiche "Mario Negri"
20157 Milan, Italy

Andrew P. Goldberg
University of Washington School of Medicine
Department of Medicine
Seattle, Washington 98195
and
Veterans Administration Hospital
Division of Metabolism
Seattle, Washington 98108

Frances Gotcsik
University of Rochester Cancer Center
Division of Laboratory Animal Medicine
and
Department of Pathology
University of Rochester School of Medicine
and Dentistry
Rochester, New York 14642

K-J. Gräff
Department of Endocrine Pharmacology
Schering AG Berlin/Bergkamen
1000 Berlin 65, West Germany

Frank E. Greene
The Milton S. Hershey Medical Center
The Pennsylvania State University
Hershey, Pennsylvania 17033

G. Guiso
Istituto di Ricerche Farmacologiche "Mario Negri"
20157 Milan, Italy

Chhanda Gupta
The Milton S. Hershey Medical Center
The Pennsylvania State University
Hershey, Pennsylvania 17033

William Hansel
Department of Animal Science
Cornell University
Ithaca, New York 14853

Robert A. Hatcher
Emory University Family Planning Program
Emory University School of Medicine
Atlanta, Georgia 30322

William R. Hazzard
University of Washington School of Medicine
Department of Medicine
Seattle, Washington 98195
and
Northwest Lipid Research Clinic
Seattle, Washington 98104
and
Harborview Medical Center
Seattle, Washington 98104

J. Joanne Hoover
University of Washington School of Public Health and Community Medicine
Department of Biostatistics
Seattle, Washington 98195

Samson Jacob
The Milton S. Hershey Medical Center
The Pennsylvania State University
Hershey, Pennsylvania 17033

A. Jori
Istituto di Ricerche Farmacologiche "Mario Negri"
20157 Milan, Italy

Hermann Kappus
Institute of Toxicology
University of Tübingen
D–7400 Tübingen, West Germany

Clifford R. Kay
Royal College of General Practitioners
Manchester Research Unit
Manchester M20 OTR, England

H. Ladinsky
Instituto di Ricerche Farmacologiche
"Mario Negri"
20157 Milan, Italy

T. J. Lin
Departments of Endocrinology and Obstet-
rics and Gynecology
Medical College of Georgia
Augusta, Georgia 30902

Yen Chiu Lin
The Milton S. Hershey Medical Center
The Pennsylvania State University
Hershey, Pennsylvania 17033

C. Longcope
Worcester Foundation for Experimental
Biology
Shrewsbury, Massachusetts 01545

V. B. Mahesh
Departments of Endocrinology and Obstet-
rics and Gynecology
Medical College of Georgia
Augusta, Georgia 30902

J. I. Mann
Department of Social and Community
Medicine
University, Oxford
Oxford, OX1 3QN, England

A. Mantovani
Istituto di Ricerche Farmacologiche
"Mario Negri"
20157 Milan, Italy

F. Martin
Department of Biochemistry
Trinity College
Dublin 2, Ireland

K. McEntee
Department of Animal Science
Cornell University
Ithaca, New York 14853

M. Mehring
Department of Endocrine Pharmacology
Schering AG Berlin/Bergkamen
1000 Berlin 65, West Germany

T. M. Mills
Departments of Endocrinology and Obstet-
rics and Gynecology
Medical College of Georgia
Augusta, Georgia 30902

M. L. Moras
Istituto di Ricerche Farmacologiche
"Mario Negri"
20157 Milan, Italy

Neal A. Musto
The Milton S. Hershey Medical Center
The Pennsylvania State University
Hershey, Pennsylvania 17033

W. Mützel
Research Laboratories of Schering AG,
Berlin/Bergkamen
1000 Berlin 65, West Germany

David Nahrwold
The Milton S. Hershey Medical Center
The Pennsylvania State University
Hershey, Pennsylvania 17033

Zuher Naib
Cytology Department
Grady Memorial Hospital
Atlanta, Georgia 30303

Baiba Norton
Institute for Steroid Research
Montefiore Hospital and Medical Center
Bronx, New York 10467
and

Department of Biochemistry
Albert Einstein College of Medicine
Bronx, New York 10461

Howard W. Ory
Family Planning Evaluation Division
Bureau of Epidemiology
Center for Disease Control
Atlanta, Georgia 30333

Juraj Osterman
The Milton S. Hershey Medical Center
The Pennsylvania State University
Hershey, Pennsylvania 17033

Frederick A. Pellegrin
Kaiser-Permanente Medical Center
Walnut Creek, California 94596

Eric Peritz
Kaiser-Permanente Medical Center
Walnut Creek, California 94596

N. Polentarutti
Istituto di Ricerche Farmacologiche
"Mario Negri"
20157 Milan, Italy

F. Ponzio
Istituto di Ricerche Farmacologiche
"Mario Negri"
20157 Milan, Italy

Savitri Ramcharan
Kaiser-Permanente Medical Center
Walnut Creek, California 94596

Carolyn Reed
University of Rochester Cancer Center
Division of Laboratory Animal Medicine
and
Department of Pathology
University of Rochester School of Medicine
and Dentistry
Rochester, New York 14642

Patricia Reichhart
University of Rochester Cancer Center
Division of Laboratory Animal Medicine
and

Department of Pathology
University of Rochester School of Medicine
and Dentistry
Rochester, New York 14642

Herbert Remmer
Institute of Toxicology
University of Tübingen
D–7400 Tübingen, West Germany

M. Salmona
Istituto di Ricerche Farmacologiche
"Mario Negri"
20157 Milan, Italy

Madhabananda Sar
Departments of Anatomy and Pharmacology
Laboratories for Reproductive Biology
University of North Carolina at Chapel Hill
Chapel Hill, North Carolina 27514

M. Sironi
Istituto di Ricerche Farmacologiche
"Mario Negri"
20157 Milan, Italy

F. Spreafico
Istituto di Ricerche Farmacologiche
"Mario Negri"
20157 Milan, Italy

Walter E. Stumpf
Departments of Anatomy and Pharmacology
Laboratories for Reproductive Biology
University of North Carolina at Chapel Hill
Chapel Hill, North Carolina 27514

F. M. Sturtevant
Searle Laboratories
G. D. Searle & Company
Chicago, Illinois 60680

A. M. Tacconi
Istituto di Ricerche Farmacologiche
"Mario Negri"
20157 Milan, Italy

A. Tagliabue
Istituto di Ricerche Farmacologiche "Mario Negri"
20157 Milan, Italy

Carl W. Tyler, Jr.
Family Planning Evaluation Division
Bureau of Epidemiology
Center for Disease Control
Atlanta, Georgia 30333

Thurma Vaughan
University of Rochester Cancer Center
Division of Laboratory Animal Medicine
and
Department of Pathology
University of Rochester School of Medicine
and Dentistry
Rochester, New York 14642

A. Vecchi
Istituto di Ricerche Farmacologiche "Mario Negri"
20157 Milan, Italy

E. Veneroni
Istituto di Ricerche Farmacologiche "Mario Negri"
20157 Milan, Italy

Patricia W. Wahl
Univeristy of Washington School of Public Health and Community Medicine
Department of Biostatistics
Seattle, Washington 98195

K. I. H. Williams
Worcester Foundation for Experimental Biology
Shrewsbury, Massachusetts 01545

Winfield T. Williams
Kaiser-Permanente Medical Center
Walnut Creek, California 94596

Pharmacology of Steroid Contraceptive Drugs
edited by S. Garattini and H. W. Berendes.
Raven Press, New York © 1977.

Oral Contraceptives—The Clinical Perspective

Clifford R. Kay

*Royal College of General Practitioners, Manchester Research Unit,
Manchester, M20 OTR, England*

The oral contraception study of the Royal College of General Practitioners started in 1968. Approximately 1,400 doctors participated, and between them they recruited for observation, between May 1968 and July 1969, 23,000 takers (pill users) and 23,000 controls. The takers and controls were matched for age, and they had to be either married or living as married. The object of the study is to compare the total reported morbidity in the takers with that of the controls. The study will continue at least until 1978.

The first major report on this study was published in 1974 and analyzed the data collected during the first 4 years of observation. In this chapter I summarize some of the more important findings.

METHOD

It is important to understand that this study is in no way a clinical trial. It is better described as a study of the natural history of two large groups of women, one of which had chosen the "pill" as a method of contraception, while the other had chosen other contraceptives or none at all. Women who choose the pill are likely to be different from those who do not. We must expect their differences to affect their respective morbidity, and so it was important to record the characteristics of all the takers and controls.

Characteristics of the Cohorts

The social status of the two groups was remarkably similar, but the takers had a higher parity. They also smoked on average 22% more cigarettes and smoked more heavily, a finding we published in 1969. The takers had a better medical history. This was due to selection—selection by the doctors in advising women with certain illnesses not to take the pill, and by the patients since women with certain illnesses have a lower fertility and a lesser need for contraception. The most extreme example of this is a woman who has had a hysterectomy.

Standardization

It would be wrong to compare the incidence of illness in the takers with that in the controls without making allowance for these differences, and this has been done by the process of standardization. The disease episode rates reported in takers and controls have been adjusted to the rate that would have occurred if takers and controls had been identical in respect to age, social status, parity, and cigarette consumption. The difference in previous medical history was allowed for usually by excluding from the analyses of a particular illness all women with a history of that illness prior to recruitment.

Calculation of Rates

For every illness reported in takers, the number of episodes of that illness is divided by the total observation period of the takers, giving a rate per thousand women-years. This rate is then standardized in the way I described and is divided by the standardized rate of the same illness in the controls. This gives the ratio of the standardized rates, i.e., the relative risk or benefit of taking the pill.

The experience of a pill user is included in the taker category only as long as she remains on the pill. Any woman who stopped the pill was included in a group of ex-takers, and their experience was analyzed separately. Generally the observations were very similar to those of the controls, and indeed they provide a useful additional control group. For the sake of simplicity, however, I do not include them here. The total period of observation at this stage of the study is approximately 35,000 women-years in takers and 42,000 women-years in controls.

Pregnancy affects the incidence of many diseases and almost certainly affects the reporting of others. Since a large number of the controls became pregnant and few pregnancies are included in the observation of takers, it would give a false impression to compare takers with controls without making allowance for pregnancy. To do this, all events reported during pregnancy or the puerperium, together with the associated period of observation, have been entirely excluded from all the data I am displaying.

Bias

One of the most important ways in which this study differs from a clinical trial is that the agent under investigation (i.e., the pill) could not be administered blindly. In other words, both doctors and their patients had to know if the pill was being used. As a result, it must be expected that the observations are biased, and it is impossible to interpret the findings without considering the likely types and extent of bias involved.

There are two main categories: diagnostic bias deriving from the doctor, and reporting bias deriving from the patient. Diagnostic bias may be considered under two main headings. It is possible that doctors may be more likely to diagnose all illness in their takers more often than in their controls because they have a special concern for their oral contraceptive users and perhaps an especially good relationship with them. In fact there is no evidence in the study that this has occurred, since in the majority of illnesses there is no important difference between the rates reported in the takers and those in the controls. However, where specific illnesses are known to be affected by use of the pill, you would expect doctors to be particularly careful to look for these conditions in pill users and to be more likely to diagnose them than in the case of nonusers. Again, there is no good evidence that this has happened, since in some instances the differences between takers and controls are much less than would have been generally expected, e.g., depression. In other instances (e.g., venous thromboembolism) the size of the risk found in this study corresponds almost exactly with that determined by different methods in the retrospective studies.

However, one type of diagnostic bias has occurred. Doctors usually give their pill users routine examinations at regular intervals, and so asymptomatic conditions are more likely to be reported for takers than for controls. The diagnosis of hypertension is a particularly important example of this screening effect.

There is evidence, however, that women who are using oral contraceptives are more likely to report illnesses than nonusers. For example, they have more opportunity to do so since they have to see the doctor to obtain their prescriptions for the pill. A random sample of takers were analyzed to determine the number of episodes of illness reported on the same day a pill prescription was issued. Eighteen percent of reported illnesses fell into this category.

An illness can be reported on the same day a pill prescription was issued in three circumstances. A woman may report her illness then because she happens to be getting her prescription on that day, or she can get her prescription because she happens to be consulting her doctor about an illness. Finally, when she is getting her prescription, she may report an illness she otherwise would never have brought to the attention of her doctor. Only reports of illness in the last category can be considered biased, and thus the amount of *bias* arising from this source must be substantially less than the total of 18% of illnesses that were reported on the prescription date.

It is more difficult to assess the reports of illness arising from the psychological reactions to the use of the pill, but it is possible to describe those illnesses most likely to be overreported in this way. They are generally the common and more trivial conditions, particularly those where the diagnosis is ill-defined, as well as those which are frequently never reported to doctors, e.g., colds, headaches, and migraine. It must be obvious that gynecological disorders are also more likely to be reported by oral contraceptive users than by nonusers.

It is important to realize that all forms of diagnostic and reporting bias lead predominantly to overreporting in takers. This means that adverse effects of the pill tend to be exaggerated and beneficial effects to be reduced. This must be borne in mind when the results are interpreted.

Magnitude of Bias

The total number of reported episodes of illness in takers was 66,285 and in controls 66,253, making the ratio of standardized rates 1.19 ($p < 0.01$). The ratio shows that 19% more episodes of illness were reported in the takers than in the controls. Out of several thousand morbidity categories analyzed, only a very small proportion showed any evidence of a pharmacological relationship to the pill. Thus the overall excess of 19% of episodes reported in takers must be predominantly due to bias. Indeed it is reasonable to assume that 19% is the average bias prevailing throughout the study. In some illnesses the bias is much less, and in others it is certainly much more, but the 19% difference is a useful guideline for assessing the amount of bias likely to be present in the reporting of any particular illness.

Presentation of Data

These data are important for another reason, since they show the way in which I present all the morbidity data. The relative risk or benefit of pill usage is recorded as the *ratio* of the rates, and its level of statistical significance is also reported in each case. In order to give you some idea of the confidence that can be placed in this ratio, the *number* of episodes reported for takers and controls is also shown.

CRITERIA FOR DETERMINING PHARMACOLOGICAL EFFECT

How then do we decide whether a reported difference between takers and controls is due to bias or to the pharmacological effect of the pill? First we consider the size of the difference. In general, a big difference is more likely than a small difference to be due to a pharmacological effect. Next we consider if the difference could have occurred by chance, and this is assessed by use of a statistical test. It is easy to exaggerate the importance of statistical tests, and in this study in particular, where large numbers of episodes are reported, the test often gives highly significant results for small differences that can be largely explained by bias. We already considered how bias can be assessed, but it is particularly valuable if differences can be shown within the taker group, where the biases arising between takers and controls do not of course apply.

In theory, a clear relationship to the estrogen or progestogen dose is very good evidence of a pharmacological effect. In practice, the problem is extremely complicated, since there are two types of estrogen and eight or nine different progestogens, each of which has a different potency. This means that a simple comparison of dosage cannot be wholly convincing. However, since in most diseases there is no evidence of any relationship to dosage, it has been assumed that where a relationship is evident it increases the likelihood that the pill is having some pharmacological influence on the illness being considered. No *greater* importance can be attached to the observation.

If the incidence of a particular illness shows a relationship to the length of time the oral contraceptive has been in use, the possibility that the pill is having a pharmacological influence is increased. Care must be taken, however, to exclude the possibility that there has been a change in the incidence of the condition in the community during the period of observation, and this is determined by examining changes in incidence occurring during the study in the controls. Furthermore, some apparent changes of incidence in takers can be due to changes in the diagnostic habits of the participating doctors rather than the effect of the pill, and this has happened in the reporting of hypertension.

Finally, we must take into account the results from other studies. Any apparent, newly discovered effect of the pill must be advanced with great caution; but if the observations are in close agreement with those of other studies, they can be presented with much greater confidence.

Therefore, with some idea of the methods used and the ways in which the results have been interpreted, we can now examine in detail the observations reported to us about the illnesses experienced by the takers and controls. I present these generally in the order in which they occur in the International Classification of Diseases.

ILLNESSES REPORTED BY TAKERS AND CONTROLS

General Infections

Some commonly occurring infections (Table 1) have an increased rate of reporting in the takers. Chickenpox is an unpleasant and well-defined condition when it occurs in an adult. It is unlikely to be subject to biased reporting, and it shows the greatest excess of this group of diseases. Herpes simplex and rubella are much less serious illnesses, and the diagnosis may often be uncertain, so they are much more likely to be biased. The same remarks apply to mumps, Bornholm disease, and infectious mononucleosis; but here in addition the differences observed are not statistically significant. Taken together, however, they suggest the possibility that some virus infections may be increased in pill users, although the evidence that chickenpox is influenced by use of the pill is somewhat stronger.

Chickenpox and Parity

The relationship to parity (Fig. 1) in the takers did not occur in the controls. Chickenpox is less likely to occur in takers as the family size increases, and this

TABLE 1. *General infections*

Infection	Takers	Controls	Ratio
Chickenpox	35	23	1.81 ($p < 0.05$)
Herpes simplex	145	123	1.54 ($p < 0.01$)
Rubella	102	74	1.49 ($p < 0.01$)
Mumps	63	59	1.40
Bornholm disease	12	8	1.61
Infectious mononucleosis	18	13	1.48

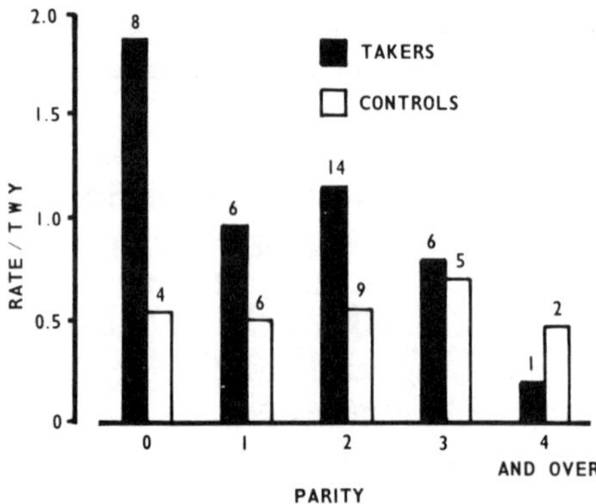

FIG. 1. Chickenpox and parity.

could be explained by the theory that the pill diminishes immunity to chickenpox developed during childhood. This diminished immunity would, however, be boosted in an adult if her children were infected; and the larger the number of children, the greater is the chance that a mother's immunity would be increased. Thus takers who had a large family before they were recruited to the study are likely to have a higher immunity to chickenpox than those with a smaller family. It is very unlikely that this parity difference in takers could be due to bias, which strengthens the view that the pill has a pharmacological influence on the incidence of chickenpox. Moreover, as I suggested, it may have some effect on the incidence of other general infections, although this is unlikely to be of any great practical importance.

Cancer

It is too early yet to come to any conclusions about the relationship of pill usage to cancer (Table 2). The number of cases reported is quite small, but there is no evidence so far, either from this or other studies, that the risk of cancer is increased by the use of oral contraceptives.

TABLE 2. *Neoplasms*

Neoplasm	Takers	Controls	Ratio
Malignant neoplasm			
Breast	11	16	1.08
Cervix uteri	2	4	0.47
Benign neoplasm of breast			
(Fibroadenosis)	290	463	0.80 ($p < 0.01$)
Other benign neoplasms			
Fibroids	28	114	0.41 ($p < 0.01$)
Ovarian cyst	21	69	0.37 ($p < 0.01$)

Benign Breast Disease

On the other hand, it is virtually certain that the pill gives some protection against benign neoplasms of the breast (Table 2). There is a 20% reduction in pill users, which is statistically highly significant. Bearing in mind that bias tends to obscure beneficial effects of the pill, it is reasonable to assume that the pill has a greater protective effect than these statistics indicate; in fact, two retrospective studies suggest that the pill reduces the incidence of benign breast disease by approximately half. This seems to be associated with the progestogen component of the pill (Fig. 2), although we must remember the confusing effect of the different potencies of the progestogens. Figure 3 shows that the protective effect becomes obvious only after approximately 2 years of pill use, which is in agreement with the findings of a retrospective survey.

Other Benign Neoplasms

The other common benign neoplasms are fibroids and ovarian cysts (Table 2). The low rate of fibroids in takers is largely due to selection. The number of controls with a history of fibroids before recruitment was five times as great as the rate recorded for takers; this is almost certainly because fibroids predispose to infertility and so there is a lesser need for contraceptives. We thus have no reason to conclude that the pill reduces the incidence of fibroids.

On the other hand, very little of the low rate of ovarian cysts reported in takers is due to selection, since the history in takers and controls prior to recruitment was similar. Of course the main effect of the pill is to prevent the maturation of graafian follicles, and so it was to be expected that the occurrence of follicular cysts in pill users would be greatly reduced. This can almost certainly be counted as one of the beneficial effects of the pill.

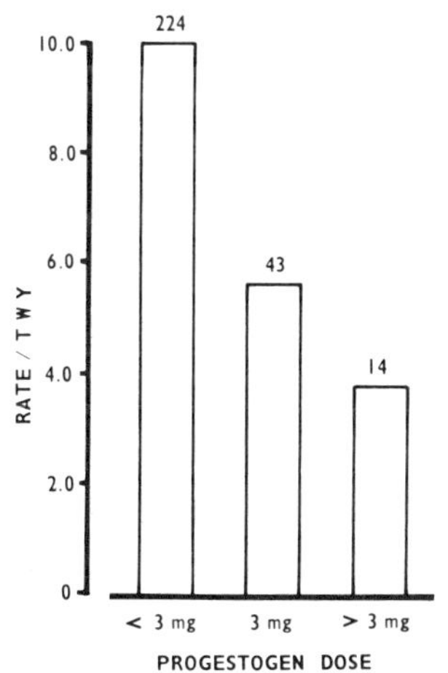

FIG. 2. Fibroadenosis of the breast.

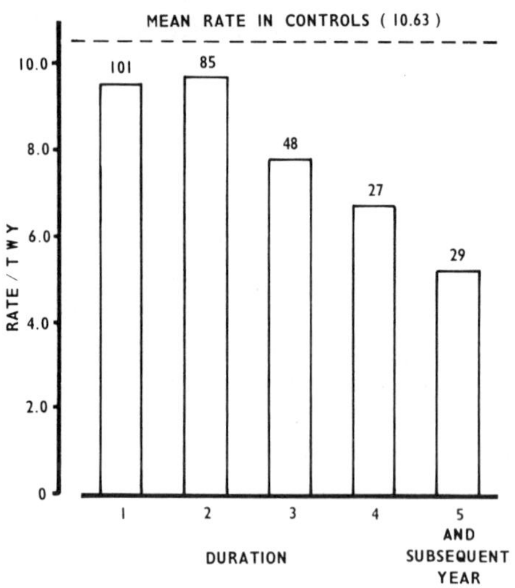

FIG. 3. Fibroadenosis of the breast.

Anemias

Oral contraceptives protect against iron deficiency anemia and conditions described simply as anemia (Table 3). (Almost all of these are of the iron deficiency type also.) This effect is mainly due to the markedly reduced menstrual loss when taking the pill, but there are changes in iron metabolism in pill users which suggest that there may be a more direct effect in addition. There is evidence from several studies that women who use oral contraceptives have lower levels of vitamin B_{12} and folic acid in their serum, but these results confirm that there is no evidence whatsoever that this increases the likelihood of the development of macrocytic anemias.

Endocrine Disease

There is no evidence that the pill affects the development of any endocrine disorder (Table 4), and it is particularly encouraging to see that this also applies to diabetes, although the number of cases is still small. All these data refer to women who developed these disorders for the first time after recruitment to the

TABLE 3. *Anaemias*

Anemia	Takers	Controls	Ratio
Iron deficiency	191	425	0.58 ($p < 0.01$)
Unspecified	323	509	0.76 ($p < 0.01$)
Macrocytic	7	15	0.58

TABLE 4. *Endocrine disorders*

Disorder	Takers	Controls	Ratio
Simple goiter	22	25	1.00
Thyrotoxicosis	33	51	0.72
Myxedema	4	11	0.43
Diabetes	6	8	0.88
Premenstrual tension	220	391	0.71($p < 0.01$)

study. This correction has not been applied to the reports of premenstrual tension where all diagnoses are included, even if they were repeated several times. As expected, oral contraceptives reduce the incidence of premenstrual tension, but the effect is probably less than most people believe.

Psychosis and Depression

There is no indication here (Table 5) or evidence from other studies that oral contraceptives have any effect on the incidence of psychoses.

It is widely believed that the pill causes depression. This term usually means neurotic or reactive depression, and so it may come as a surprise that the number of reports of depression was only 30% higher in the takers than in the controls (Table 5). Even that excess is unlikely to be due entirely to the pharmacological action of the sex steroids.

Depression is a particularly good example of the type of illness that would be subject to above-average bias. It is common, usually not serious, and frequently never reported to doctors. It is also highly subjective. There is no evidence in the study data that the incidence of depression in takers is related to estrogen

TABLE 5. *Psychoses, neuroses, and neurological disorders*

Disorder	Takers	Controls	Ratio
Psychosis			
Schizophrenia	9	15	0.85[a]
Endogenous depression	109	149	0.85[a]
Neurosis			
Depressive neurosis	3,354	2,969	1.30[b]
Loss of libido	372	86	4.54[b]
Neurological disorder			
Epilepsy	9	5	2.64
Migraine	1,082	640	1.99[b]
Tension headache	258	231	1.30[a]
Headache	1,760	631	3.02[b]
Brachial neuritis	50	29	1.92[b]

[a] $p < 0.05$.
[b] $p < 0.01$.

or progestogen dosage, or to duration of use of the pill. Evidence from other studies where a properly controlled double-blind crossover technique has been used suggests that the pill does not cause any material depression.

One study, however, suggested that women who are on the pill are more likely to be severely depressed than they would have been if they were not taking it. Again, our data fail to support this. The rate of hospital admissions for treatment of depression is not significantly greater in the takers than it is in the controls. Thus the reported excess of depression in Takers could be entirely due to bias. This is important because depression is the illness most frequently recorded as a reason for stopping the pill.

Libido

There is a similar lack of evidence that the excess of reports of loss of libido (Table 5) is due to a pharmacological effect of the pill. However, here we must take into account the fact that loss of libido was reported 4.5 times as often by the takers as by the controls. On the other hand, the likelihood of bias is even greater than with depression, since sexual problems are clearly much more likely to be mentioned by a patient when she is discussing contraception than at other consultations. Moreover, the pill is often started for the first time after a pregnancy, and loss of libido may be related more to the recent pregnancy than to the use of the pill. The best that we can conclude is that pill users *complain* frequently of loss of libido, but that there is no good evidence that this is *caused* by the pill.

Neurological Disorders

The reports of epilepsy (Table 5) consist only of new cases diagnosed for the first time during the period of observation. The numbers are small, and the difference between takers and controls is not statistically significant. However, it is very unlikely that there is any material bias in the reports, so there is a strong suspicion that the pill may be associated with an increased incidence of epilepsy. We need more data and other controlled studies to clarify the issue.

Although the reports of migraine, tension headaches, and other headaches are all increased in Takers, there is no supporting evidence that this is due to a pharmacological effect of the oral contraceptives. The amount of biased reporting is likely to be large, and it is well known that headache is one of the commonest placebo reactions in any drug trial.

Brachial neuritis is a curiosity. I am not sure what the diagnosis means, and perhaps the most curious feature is that the rate is 2.5 times greater in the ex-takers than it is in the controls. No reference to its association with oral contraceptive usage has been found in any of the literature. Perhaps someone reading this will offer a solution.

Cerumen

Another curiosity, but an explicable one, is that the pill significantly reduces reports of wax in the ears by 24%. Since oral contraceptives are known to reduce the secretion of sebum, this should come as no surprise. Most studies suggest that it is the result of the estrogen component of the pill.

Hypertension

Now we come to what I believe is the most important problem associated with the use of oral contraceptives—the development of hypertension. Any direct comparison of the rates reported in takers with that in controls is misleading (Table 6), since takers have their blood pressure checked at regular intervals whereas the controls do not. We are therefore getting diagnoses from the takers as a result of a screening procedure.

Although we must ignore the results reported from the controls, there is still some important and useful information to be gleaned from this study. Figure 4 shows that hypertension in oral contraceptive users appears to be related to the progestogen dose. No other study has found this relationship, and because of the problem of interpreting the effect of different potencies of the various progesto-

TABLE 6. *Vascular disease*

Disease	Takers	Controls	Ratio
Essential hypertension	236	105	2.59[a]
Coronary artery disease			
Acute infarction	5	1	5.22
Other acute	1	2	2.52
Chronic ischemic	3	1	3.55
Angina pectoris	8	8	1.03
Total	17	12	1.80
Cerebrovascular disease	16	4	4.10[b]
Venous thrombosis			
Superficial (leg)	106	87	1.48[c]
Deep (leg)	41	8	5.66[b]
Hospital admissions	10	3	4.84[c]
Other and unspecified	20	9	2.14[c]
Total	167	104	1.87[b]
Other vascular disease			
Raynaud's syndrome	40	16	3.09[b]
Chilblains	134	114	1.48[c]
Capillaries	6	4	2.10
Allergic purpura	8	4	2.47
Spontaneous bruising	12	5	3.14[c]

[a] See text for interpretation.
[b] $p < 0.01$.
[c] $p < 0.05$.

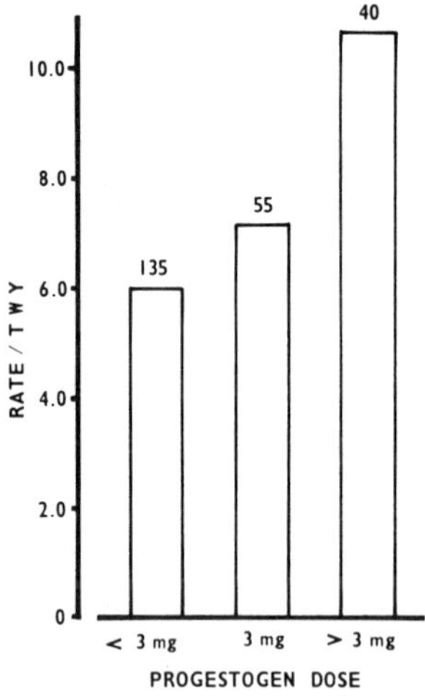

FIG. 4. Hypertension.

gens, this view can be advanced only very tentatively. We found no evidence at all that hypertension was related to the estrogen component.

Estrogen is known to affect the renin-angiotensin-aldosterone system. Indeed all oral contraceptive users show these changes, but they occur quite independently of the development of hypertension. This means that there must be some other mechanism which results in hypertension in a minority of oral contraceptive users, and it is this, as yet undiscovered mechanism which may be mediated by the progestogen component.

There is a well-marked relationship to duration of use of the pill (Fig. 5).

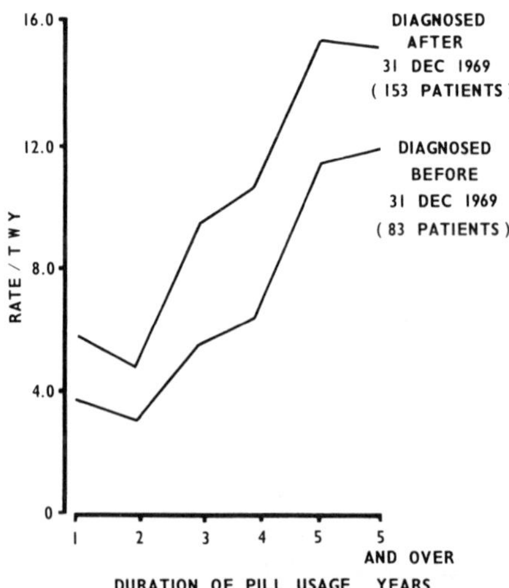

FIG. 5. Hypertension.

Physicians tended to diagnose hypertension more frequently as the study progressed, so here we have considered separately the diagnoses made before Dec. 31, 1969 and those made afterward. The effect of duration of use is quite clear in both cases, and the higher rates reported after December 1969 are almost certainly due to increasingly intensive screening by physicians as they became more and more aware of the problems.

These results are, of course, based only on first diagnoses of hypertension during the period of observation. Over the same period of time there was no increased incidence of reporting of hypertension in the controls.

The development of hypertension in oral contraceptive users is also strongly related to the age of the patient (Fig. 6). In fact, the incidence in women 35 years

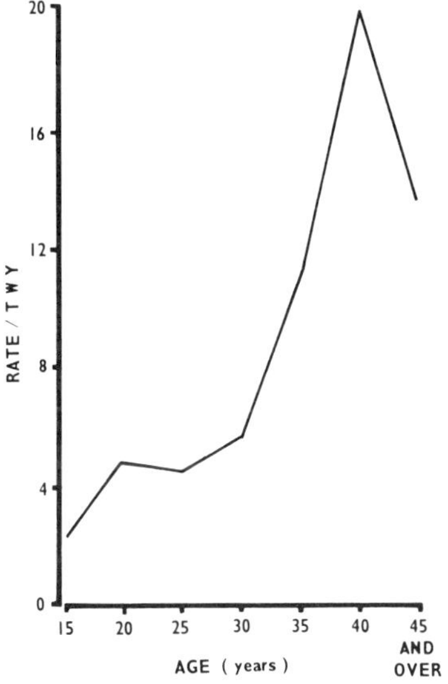

FIG. 6. Hypertension in relation to age in 236 patients. Corrected for parity. Under 35 years: 4.72/TWY. Over 35 years: 13.45/TWY.

of age and over is three times that of younger women. This age relationship has also been shown in other studies.

Fortunately the experience of most observers is that pill-induced hypertension is reversible after the pill is stopped. We have no data on reversibility in this study.

Coronary Artery Disease

The pill causes changes in the serum lipids that resemble the patterns seen in men and which seem to be associated with arteriosclerosis. This raises the possibility that the use of oral contraceptives might be associated with an increased incidence of coronary artery disease. Although suspicion is high, the relationship had not been proved when our report was published, and the number of cases reported in our study is too small to justify any conclusions (Table 6).

Cerebrovascular Disease

The case for cerebrovascular disease, however, is much clearer (Table 6). An increased risk associated with pill usage was found in all four major retrospective studies, and the results of these studies give the best estimate of risk as a sixfold increase. Recently a collaborative study from the United States showed a ninefold increase of thrombotic stroke and a doubling of risk of hemorrhagic stroke. Our own data, although small in number, are statistically highly significant and are consistent with these previous observations.

Venous Thrombosis

The numbers in Table 6 referring to venous thrombosis represent the first diagnosis of this disorder in women with no predisposing cause, i.e., no previous history of venous thrombosis, no recent surgical operations, and no severe debilitating illness. Events occurring during pregnancy and the puerperium are also excluded, as they are from all the other data presented.

The risk of deep thrombosis of the leg is 5.66 times greater in oral contraceptive users than nonusers. This difference is statistically highly significant and is the first confirmation from a prospective study of similar findings in retrospective studies. Superficial thrombosis is increased only approximately 50% in pill users. The main retrospective studies of deep vein thrombosis have been done on hospital cases. Here again our data (Table 6) are in close agreement with those of the previous studies.

In December 1969 the British Committee on Safety of Drugs issued a statement that they accepted evidence that the incidence of venous thrombosis in pill users was related to the dose of estrogen. They estimated that changing to a 50-μg dose of estrogen from a higher dose would result in a 25% reduction of deep vein thrombosis. Our results are in almost exact agreement with that estimate.

The risk of deep vein thrombosis attributable to the pill calculated from our study data is 81 in 100,000 oral contraceptive users per year for those women taking oral contraceptives with a 50-μg dose of estrogen, and 112 in 100,000 women per year for those using pills containing a higher dose. As in other studies we found that the incidence of neither superficial nor deep vein thrombosis was related to duration of pill usage.

Other Vascular Diseases

Table 6 also shows the possible effect of the pill on the microcirculation. Of the three conditions where the difference between takers and controls is statistically significant, chilblains and spontaneous bruising are the sort of vague common illnesses which are probably liable to a considerable degree of bias, but Raynaud's syndrome is a clear-cut diagnosis and an uncomfortable condition which most women would be expected to report to their doctors. Thus there is no reason to believe that it would be subject to an above-average bias, and the result suggests that its incidence is increased as a result of a pharmacological effect of the pill. However, as this observation has not been reported from any other studies, it requires confirmation.

Gallbladder Disease

An association of pill usage with an increased incidence of gallbladder disease has been reported from the United States from a collaborative study centered in Boston. The results here (Table 7) represent the number of women who were

TABLE 7. *Gallbladder disease*

Disease	Takers	Controls	Ratio
Cholelithiasis	49	41	1.37
Cholecystitis	53	46	1.28
Total	102	87	1.32

diagnosed either as having gallstones *or* cholecystitis, and therefore the total of these two diseases represent different women, each of whom was suffering from gallbladder disease. The increased rate in takers is not statistically significant; but since it supports the findings of the Boston study and there is other evidence here of a pharmacological effect of the pill, it seems reasonable to consider the results in more detail. Figure 7 shows that there is a well-defined relationship to the dose of the progestogen.

Cholecystitis shows no relationship to the length of time the pill has been in use, but the formation of gallstones is related (Fig. 8). Obviously gallstones take time to develop, and it is not surprising that the effect does not seem to be apparent until after 2 years of use of the pill, reaching what is probably a maximum incidence after the fifth year when the rate is approximately twice that

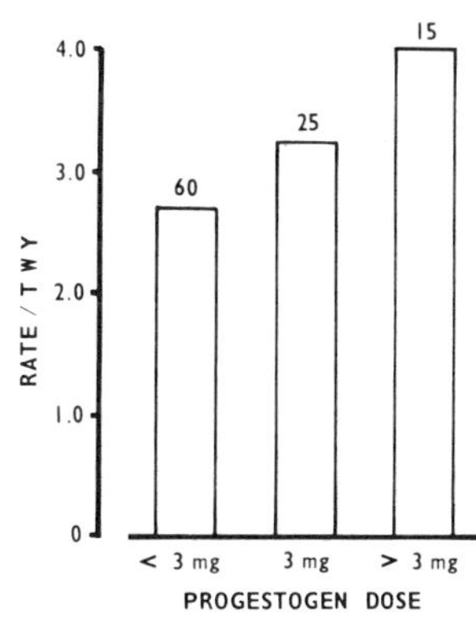

FIG. 7. Gallbladder disease.

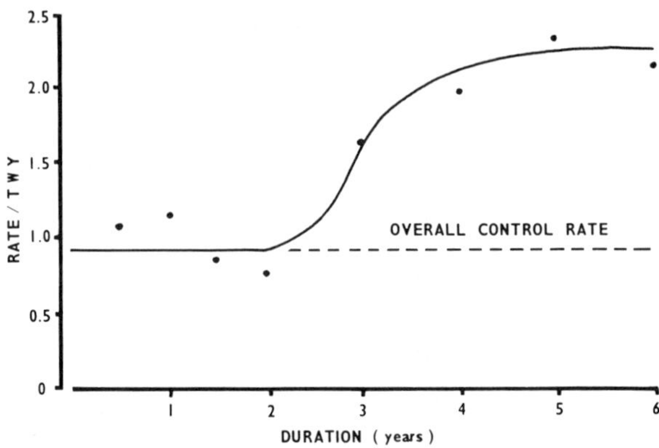

FIG. 8. Gallstone diagnosis in relation to duration of pill usage.

of the controls. The pill is known to reduce the excretion of bile from the liver, and if there is a reduction in the concentration of bile salts and lecithin, cholesterol tends to be precipitated, giving rise to cholecystitis and gallstones.

Urinary Tract Infections

There is a strong clinical impression that women on the pill have many urinary tract infections. Thus the results in Table 8 are slightly surprising in that they show only a moderate excess in the takers. However, the reports are unlikely to be seriously biased because if bias were in operation you would expect that the least well-defined diagnosis would show the greatest difference between takers and controls, and the most specific would show the least. In fact, the opposite has occurred. Furthermore, there is a relationship to the estrogen dosage (Fig. 9), and other studies tend to support the view that there is an increased risk of urinary infection when using the pill.

Vaginal Discharge

All the causes of vaginal discharge (Table 9) are increased in takers, but there is likely to be substantial diagnostic and reporting bias since Pill users have more frequent vaginal examinations than nonusers as well as ample opportunity for

TABLE 8. *Urinary tract disorders*

Disorder	Takers	Controls	Ratio
Pyelitis	396	287	1.54 ($p < 0.01$)
Cystitis	1,980	1,885	1.22 ($p < 0.01$)
Urinary infection	883	897	1.12
Dysuria	87	99	1.08

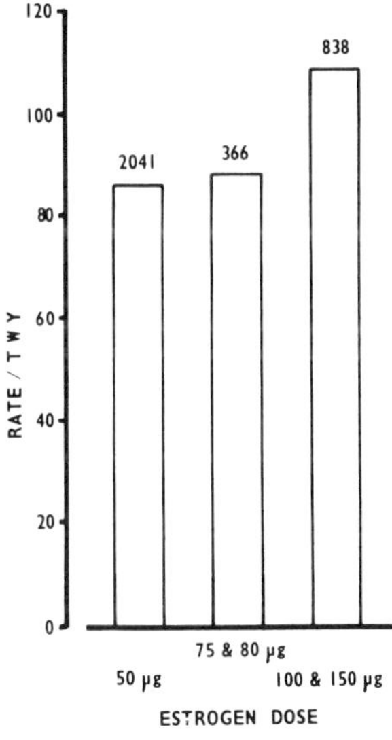

FIG. 9. Urinary tract infection.

TABLE 9. *Vaginal discharge*

Cause of discharge	Takers	Controls	Ratio
Cervicitis	209	144	1.59[a]
Erosion	821	481	1.89[a]
Vaginitis	671	524	1.47[a]
Moniliasis	1,115	661	1.98[a]
Trichomonas	572	397	1.65[a]
Leukorrhea	914	752	1.39[a]
Pruritus ani	91	105	1.21
Pruritus of genital organs	541	349	1.91[a]
Bartholin's cyst	29	35	1.03

[a] $p < 0.01$.

discussing gynecological complaints. Only in the case of cervicitis is there supporting evidence of a pharmacological influence. There is a relationship to the progestogen dose and it increases in incidence over the years; hence it is reported during the sixth year of use three times as often as during the first year. Hospital admissions for the treatment of cervicitis are 50% higher in the takers than in the controls. The evidence from other studies is contradictory, although there is more support for the effect of the pill on an increased reporting of monilia than for the other conditions.

Menstrual Disorders

The pill obviously has a beneficial effect on menstrual disorders (Table 10), with a reduction in menstrual loss and a particularly dramatic effect on the

TABLE 10. *Menstrual disorders*

Disorder	Takers	Controls	Ratio
Scanty menstruation	154	59	2.97[a]
Menorrhagia	430	1,004	0.52[a]
Dysmenorrhea	130	454	0.37[a]
Epimenorrhea and polymenorrhea	66	102	0.83
Irregular menstruation	180	336	0.65[a]
Intermenstrual bleeding	106	178	0.72[a]
Other menstrual disorders	80	132	0.70[b]

[a] $p < 0.01$.
[b] $p < 0.05$.

incidence of dysmenorrhea. Pills containing the lowest doses of estrogen and progestogen result in the least amount of withdrawal bleeding.

Eczema and Related Disorders

There is a suggestion here that the eczemas are commoner in pill users than in the controls (Table 11). The excess may not be due to substantially biased

TABLE 11. *Dermatoses*

Disorder	Takers	Controls	Ratio
Eczema and related disorders			
Seborrheic dermatitis	88	86	1.24
Infantile eczema and related conditions	22	14	1.99
Eczema and dermatitis due to detergents	45	36	1.52
Eczema and dermatitis due to drugs	19	11	2.17[a]
Photosensitivity	23	7	4.26[b]
Other eczema and dermatitis due to other specific agents	104	80	1.50[a]
Other eczema and dermatitis due to unspecified cause	1,323	1,276	1.24[b]
Localized neurodermatitis	58	46	1.59[a]
Erythemas			
Erythema multiforme	9	7	2.71
Erythema nodosum	46	17	3.18[b]
Rosacea	52	25	2.80[b]
Other erythema	20	13	1.80
Psoriasis	161	166	1.15
Pityriasis	60	51	1.39
Other skin disorders			
Alopecia	149	161	1.08
Acne	176	240	0.84
Sebaceous cyst	89	137	0.76[a]
Chloasma	81	71	1.44[a]

[a] $p < 0.05$.
[b] $p < 0.01$.

reporting, since the nonspecific category shows a smaller excess than the specific ones, and this is the opposite of the expected effect of bias.

Photosensitivity is increased more than fourfold in takers. This association has been reported before, so it seems likely that this is a rare pharmacological effect of the pill. Neurodermatitis shows a well-marked relationship to progestogen dose (Fig. 10), which increases the likelihood that we are observing a pharmacological

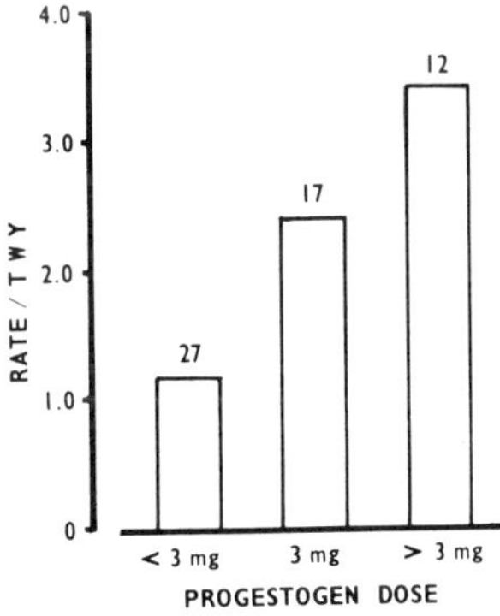

FIG. 10. Neurodermatitis.

reaction. However, as the phenomenon has not been reported elsewhere, it requires confirmation. It cannot be regarded as a serious clinical problem, however. Hence the impression is that the pill increases the sensitivity and reactivity of the skin.

Erythemas

One of the causes of erythema multiforme and erythema nodosum is a sensitivity to drugs, and there is no reason why the sex steroids should not give rise to these reactions (Table 11). Indeed, an association with pill usage has been reported before, and the results here are unlikely to be subject to an above-average degree of bias.

Rosacea also is unlikely to be subject to an unusual amount of biased reporting, but this relationship has not been reported before. Therefore we can conclude only that this is a possible reaction to the pill which requires confirmation by other studies.

Other Skin Disorders

Contrary to many reports, there is no evidence that the pill causes alopecia (Table 11). On the other hand, there is a small excess of chloasma among pill users, and this observation is unlikely to be biased.

Pill users report acne and sebaceous cysts less often than nonusers, and this beneficial effect can be explained by the reduction of sebum secretion when oral

TABLE 12. *Outcome of total pregnancies*

Pregnancy outcome	Ex-takers		Controls	
	No.	%	No.	%
All abortions	542	20.98	909	12.28
Ectopic pregnancy	4	0.15	11	0.15
Stillbirth	20	0.97	89	1.36
Abnormality in baby	78	3.80	236	3.60
Single birth	2,022	98.54	6,416	97.88
Multiple birth	30	1.46	139[a]	2.12
Total births	2,052		6,555	
Total pregnancies	2,583		7,405	

[a] One set of triplets.

contraceptives are used. This is the same mechanism that results in fewer reports of wax in the ears from takers.

Outcome of Pregnancy

Now we come to a different aspect of pill usage—its effect on future pregnancies and future fertility. This series of nearly 2,600 pregnancies occurring after use of the pill (Table 12) may not be large enough to exclude all possible adverse effects, but it is encouraging. There are no material differences between the pregnancies in the ex-takers and those in the controls, except for total abortions. This includes induced and spontaneous abortion.

If, however, we examine the abortion rate in ex-takers in planned and unplanned pregnancies separately (Table 13), we see that the rate in those who wanted the pregnancy is almost exactly the same as that of the controls, whereas those who became pregnant after stopping the pill for all other reasons had an abortion rate of 31%. Obviously the abortion rate is related to the motivation of the patient and not to previous use of the pill.

Fertility

What about fertility? Figure 11 is an analysis of what happened to almost 2,300 women who stopped the pill because they wanted to have a baby. It shows the

TABLE 13. *Abortion related to reason for stopping*

Abortion	Desired pregnancy		All other reasons	
	No.	%	No.	%
All abortions	193	13.37	349	30.61
No. of pregnancies	1,443		1,140	

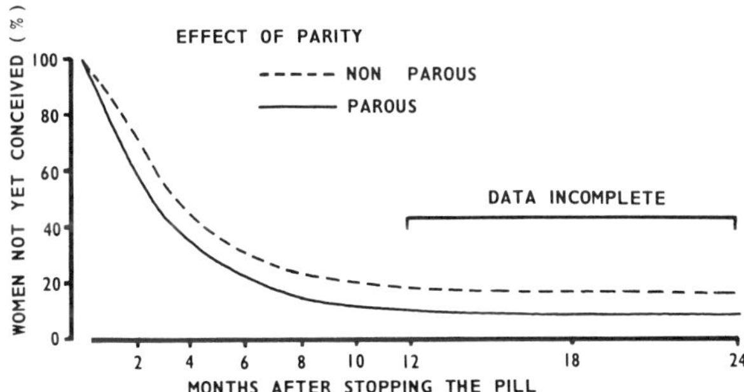

FIG. 11. Conceptions in 2,291 women who stopped the pill to become pregnant.

proportion of these women who failed to conceive month by month up to 2 years after they began attempting pregnancy. By the end of 2 years, the number of women who failed to conceive reached the 10% level, which is accepted as the prevalence of infertility among the general population.

The fertility rate is almost certainly better than this graph suggests, since some women have changed their mind and started to use other contraceptives during this time, and during the second year some pregnancies will certainly have occurred which had not been entered into the computer at the time the data were analyzed.

One snag about these results is that we have no comparable data from the controls. It is possible to present the data, however, in such a way that they can be properly interpreted without the use of controls (Fig. 12). If you take a population of women of average fertility who are attempting pregnancy and plot the conception rates month by month, the most fertile get pregnant quickly. The

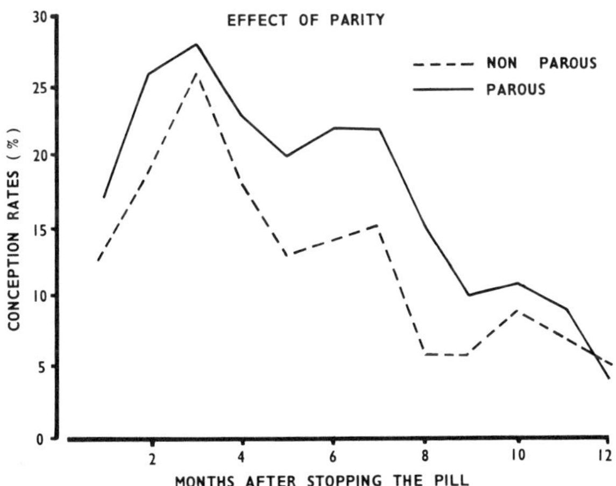

FIG. 12. Monthly conception rates after stopping the pill in 2,291 women desiring pregnancy.

remaining nonpregnant group contains an increasing proportion of infertile women, as those who are fertile conceive and are selected out. In other words, the fertility of the whole nonpregnant population, as measured by conception rates, is highest during the first month and drops steadily during each succeeding month.

Here we plotted the monthly conception rates in the ex-takers attempting pregnancy. The fertility actually increases for the first 3 months, which is almost certainly due to the fact that a proportion of the women are recovering from a temporary subfertility due to the pill. This slight delay in the return of full fertility in some women was also suggested in an American study. We cannot explain the second and third peaks, but they may be due to chance. I must emphasize, however, that in spite of the delay, Figure 12 provides good evidence that the ex-takers catch up and that their fertility by the end of 2 years is not depressed.

Continuation Rates

Among many other analyses included in the report, we examined the way in which the pill has been used and, possibly, misused. As many as 27% of women had given up the pill at the end of the first year, even though they still needed contraception; this result is better than that reported in most studies. The most common reason for giving up in these circumstances is the development of some illness attributed to the pill, although the evidence of any association on the basis of our findings is extremely doubtful.

The use-effectiveness of the pill calculated over the 4 years observation was 0.34 unwanted pregnancies per hundred women years of use.

Effect of the Pill on Disease Reporting

The object of the study was to obtain a comprehensive view of the effect of the pill on health, and Table 14 shows the grand total of episodes of morbidity reported. One interesting and surprising point is that when we bring into the calculations the illnesses associated with pregnancy in the controls it makes very little difference to the relative rates in takers and controls. This is because al-

TABLE 14. *Grand total of reported morbidity*

Pregnancy factor	Takers		Controls		Ratio
	No.	Standard-ized rate (TWY)	No.	Standard-ized rate (TWY)	
Excluding pregnancy	66,285	2,057.35	66,253	1,724.53	1.19 ($p < 0.01$)
Including pregnancy	66,544	1,866.68	73,128	1,546.64	1.21 ($p < 0.01$)

though pregnancy increases the incidence of some illnesses it protects against others and probably reduces the *reporting* of many diseases.

Using the total reported episode rate in takers and controls, we find that takers report on average six episodes of illness every 3 years, and the controls report an average of five. The extra episode of illness, however, is not due to the pill. As we saw earlier, this 19% or 20% excess is almost certainly predominantly due to biased reporting.

THE PILL—GOOD OR BAD?

We know that the pill has some adverse associations and some beneficial ones. How can we balance one against the other? In fact, this is extremely difficult to achieve, but I attempted it in Fig. 13. This shows the differences in the rate of reporting between takers and controls in all those conditions where there seems to be an association with pill usage. I subdivided these into probable and possible associations, but it is not possible in this type of diagram to allow for the varying effect of bias, so I indicated separately those conditions in which bias is likely to be substantial. Now if we exclude these conditions of high bias (i.e., migraine

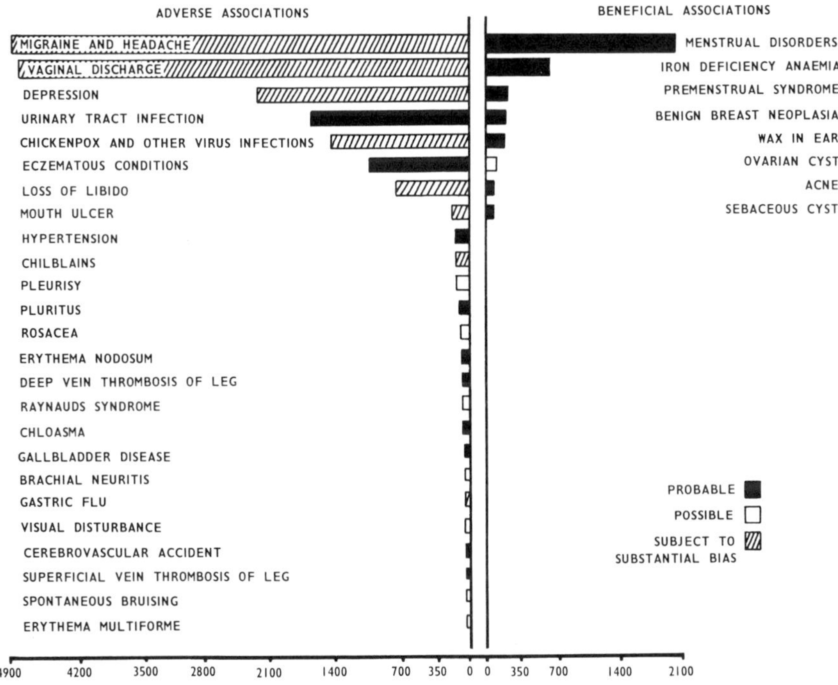

FIG. 13. Oral contraceptives: advantages and disadvantages. Differences in frequency of reporting between takers and controls. Rates/100,000 takers/year.

and headache, vaginal discharge, depression, virus infections, and loss of libido), the beneficial associations begin to balance the adverse ones. Obviously this is not a completely valid comparison because it can give no satisfaction to a pill user to know that her risk of developing hypertension is numerically similar to the benefit she will get from a reduction of wax in her ears, but I think it helps to put into perspective the very small risk of the more serious adverse associations of oral contraceptive usage. If, in addition, we bear in mind that there is no evidence that the pill has any adverse effect on future pregnancies or future fertility, I believe most well-informed women would conclude that the risks of using the pill are well worth taking. The results of much longer observation may, of course, modify this view.

ACKNOWLEDGMENTS

We are deeply grateful to the 1,400 general practitioners who are contributing the data for this survey. The study is supported by a major grant from the Medical Research Council. The costs of the pilot trials and current supplementary expenditure have been met by the Research Foundation Board of the Royal College of General Practitioners. The Board gratefully acknowledge the receipt of funds for research into oral contraception from Organon Laboratories Ltd., Ortho Pharmaceutical Corp., Schering Chemicals Ltd., G. D. Searle & Co. Ltd., Syntex Pharmaceuticals Ltd., and John Wyeth & Brother Ltd.

BIBLIOGRAPHY

Royal College of General Practitioners (1974): *Oral Contraceptives and Health.* Pitman Medical, London. (This contains an extensive bibliography.)

Pharmacology of Steroid Contraceptive Drugs
edited by S. Garattini and H. W. Berendes.
Raven Press, New York © 1977.

Some New Aspects of the Mechanism of Action of Steroid Hormones Implicated in the Control of Fertility

Etienne-Emile Baulieu

Unité de Recherches sur le Métabolisme Moléculaire et la Physio-Pathologie des Stéroides de l'Institut National de la Santé et de la Recherche Médicale, Département de Chimie Biologique, Faculté de Médecine Paris-Sud, 94270 Bicêtre, France

Hormones are informational molecules. These chemical messengers must find, at the target cell level, specific recognition mechanism(s) for selecting them appropriately from all other components of the *milieu intérieur*. These recognition mechanisms, which involve binding sites (*r* in Fig. 1) of very high affinity [dissociation constant (K_D) between 0.01 and 10 nM, adjusted to the low concentration of hormones in the plasma] and strict (stereo) specificity, constitute the primary function of receptors. Parenthetically, the catalytic sites of enzymes also display specificity, but the affinity is 10^4 to 10^6 times lower than that of the hormone receptor binding sites, since substrates such as sugars, amino acids, or lipids, consumed mainly for energy purposes, are found in higher concentrations and are transformed into products. In contrast, the interaction of hormones with their receptors does not alter their chemical composition *per se:* It is a purely "physical" phenomenon.

RECEPTORS: DEFINITION AND STUDIES

Specific binding, even of high affinity, does not define a receptor completely. There are other proteins, particularly in the plasma, which bind hormones rather tightly and specifically (e.g., in the human, transcortin for cortisol and progesterone, and SBP-steroid binding plasma protein for estradiol and testosterone); even if these "transport" proteins are of still obscure *raison d'être,* they are certainly *not* receptors. Indeed the full meaning of the word receptor implies responsibility for interpretation of the received signal (hormone) in terms of cellular response. The binding of the hormone leads to activation of the "executive" site (*e* in Fig. 1) of the receptor, interacting in turn with an "acceptor" component(s) of the cellular machinery which is set up to initiate a cascade of effects known as the overall hormonal response. At the molecular level there is transduction between the *r* and the *e* sites, implying an allosteric transition of the receptor protein. At the organizational (cellular) level, the receptor is the last molecular entity with which the hormone interacts to trigger the response; afterward it may (and indeed

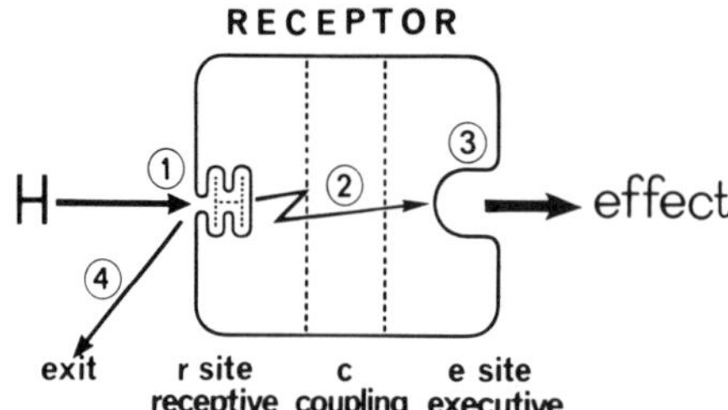

FIG. 1. Steroid hormone receptor. H represents any steroid hormone. It binds to the "receptive" site (1) with high affinity, and there is transduction (2), coupling the hormone binding to activation of the "executive" site (3). The latter may interact with another macromolecule or catalyze some reaction. When this effect is switched on, the hormone has nothing else to do than to leave (4).

does) leave, as indicated by the permanent renewal of hormone in target cells (justifying the continuous hormonal secretion in the intact organism) (1).

Early experiments of Jensen and Jacobson (2) and of Glasscock and Hoekstra (3) demonstrated the selective concentration and retention of radioactive estrogens in their target organs. Further studies during the mid-1960s by the groups of Jensen (4), Gorski (5,6), Segal (7), and our laboratory (8–10) established the proteinaceous nature and the intracellular localization of estrogen receptors, the first hormonal receptors to be demonstrated and characterized. Thereafter similar results were obtained with all steroid hormones of sexual (progesterone and androgens) and adrenal origin (for a decade of research, see ref. 11). The entry of steroids into cells and then the intracellular presence of their receptors contrasts with the location of specific binding to plasma membranes found subsequently for most polypeptidic hormone receptors. A part of the "executive" activity of these membrane receptors is to activate the membrane-bound enzyme adenyl cyclase and to increase cyclic AMP, a second messenger for the cell response. Cyclic AMP does not play a role in triggering the cellular response to steroid hormones.

That the intracellular steroid binding proteins are "real" receptors is likely, but this has not been formally demonstrated since the acceptor to which the receptor executive site corresponds has not been defined in molecular terms. There are three very strong but circumstantial arguments and a fourth which is more direct: (a) There is satisfactory parallelism between the affinities of different steroids (or even of nonsteroidal derivatives) of a given series for the receptor, and their biological activities (weak estrogens have low affinity). Such a correlation does not hold with transport plasma proteins. (b) Receptors are present in target organs although undetectable in normal nontarget organs and in genetically nonresponsive tissues (androgen target organs in the testicular feminizing syndrome). (c) After entry into the cell by a process poorly understood (12), the hormone binds to the receptor, which is found in the cytoplasm, and provokes a change in its properties (4,6); this is termed acidophilic activation (13) and makes the hormone-receptor complex capable of interacting with a variety of polyanions, notably DNA. This effect is probably related to the secondary location of the hormone-receptor complex in the cell nucleus (4,6,14), also designated "neonuclear" receptor (15) (Fig. 2). The final nuclear localization of the steroid hormone agrees well with biochemical studies of the hormonal response, which

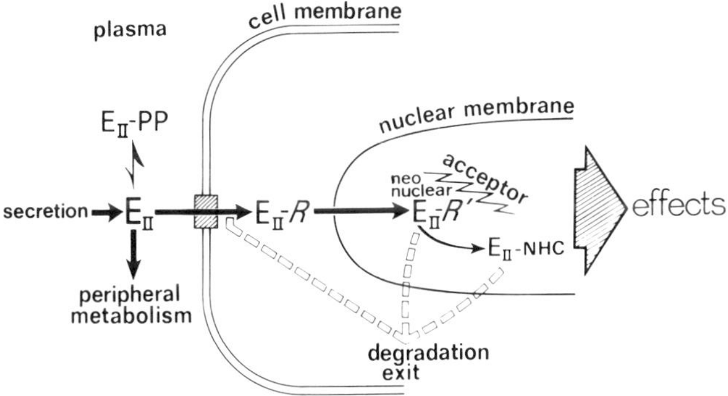

FIG. 2. Natural history of estradiol. Estradiol (E_{II}), taken as a representative steroid hormone, is secreted and circulates in the plasma, mostly bound to specific plasma protein (PP). It is subjected to degradative peripheral metabolism. It is currently believed that free E_{II} enters the cell, perhaps through a membrane-specific step as indicated on the graph. Binding to the receptor (R) leads to its transconformation (R becomes R') and translocation of the complex to a neonuclear position, with binding to an "acceptor" still undefined. The possible role of high-affinity chromatin protein (NHC) is noted here and discussed elsewhere (1). At any moment of its cellular life, estradiol may be degraded and/or released from the cell.

indicates the fundamental importance of gene transcription (again, molecular details are still unknown). (d) In a series of experiments initially developed in our laboratory (16,17), the nuclear gene-transcribing machinery of nonstimulated tissue has been exposed to preparations containing receptor-steroid complexes. There is a hormone-dependent, cytosol-dependent increase in RNA synthesis, a result which, whatever the limitations seen from the molecular biology point of view (1,18), may directly indicate a function for the receptors.

These considerations are basic to the belief that the specific proteins selectively binding the corresponding hormones of a given tissue are receptors, capable of recognition and operational in message execution. Therefore it is tempting to ask if their qualitative and quantitative evaluation may be of practical value in better understanding hormone "receptivity," and consequently if their pharmacological manipulation contributes to better control of cellular functioning in the intact living organism.

The technicalities of these studies involve: (a) correct delineation of specific binding from nonspecific binding (albumin and many other proteins bind all steroids indistinctly with an affinity corresponding to $K_D \geqslant 10^{-5}$M); (b) measurement of the binding affinity and determination of the number of sites per tissue unit (e.g., milligrams of protein or DNA); (c) survey of binding characteristics with different hormonal derivatives and of molecular properties (e.g., sensitivity to SH-blocking agents), not only to assess the proteinaceous nature of the binding but also to differentiate between receptors and plasma proteins (see also ref. 19); (d) evaluation of the available binding sites (unoccupied by hormone at the time of the study and labeled directly by radioactive hormone added to the extract) and/or, often better, total binding sites taking into consideration the endogenous hormone occupying part of them and using an "exchange technique" for this purpose (20); and (e) if possible, estimation of the receptor content of the soluble part (cytosol) and of the nuclear (KCl-extractable and "insoluble") fractions of tissue homogenates. These requirements necessitate precise and rather complex analyses, and warn against "simplified" methods which may indeed be seriously misleading.

PHYSIOLOGICAL CHANGES OF RECEPTOR CONTENT AND RECEPTIVITY

Our studies in the guinea pig demonstrated that the content of progesterone receptor in the uterus varies during the estrous cycle, depending on complex hormonal control (21,22). Progesterone levels in plasma and concentration per uterine cell of the progesterone receptor (whether free or occupied by the endogenous hormone) show cyclic variations which do not parallel one another. Plasma progesterone exhibits an increase at ovulation and a prolonged high level during diestrus (luteal phase). In contrast, the uterine receptor level peaks rapidly at proestrus. However, the maximum value is not maintained long and a decrease follows, so that the receptor level is very low during the luteal phase, even though this is the period when implantation eventually takes place. Incidentally, during pregnancy the receptor concentration is similar to that found in the absence of fertilization, up to the time of implantation.

These observations suggest that, if the progesterone receptors have an obligatory involvement in egg implantation, progesterone available when its receptors are high (around ovulation) may be physiologically important. There is circumstantial evidence that this might be the case, since Deanesly (23) obtained a number of successful implantations in the guinea pig even after ovariectomy, provided ovariectomy was performed after the third day following ovulation (implantation takes place on the seventh postovulatory day).

The increase of progesterone receptor during proestrus is probably attributable to estrogens, and in castrated animals estradiol provokes an important augmentation of binding sites. Such an increase of receptors (suppressible by protein and RNA synthesis inhibitors) (Fig. 3) may be the molecular mechanism of the classic priming of progesterone action by previously administered estradiol (24). The apparent decay of the progesterone receptor induced by estradiol in noncycled (castrated) animals corresponds to a half-life of at least 5 days and does not explain the rapid decrease during the cycle. However, in this model situation where hormonal manipulations are performed easily, progesterone can be injected when receptor is maximum, and indeed it accelerates the decay of binding sites, only 20% remaining measurable after 1 day (22). Therefore during the guinea pig estrous cycle, it is logical to attribute the rapid decrease in the number of progesterone receptors after proestrus to the progesterone of the first luteal peak and possibly to that of the early part of the second peak (Fig. 3). During the diestrous period the progesterone receptor level is even lower than that

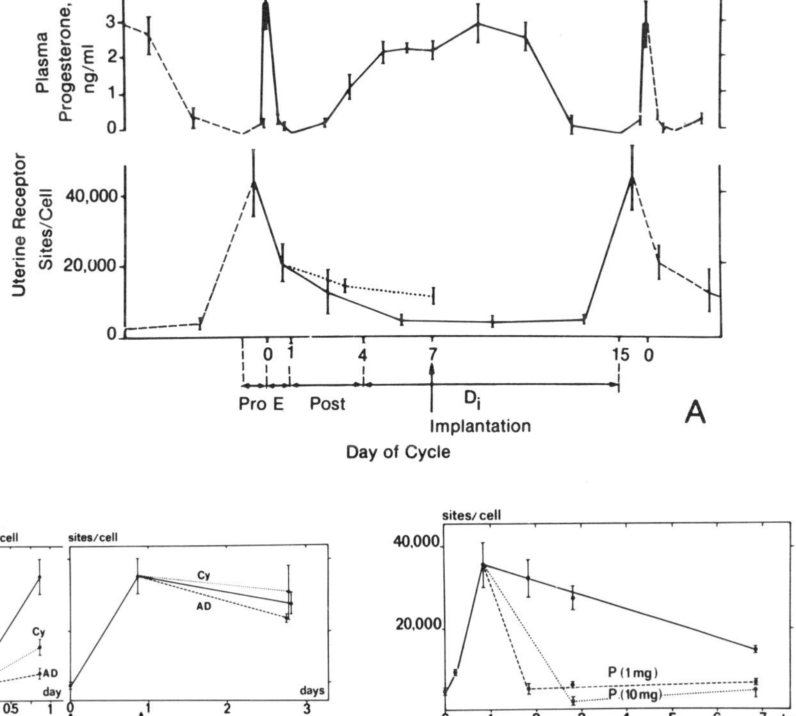

FIG. 3. Changes and hormonal control of progesterone receptor in guinea pig uterus. A: Plasma levels of progesterone over the cycle, and concentration per cell of its uterine receptor. Pro, proestrus. E, estrus. Post, postestrus. Di, diestrus. The case of pregnancy is indicated (. . .). B: Estrogen induction of progesterone receptor in castrated guinea pig uterus. Maximum is approximately 1 day after injection of estradiol (E_2). The negative effects of protein and RNA synthesis inhibitors (Cy and Ad) are shown. The prolonged apparent disappearance of the receptor (half-life 5 days) is shown on the right panel and would not account for the physiological decrease of the receptor observed during the cycle between days 0 and 4. C: Progesterone (P) injected when the receptor is maximum (as in b) accelerates decay of the receptor and therefore may be implicated in its physiological control.

measured in castrated animals not treated by hormone, a fact still poorly understood that some "negative" effect of progesterone might explain. Such results suggest that the high level of progesterone receptor at midcycle may be a target for pharmacological inactivation in order to intercept processes leading to blastocyst implantation. To date, none of the related preliminary observations in humans argue against the possibility of midcycle contraception (25). Estrogen and progesterone receptors are found in human endometrium and undergo variations during the menstrual cycle which are similar to those observed in laboratory animals (25a) (Table 1). Whereas blood progesterone shows only a small increase

TABLE 1. *Receptor concentration and the menstrual cycle phases*

Menstrual cycle phases	Total receptor concentration (fmoles/mg DNA) (mean ± SE)		Cytosol receptor/ nuclear receptor	
	Estradiol	Progesterone	Estradiol	Progesterone
I (days 0–5)	1,144 ± 186	1,100 ± 194	0.95	2.60
II (days 5–10)	2,136 ± 524	1,139 ± 258	0.34	1.70
III (days 10–15)	1,966 ± 385	2,528 ± 537	0.46	2.20
IV (days 15–20)	453 ± 85	1,045 ± 261	0.63	0.77
V (day 20–end)	481 ± 79	758 ± 156	1.21	2.07

at midcycle, there is a relatively high concentration of the hormone in the uterus (J. Ferin, *personal communication*).

Other recent work shows that the uterine estrogen receptor undergoes changes during early pregnancy in the rat (26) (Fig. 4). The plasma estradiol and progesterone levels are elevated. The concentrations of cytosol estradiol receptor were measured separately in the myometrium and the endometrium. There are always

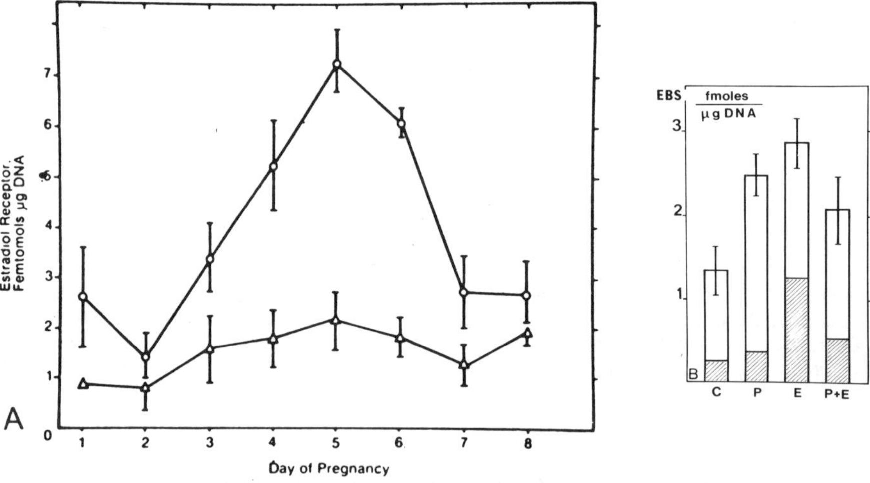

FIG. 4. Changes and hormonal control of estradiol receptor in rat uterus during early pregnancy. A: Concentration of endometrium *(top line)* and myometrium *(bottom line)* estradiol receptor during early pregnancy. B: Estradiol receptor in castrated rats' endometrium *(open bars)* and myometrium *(cross-hatched bars)* in control animals and after various hormonal regimens. It can be observed that (a) estradiol (E) increases receptor in both endometrium and myometrium; (b) progesterone (P) increases estradiol in endometrium but not in myometrium; (c) progesterone abolishes the estradiol-induced increase of myometrium receptor. Therefore simultaneous administration of P + E gives a picture similar to that observed during early pregnancy (3–6 days) when both hormones are increased in the plasma.

more binding sites per DNA units in the latter; they increase markedly in the endometrium after the third day, with a maximum appearing by 5–6 days, whereas the change is modest in myometrium. Implantation in the rat takes place on the fifth day and is not possible either before or after a narrow critical period (27). On the basis of increased estradiol and progesterone concentrations in the blood during early pregnancy, hormones were given to castrated (at day 2 of pregnancy) rats after 3 weeks without treatment. The estrogen-induced increase of estradiol receptor in both endometrium and myometrium is not unexpected. However, it is remarkable that progesterone increases the estrogen receptor in the endometrium (not significantly in the myometrium), whereas when given with estradiol it abolishes the receptor increase provoked by the latter in the myometrium. The relative concentrations of receptor in endometrium and myometrium are remarkably similar in both the physiological circumstances and the progesterone plus estrogen model. The antagonistic effect of progesterone on estradiol receptor induction in the myometrium may favor implantation by decreasing the estrogen-dependent sensitivity to catecholamines and prostaglandin $F_{2\alpha}$ (28).

In conclusion, physiological and hormone-induced changes of receptor concentrations have been demonstrated and will probably be further observed in a variety of tissues and circumstances (including development) (29,30). Indeed recent work with insulin and growth hormone receptors (31) enlarges the concept to nonsteroid hormones. Detailed studies of the relationship between receptor concentration and hormone action are now necessary, as are analyses of qualitative changes (modification of hormone specificity, difference in receptor-genome interactions), which may also occur and be of great importance.

DIFFERENT RECEPTORS FOR THE SAME HORMONE IN DIFFERENT TARGET CELLS

It is not known if the receptor for the same hormone is the same in different target tissues. For instance, is estradiol receptor identical in the endometrium and in the cervical mucosa, or in normal and pathological mammary glands, or in the hypothalamus and the anterior pituitary?

There is already one example showing that a given hormone circulating in the blood may be active in different target tissues through different receptors. The case is relatively easy to demonstrate since testosterone is active in target cells either as testosterone itself [in muscles, levator ani or skeletal (32,33); and in kidney (34)] or after transformation into metabolites such as androstanolone (dihydrotestosterone) in ventral prostate and seminal vesicles (35–37), or as estrogen(s) in the hypothalamus (38). These results suggest a difference between tissues engaged in responding to the same blood testosterone hormone, and such a diversity may be of pharmacological interest, since it may be possible to obtain dissociated activities for various androgens; indeed empirical attempts to separate anabolic properties from virilizing effects of steroids are well known.

DIFFERENT RECEPTORS FOR DIFFERENT HORMONES IN THE SAME CELLS

That estradiol can induce the progesterone receptor (see above) suggests that uterine cells which synthesize it also contain an estradiol receptor. Evidence for two receptors per cell comes from the analysis of cloned cells (MI_1) from a mammary tumor SHI–115 in mice, the growth of which is androgen-dependent, an effect that estrogens antagonize. There are two receptors in these (single type, hopefully) cells: an E (estrogen) and an A (androgen) receptor, binding estradiol and testosterone, respectively, with very high affinity (39). The E receptor does not bind testosterone, whereas the A receptor binds estradiol with relatively high affinity, although lower than that of the E receptor (Table 2). Therefore, referring

TABLE 2. *Presence of two steroid hormone receptors in S-115 mi_1 cells*

Steroid hormone	Androgen receptor	Estrogen receptor
Testosterone	++++	0
Estradiol	++	++++
Diethylstilbestrol	0±	++++

+, relative affinity of the two receptors for different ligands.

to the antiandrogenic effect of estradiol, the problem is to know whether it "passes" through a competitive binding for the A receptor, which would not be "activated" as with testosterone, or if it implicates the E receptor, which either would carry an antagonistic order to a particular site of the genome or would compete with the A receptor for its acceptor site.

DIFFERENT RECEPTORS FOR THE SAME HORMONE IN THE SAME CELL

Incidentally, since in the previous observations it is reported that estradiol binds to both the E and A receptors, this is evidence that two different receptors can bind the same steroid depending on the concentration: When estradiol is low, the higher-affinity E receptor is first occupied, whereas at a higher estradiol concentration the A receptor also begins to be saturated. If the effects promoted by the E receptor-estradiol and A receptor-estradiol complexes are opposite, we may observe a dose-response curve going up initially with increasing concentrations, until values at which the A receptor-estradiol complexes become operative and invert the slope, reproducing a pattern of pharmacological response that is well known but until now not well explained.

It was also remarked that diethylstilbestrol (DES), a nonsteroidal estrogen, binds to the E receptor similarly to the estradiol itself, whereas its interaction with the A receptor is very weak. DES has been known as a perfect estrogen when its activity is tested on the uterus; it is also a widely used compound in cancer therapy (40). Indeed the reported observation suggests that one can dissociate estradiol and DES effects: The presence of E and A receptors binding estradiol can explain a change of slope when estradiol concentration increases; the binding of DES by the E receptor alone leads to the prediction that this change of slope will not be seen with DES.

NEW THERAPEUTIC APPROACHES: RECEPTORS AND RECEPTIVITY, DISSOCIATION OF EFFECTS, AGONISM AND ANTAGONISM

From the above reported data, it follows that one can now re-examine—on biophysical grounds instead of on the basis of global observations—a series of pharmacological concepts of primary therapeutic importance. Receptivity to a given hormone may indeed depend on the amount of the corresponding receptor in target cells. The nonresponse of secondary sex organs to testosterone in the testicular feminizing syndrome (41) and in lymphoma cell mutants resistant to corticosteroid (42) are interesting examples, since no receptor is found in these tissues. There are also good correlations between the hormonal response of breast cancer and the estradiol receptor content (43), and of lymphoblastic leukemia and corticosteroid receptors (44)—results which are of obvious theoretical and practical interest. It remains to be demonstrated if subtle pharmacological manipulations will be of therapeutic and practical interest, as proposed above in the case of contraception.

The induction of steroid receptor by steroid hormones is of great value for explaining "priming," a sort of synergism acquired over a well-defined time sequence. The negative influence of steroids on receptor induction (26), conversely, is a way to explain certain antagonisms between hormones, while other possibilities are the simultaneous presence of different receptors (39) or their competition for the same receptor (45).

Finally, the case is made that one can dissociate responses ordinarily (physiologically) linked by the very nature of a natural circulating hormone. We have seen that testosterone effects are mediated by different steroidal products in target cells, and that all estradiol effects may not be shared by the synthetic DES. These results may lead to new therapeutic advances.

Regulatory proteins, the steroid hormone receptors, provide some of the most advanced models for rational physicochemical and physiological approaches to pharmacological and therapeutic problems. Their purification and complete characterization will undoubtedly lead to even more progress in clinical medicine.

ACKNOWLEDGMENTS

From many references, it is clear that I am indebted to my colleagues for their competent collaboration. The work has been supported partially by the Ford Foundation and the Délégation Générale à la Recherche Scientifique et Technique. I thank Dr. R. Sutherland for help in writing this manuscript.

REFERENCES

1. Baulieu, E-E. (1973): A 1972 survey of the mode of action of steroid hormones. In: *Proceedings of the 4th International Congress of Endocrinology,* edited by R. O. Scow. ICS 273. Excerpta Medica, Amsterdam.
2. Jensen, E. V., and Jacobson, H. I. (1962): Basic guides to the mechanism of estrogen action. *Recent Prog. Horm. Res.,* 18:387–314.
3. Glasscock, R. F., and Hoekstra, W. G. (1959): Selective accumulation of tritium-labelled hexoestrol by the reproductive organs of immature female goats and sheep. *Biochem. J.,* 72:673–682.
4. Jensen, E. V., Suzuki, T., Kawashima, T., Stumpf, W. E., Jungblut, P. W., and De Sombre, E. E. (1968): A two-step mechanism for the interaction of oestradiol with the rat uterus. *Proc. Natl. Acad. Sci. USA,* 59:632–638.
5. Toft, D., and Gorski, J. (1966): A receptor molecule for estrogens: Isolation from the rat uterus and preliminary characterization. *Proc. Natl. Acad. Sci. USA,* 55:1574–1581.
5a. Toft, D., Shyamala, G., and Gorski, J. (1967): A receptor molecule for estrogens: Studies using a cell free system. *Proc. Natl. Acad. Sci. USA,* 57:1740–1743.
6. Gorski, J., Toft, D., Shyamala, G., Smith, D., and Notides, A. (1968): Hormone receptors: Studies on the interaction of estrogen with the uterus. *Recent Prog. Horm. Res.,* 24:45–80.
7. Talwar, G. P., Segal, S. J., Evans, A., and Davidson, O. W. (1964): The binding of estradiol in the uterus: A mechanism for derepression of RNA synthesis. *Proc. Natl. Acad. Sci. USA,* 52:1059–1066.
8. Alberga, A., and Baulieu, E. E. (1965): Concentration élective de l'oestradiol dans l'endomètre chez la ratte. *C. R. Acad. Sci. Paris,* 261:5226–5228.
9. Baulieu, E. E., Alberga, A., and Jung, I. (1967): Récepteurs hormonaux: Liaison spécifique de l'oestradiol à des protéines utérines. *C. R. Acad. Sci. Paris,* 265:354–357.
10. Baulieu, E. E., Alberga, A., Jung, I., Lebeau, M. C., Mercier-Bodard, C., Milgrom, E., Raynaud, J. P., Raynaud-Jammet, C., Rochefort, H., Truong, H. and Robel, P. (1971): Metabolism and protein binding of sex steroids in target organs: An approach to the mechanism of hormone action. *Recent Prog. Horm. Res.,* 27:351–419.
11. Raspé, G., editor (1971): *Advances in the Biosciences,* Vol. 7. Pergamon Press-Vieweg, Oxford.
12. Milgrom, E., Atger, M., and Baulieu, E. E. (1973): Studies on estrogen entry into uterine cells and on estradiol-receptor complex attachment to the nucleus. Is the entry of estrogen into uterine cells a protein-mediated process? *Biochim. Biophys. Acta,* 320:267–283.
13. Milgrom, E., Atger, M., and Baulieu, E. E. (1973): Acidophilic activation of steroid hormone receptors. *Biochemistry,* 12:5198–5205.
14. Fanestil, D. D., and Edelman, I. S. (1966): Characteristics of the renal nuclear receptors for aldosterone. *Proc. Natl. Acad. Sci. USA,* 56:872–879.
15. Rochefort, H., and Baulieu, E. E. (1968): Récepteurs hormonaux: Relations entre les "récepteurs" utérins de l'oestradiol, "8 S" cytoplasmique at "4 S" cytoplasmique et nucléaire. *C. R. Acad. Sci. Paris,* 267:662–665.
16. Raynaud-Jammet, C., and Baulieu, E. E. (1969): Action de l'oestradiol in vitro: Augmentation de la biosynthèse d'ARN dans les noyaux utérins. *C. R. Acad. Sci. Paris,* 268:3211–3214.
17. Mohla, S., DeSombre, E. R., and Jensen, E. V. (1972): Tissue-specific stimulation of RNA synthesis by transformed estradiol-receptor complex. *Biochem. Biophys. Res. Commun.,* 46:661–667.
18. Baulieu, E. E., Alberga, A., Raynaud-Jammet, C., and Wira, C. R. (1972): New look at the very early steps of oestrogen action in uterus. *Nature [New Biol.],* 236:236–239.
19. Milgrom, E., and Baulieu, E. E. (1970): Progesterone in the uterus and the plasma. II. The role

of hormone availability and metabolism on selective binding to uterus protein. *Biochem. Biophys. Res. Commun.* 40:723–730.

20. Anderson, J., Clark, J. H., and Peck, E. J. (1972): Oestrogen and nuclear binding sites: Determination of specific sites by ^{3}H-oestradiol exchanges. *Biochem. J.*, 126:561–567.

21. Milgrom, E., Atger, M., Perrot, M., and Baulieu, E. E. (1972): Progesterone in uterus and plasma. VI. Uterine progesterone receptors during the estrus cycle and implantation in the guinea pig. *Endocrinology*, 90:1071–1078.

22. Milgrom, E., Luu Thi, M., Atger, M., and Baulieu, E. E. (1973): Mechanisms regulating the concentration and the conformation of progesterone receptor(s) in the uterus. *J. Biol. Chem.*, 248:6366–6374.

23. Deanesly, R. (1960); Implantation and early pregnancy in ovariectomized guinea-pigs. *J. Reprod. Fertil.*, 1:242–248.

24. Courrier, R. (1950): Interactions between estradiol and progesterone. *Vitamins Horm.*, 8:179–214.

25. Baulieu, E. E. (1975): Antiprogesterone effect and mid-cycle (periovulatory) contraception. *Eur. J. Obstet. Gynecol. Reprod. Biol.*, 4:161–166.

25a. Bayard, F., Damilano, S., Robel, P., and Baulieu, E-E. (1975): Récepteurs de l'oestradiol et de la progestérone dans l'endomètre humain au cours du cycle menstruel. *C. R. Acad. Sci. Paris*, 281:1341–1344.

26. Mester, J., Martel, D., Psychoyos, A., and Baulieu, E. E. (1974): Hormonal control of oestrogen receptor in uterus and receptivity for ovoimplantation in the rat. *Nature (Lond.)*, 250:776–778.

27. Psychoyos, A. (1973): Hormonal control of ovoimplantation. *Vitamins Horm.*, 31:201–256.

28. Baudouin-Legros, M., Meyer, P., and Worcel, M. (1974): Effects of prostaglandin inhibitors on angiotensin, oxytocin and prostaglandin $F_{2\alpha}$ contractile effects on the rat uterus during the oestrous cycle. *Br. J. Pharmacol.*, 52:393–399.

29. Clark, J. H., and Gorski, J. (1970): Ontogeny of the estrogen receptor during early uterine development. *Science*, 169:76–78.

30. Michel, G., Jung, I., Baulieu, E. E., Aussel, C., and Uriel, J. (1974): Two high affinity estrogen binding proteins of different specificity in the immature rat uterus cytosol. *Steroids*, 24:437–449.

31. Gavin, J. R., Roth, J., Neville, D. M., De Meyts, P., and Buell, D. N. (1974): Insulin-dependent regulation of insulin receptor concentrations: A direct demonstration in cell culture. *Proc. Natl. Acad. Sci. USA*, 71:84–88.

32. Jung, I., and Baulieu, E. E. (1972): Testosterone cytosol receptor in the rat levator ani muscle. *Nature [New Biol.]*, 237:24–26.

33. Michel, G., and Baulieu, E. E. (1974): Récepteur cytosoluble des androgènes dans un muscle strié squelettique. *C. R. Acad. Sci. Paris*, 279:421–424.

34. Bullock, L. P., and Bardin, C. W. (1974): Androgen receptors in mouse kidney: A study of male, female and androgen-insensitive (tfm/y) mice. *Endocrinology*, 94:746–756.

35. Bruchovsky, N., and Wilson, J. D. (1968): The conversion of testosterone to 5α-androstan-17β-ol-3-one by rat prostate in vivo and in vitro. *J. Biol. Chem.*, 243:2012–2021.

36. Anderson, K. M., and Liao, S. (1968): Selective retention of dihydrotestosterone by prostatic nuclei. *Nature (Lond.)*, 219:277–279.

37. Baulieu, E. E., Lasnitzki, I., and Robel, P. (1968): Metabolism of testosterone and action of metabolites on prostate glands grown in organ culture. *Nature (Lond.)*, 219:1155–1156.

38. Naftolin, F., Ryan, K. J., Davies, I. J., Reddy, V. V., Flores, F., Petro, Z., Kuhn, M., White, R. J., Tkoaka, Y., and Wollin, L. (1975): The formation of estrogens by central neuroendocrine tissues. *Recent Prog. Horm. Res.*, 31:295–319.

39. Jung-Testas, I., and Baulieu, E. E. (1974): Plusieurs récepteurs par cellule pour la même et pour différentes hormones stéroides: Conséquences pharmacologiques possibles. *C. R. Acad. Sci. Paris*, 279:671–674.

40. Huggins, C. (1967): Endocrine-induced regression of cancers. *Science*, 156:1050–1054.

41. Bullock, L. P., and Bardin, C. W. (1972): Androgen receptors in testicular feminization. *J. Clin. Endocrinol.*, 35:935–937.

42. Sibley, C. H., and Tomkins, G. M. (1974): Mechanisms of steroid resistance. *Cell*, 2:221–227.

43. Jensen, E. V., Block, G. E., Smith, S., Kyser, K., and DeSombre, E. R. (1971): Estrogen receptors and breast cancer response to adrenalectomy: Prediction of response in cancer therapy. *Natl. Cancer Inst. Monogr.*, 34:55–70.

44. Lippman, M. E., Halterman, R. H., Leventhal, B. G., Perry, S., and Thompson, E. B. (1973): Glucocorticoid binding proteins in human acute lymphoblastic leukemic blast cells. *J. Clin. Invest.*, 52:1715–1725.
45. Geynet, C., Millet, C., Truong, H., and Baulieu, E. E. (1972): Estrogens and antiestrogens. *Gynecol. Invest.*, 3:2–29.

Pharmacology of Steroid Contraceptive Drugs
edited by S. Garattini and H. W. Berendes.
Raven Press, New York © 1977.

Relative Transport of Estrogens into the Central Nervous System

Jack Fishman and Baiba Norton

Institute for Steroid Research, Montefiore Hospital and Medical Center; and Department of Biochemistry, Albert Einstein College of Medicine, Bronx, New York 10467

The physiological functions of the female sex hormones fall into two main categories depending on their site of action. In peripheral target tissue the estrogens induce biochemical and morphological changes associated with their "estrogenicity." In the central nervous system (CNS) and the pituitary the estrogens serve to regulate the secretion of pituitary hormones and their hypothalamic releasing or inhibiting factors (14). The pharmacological profile of any estrogen, whether of endogenous or exogenous origin, therefore depends to some extent on its relative distribution between the central and peripheral sites of action. Many factors participate in the availability of a material to a target organ. Among these are polarity, lipophilicity, plasma protein binding, and receptor content (2,21). In the central system an additional factor is the readiness with which the estrogen crosses the blood-brain barrier. Although there is considerable information available on the distribution of central and peripheral receptors for estrogens (12,19,20), little is known about the ability of the various estrogens to enter the CNS from the peripheral circulation. The following studies were therefore carried out to obtain a measure of the *in vivo* distribution of several estrogens in central and peripheral target and nontarget tissues.

To assess the ability of several estrogens to cross the blood-brain barriers we sought to compare them in *in vivo* experiments with estradiol under identical conditions. The procedure designed requires intravenous injection of a mixture of the tritium-labeled test compound with ^{14}C-estradiol into mature female Sprague-Dawley rats. The animals are sacrificed by cervical fracture 15 min after the injection, and samples of the blood are obtained. The pituitary and brain are removed, and the latter is sectioned into the cerebral cortex, hypothalamus, medial thalamus, corpus striatum, midbrain, cerebellum, and medulla using a modification of the method of Glowinsky and Iverson (9). Peripheral tissues dissected and examined include the diaphragm, ovaries, uterus, kidney, and liver. The isotope content of each tissue sample is determined by combustion in an Oxymat tissue oxidizer. In this procedure the $^{14}CO_2$ and ^3H_2O generated in the process are separated, trapped, and counted individually. This allows accurate determination of the content of each isotope in the tissue without the serious quenching problems associated with chemical tissue digestion. The principal advantage of the present method over those requiring solvent extraction is that it includes all of the forms in which the material is present in the tissue, many of which would fail to be extracted with organic solvents. Its disadvantage of course resides in the fact that the nature of the material with which the isotope is associated is not known. Each experiment was carried out on six animals, and the results in Table 1 are the average values. The use of mixtures of ^{14}C-estradiol and ^{3}H-labeled test compound permits comparison of the latter with the former under truly identical conditions.

In the initial experiments we sought to compare the central-peripheral distribution characteristics of the principal metabolites of estradiol with that of the parent hormone. The first step in estradiol metabolism is oxidation to estrone (5). This reaction, however, is reversible, and the present method could not be used as such for estradiol-estrone comparison. An alternative and more complex procedure was devised for this purpose, and the results will be reported in the future. The two other principal metabolites of estradiol are estriol and 2-hydroxyestrone, which are derived by irreversible processes via estrone. The distribution of these two endogenous estrogens has assumed particular interest in view of recent developments. Estriol, which has long been thought to be an impeded estrogen with only slight uterotropic activity (11), has now been demonstrated to be fully equivalent to estradiol in its action on peripheral target sites (1). On the other hand, 2-hydroxyestrone, whose *in situ* biosynthesis from estradiol in the brain has been demonstrated (6–8), is apparently an ineffective uterotropic agent (10), although it does have significant CNS activity (17). We therefore examined the blood-brain transport of these two compounds versus estradiol. In addition,

TABLE 1. *Ratio of two isotopes in various tissues after intravenous injection*

Tissue	Estriol-[3]H / Estradiol-[14]C	2-Hydroxyestrone-[3]H / Estradiol-[14]C	17α-Ethynylestradiol-[3]H / Estradiol-[14]C
Dose	1.00	1.00	1.00
Blood	1.57	4.03	1.39
Cerebral cortex	0.83	0.74	2.06
Hypothalamus	0.79	0.81	2.15
Medial thalamus	0.75	0.76	2.90
Corpus striatum	0.82	0.78	2.51
Midbrain	0.59	0.61	3.46
Cerebellum	0.64	0.74	2.69
Medulla	0.47	0.61	2.11
Pituitary	1.20	1.10	1.32
Ovaries	1.27	0.75	1.35
Uterus	1.33	0.89	1.10
Kidney	1.65	4.06	1.20
Liver	0.77	0.63	0.95

In each experiment six adult female Sprague-Dawley rats at no particular stage of the cycle were injected intravenously with the isotope mixture representing estradiol-^{14}C and the tritium-labeled test compound. The results are the ratio of the two isotopes (^{3}H/^{14}C) present in the tissue.

we studied in the same manner the transfer of 17α-ethynylestradiol, a synthetic estrogen that is a component of many oral contraceptive compositions.

The results of these experiments are recorded in Table 1. They are given in terms of the isotope ratios present in the tissues with the values normalized to a dose ratio of 1. It must be emphasized that the radioactivity includes both substrates and any of their metabolites, and that the identity of the compounds bearing the respective isotope is uncertain. For purposes of simplicity, only the substrate originally associated with isotope is used in the discussion.

In the estriol experiment the isotope ratio of the blood is considerably greater than 1.0; this is evidence that there is more circulating estriol than estradiol, and it implies a faster clearance of the latter. This is reflected in the $<$1.0 isotope ratio in the liver (the major site of metabolism), indicating a greater concentration of estradiol than estriol in this organ. The central tissues uniformly have an isotope content with a ratio $<$1.0. This is clear evidence that estriol has greater difficulty in crossing the blood-brain barrier than estradiol or its products. There does not appear to be any great or significant variation of isotope ratio between the various brain areas. At first this may be considered surprising because of the demonstrated preponderance of estradiol receptors in the hypothalamus (13), suggesting that this tissue should reflect a greater estradiol content and hence a ratio lower than the cerebellum or cerebral cortex. It must be recognized, however, that much of the radioactivity injected as estradiol reaches the brain as estrone or other metabolites; hence the relative excess of estradiol in specific central sites is masked so that it may not be detected by this procedure. In addition, the affinity of estriol for the estrogen receptor (15) further tends to blur the distinction between receptor-rich and receptor-poor central areas. The pituitary, which has its own blood supply, shows a distinct difference from the central tissue in that its isotope ratio is greater than that of the dose, implying its greater accessibility to the estriol component. The ratio of 1.20, however, is lower than that in the circulating plasma, suggesting that the estrogen receptor content in the pituitary (3,4) is exerting its influence to concentrate estradiol relative to the plasma. A similar situation apparently exists in the uterus, a principal target tissue. From these results it may be tentatively concluded that, aside from other factors such as conjugation or metabolism, estriol is more available to peripheral than to central estrogen target sites and hence can be expected to be a more potent uterotropic agent than a gonadotropin-regulating hormone.

The results of the 2-hydroxyestrone experiment reveal that this material is cleared from plasma much more slowly than estradiol, with the blood isotope ratio being four times that of the dose. This discrepancy is again partially reflected in the 0.6 isotope ratio found in the liver, implying a more rapid metabolism of estradiol. The central tissues examined again reveal a much greater entry of estradiol relative to 2-hydroxyestrone. No significant differences in the isotope ratios of the several brain sections were encountered. The arguments used previously with estriol can be applied in this instance also to explain this invariance, particularly since 2-hydroxyestrone has also been demonstrated to be an effective ligand for the brain estrogen receptor (4). The pituitary isotope ratio content of 1.10 is significantly higher than that of the brain, being close to that of the dose but greatly lower than that in circulating blood. This reflects greater access to the pituitary for the 2-hydroxyestrone because of the absence of the blood-brain barrier. Interestingly, the uterus isotope ratio of 0.9 indicates a greater estradiol content than the pituitary, suggesting that the latter tissue may have a particular affinity for 2-hydroxyestrone or one of its products. This may be related to the demonstrated positive feedback action on LH release of the catechol estrogen (17). The limited access of 2-hydroxyestrone to the central tissues need not imply a lack of activity for this estrogen at these sites because, unlike estriol, it can be synthesized in the brain from estradiol (6–8). Indeed, it may be speculated that, similar to estradiol, which can also be biosynthesized in the CNS (18), the catechol estrogen may be bifunctional in the CNS depending on whether it reaches the CNS target from the peripheral circulation or is generated at the site. Although 2-hydroxyestrone can bind to the uterine estrogen receptor (16), its relatively low content in this organ suggests that it does not compete well for these sites with the endogenous or coinjected estradiol.

A drastically different result was obtained in the ethynylestradiol experiment. In this case too the plasma ratio indicates a more rapid clearance of estradiol component, although the ratio of 1.39 is the lowest encountered in all three experiments. The isotope ratio of the central tissues, however, reveals a clear and significantly greater penetration of ethynylestradiol relative to estradiol. There are significant differences in the isotope ratio of the various brain sections, but their meaning is currently unclear. In contrast, the pituitary and uterus isotope ratios reflect that of the blood, suggesting an even competition for these sites by the two components of the injected mixture. The ease of access of ethynylestradiol to the central tissues may be responsible for its effectiveness as the estrogenic component of the oral contraceptive preparations since even after attrition following oral ingestion enough of the material can enter the brain to perform its function.

Even though the relative blood-brain barrier crossing of the three compounds discussed here may have been predicted on the basis of their lipophilic index, the results obtained also include their respective metabolites and are therefore much more revealing. The experiments described represent the first application of this methodology to the problem; other studies already under way or contemplated are expected to reveal more about the complex problem of central versus peripheral action of various natural and synthetic estrogens. It is hoped that compounds can be obtained whose action will be limited to only one of the two sites of action via selective constraints on their access to the brain or peripheral tissues. Such compounds may be expected to have obvious and important clinical application.

REFERENCES

1. Anderson, J. N., Peck, E. J., and Clark, J. H. (1975): Estrogen-induced uterine responses and growth: Relationship to receptor estrogen binding of uterine nuclei. *Endocrinology,* 96:160.

2. Biagi, G. L., Barbara, A. M., Gondolfi, O., Guevra, M. C., and Contelli-Forti, G. (1975): R_m values of steroids as an expression of their lipophilic character in structure-activity studies. *J. Med. Chem.*, 18:873.
3. Davies, I. J., Naftolin, F., Ryan, K. J., Fishman, J., and Sui, J. (1975): The affinity of catechol estrogens for estrogen receptors in the pituitary and anterior hypothalamus of the rat. *J. Endocrinol.*, 97:554.
4. Davies, I. J., Siu, J., Naftolin, F., and Ryan, K. J. (1975): *Adv. Biosci.*, 14:89.
5. Fishman, J. (1963): Role of 2-hydroxyestrone in estrogen metabolism. *J. Clin. Endocrinol. Metab.*, 23:207.
6. Fishman, J., Naftolin, F., Davies, I. J., Ryan, K. J., and Petro, Z. (1976): Catechol estrogen formation by the human fetal brain and pituitary. *J. Clin. Endocrinol. Metab.*, 42:177.
7. Fishman, J., and Norton, B. (1975): Brain catechol estrogens—formation and possible function. *Adv. Biosci.*, 15:123.
8. Fishman, J., and Norton, B. (1975): Catechol estrogen formation in the central nervous system of the rat. *Endocrinology*, 96:1054.
9. Glowinski, J., and Iverson, L. L. (1966): Regional studies of catecholamines in the rat brain. I. The disposition of [³H] norepinephrine, [³H] dopamine and [³H] dopa in various regions of the brain. *J. Neurochem.*, 13:655.
10. Gordon, S., Cantrell, E. W., Cekleniak, W. P., Albers, H. J., Manner, S., Stolar, S. M., and Bernstein, S. (1964): Steroid and lipid metabolism: The hypocholesteremic effects of estrogen metabolites. *Steroids*, 4:267.
11. Huggins, C., and Jensen, E. F. (1955): The depression of estrone-induced uterine growth by phenolic estrogens with oxygenated functions of positions 6 or 16: The impeded estrogens. *J. Exp. Med.*, 102:335.
12. Jensen, E. V., and DeSombre, E. R. (1973): Estrogen-receptor interactions. *Science*, 182:126.
13. Kato, J. (1973): Localization of oestradiol receptors in the rat hypothalamus. *Acta Endocrinol. (Kbh.)*, 72:663.
14. King, R. J. B., and Mainwaring, W. I. P. (1974): *Steroid Cell Interactions.* University Park Press, Baltimore.
15. Korenman, S. G. (1969): Comparative binding affinity of estrogens and its relation to estrogenic potency. *Steroids*, 13:163.
16. Martucci, C., and Fishman, J. (1976): Uterine estrogen receptor binding of catechol-estrogens and of estetrol (1,3,5(10)-estratriene-3,15α,16α,17β-tetrol). *Steroids*, 27:325.
17. Naftolin, F., Morishita, H., Davies, I. J., Rodd, R., Ryan, K. J., and Fishman, J. (1975): 2-Hydroxyestrone induced rise in serum luteinizing hormone in the immature male rat. *J. Biochem. Biophys. Res. Commun.*, 64:905.
18. Naftolin, F., Ryan, K. J., and Petro, Z. (1973): Aromatization of androstenedione by the anterior hypothalamus of adult male and female rats. *Endocrinology*, 90:295.
19. Pfaff, P., and Keiner, M. (1975): Atlas of estradiol-concentrating cells in the central nervous system of the female rat. *J. Comp. Neurol.*, 151:121.
20. Vreeburg, J. T. M., Schretkin, P. J. M., and Baum, M. S. (1975): Specific, high-affinity binding of 17β-estradiol in cytosols from several brain regions and pituitary of intact and castrated adult male rats. *Endocrinology*, 97:969.
21. Westphal, U. (1971): *Steroid-Protein Interactions.* Springer-Verlag, Berlin.

Pharmacology of Steroid Contraceptive Drugs
edited by S. Garattini and H. W. Berendes.
Raven Press, New York © 1977.

Sites of Action of Contraceptive Drugs in the Central Nervous System

Walter E. Stumpf and Madhabananda Sar

Departments of Anatomy and Pharmacology, Laboratories for Reproductive Biology, University of North Carolina at Chapel Hill, Chapel Hill, North Carolina 27514

Considerable evidence suggests central action of contraceptives, not only with respect to the modulation of gonadotropin secretion but also behavior, electrical neuronal activity, and various autonomic functions. The contraceptive action of the "pill" is thought to be mediated through the central nervous system and pituitary, as well as through direct effects on peripheral reproductive tissues. Most of the currently used contraceptive pills prevent ovulation by suppressing the preovulatory surge of gonadotropin secretion. This central effect is due to the estrogenic or progestogenic nature of the components and can be mediated by a component alone or in combination.

Since the components of the combined and sequential pills are congeners of the endogenous hormones estradiol and progesterone, the sites of action of these analogs can be expected to be similar to those of the natural hormones. However, differences in absorption, distribution, binding affinity, metabolism, and excretion must be expected. Furthermore, the progestational component of many preparations shows chemical and functional relationships to androgenic and/or estrogenic steroids. Thus binding characteristics in the brain may not be identical to those of the related "primary" natural steroid. Indeed, experimental evidence has been provided that differences exist in binding affinity of synthetic contraceptives (2). Therefore extrapolations between compounds of one group of related steroids can be made only with reservation.

The organ distribution of several of the synthetic contraceptives has been reported in the literature (1,5,27,28). Although evidence is available from radioassay studies and whole-body autoradiography about uptake of contraceptives in the brain, no data are provided on the selective cellular and subcellular distribution of these compounds. This may be due to lack of available labeled compounds with high specific activity.

For this reason, and since it can be expected that the synthetic estrogenic and progestagenic steroids compete for receptors of gonadal steroids, the topographical distribution of estrogen and progestin target cells in the mammalian brain are reviewed. Both the mature and developing brain are considered with regard to the known activational effects of these compounds on the mature brain and the permanent organizational effects on the fetal or neonatal brain.

In our laboratory experiments were performed with ³H-estradiol and ³H-progesterone, using dry-mount and thaw-mount autoradiography. The labeled material was injected either intravenously or subcutaneously at a physiological or near-physiological dose: 0.1–0.5 μg/100 g body weight for ³H-estradiol-17β and 0.5–1.0 μg/100 g body weight for ³H-progesterone. The specific activity ranged between 80 and 100 Ci/mM. The animals, including various species of rodents, primates, and lower vertebrates, were killed 15 min to 2 hr after the injection, and tissues were excised and prepared for autoradiography. The

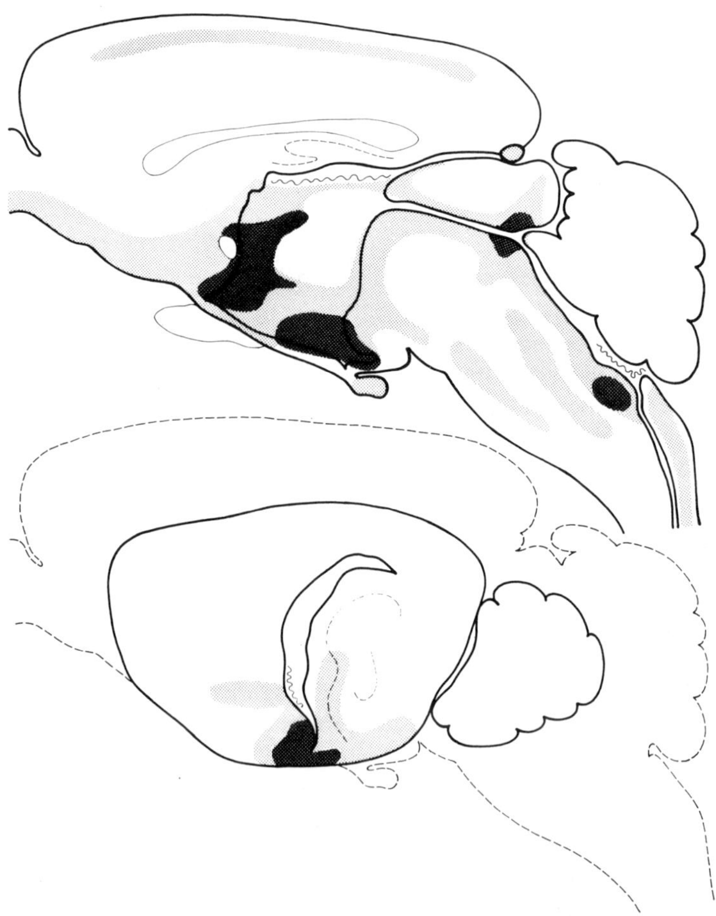

FIG. 1. Estrogen target cell distribution in rodent brain based on the autoradiographic localization of ³H-estradiol-17β; projected on sagittal planes and showing relationships to the third and fourth ventricles and aqueduct **(top)** and the lateral ventricle **(bottom)**. The dark and light stippling corresponds to high and intermediate-low concentration of steroid hormone in nuclei of nerve cells.

specificity of the results was established through competition studies. Details of the techniques appear elsewhere (21).

³H-ESTRADIOL

³H-Estradiol concentrates in nuclei of neurons with varying intensity similar to the nuclear concentration seen in the uterine tissues. Ependymal cells are essentially unlabeled, except for a few specific regions. Glial cells are unlabeled, except perhaps for specialized "glial" cells in various ventricular recess organs. In all of the vertebrate species studied, estrogen target neurons were found widespread in many parts of the brain and pituitary (3,7,11,13–17,19–26). Regions of highest accumulation of estrogen-concentrating cells are the preoptic and basal hypothalamus and the amygdala. Medium-intensity nuclear uptake is seen in the olfactory tubercle, midbrain, pons, and medulla oblongata. Weak nuclear concentration of radioactivity is observed, in addition to the above areas, in phylogenetically old parts of the cortex (allocortex) and in the anterior thalamus and epithalamus. It is noteworthy that estrogen-concentrating cells accumulate within or in close proximity to the ventricular recess organs, such as the optic recess organ, the subfornical organ, the infundibulum, the pineal, the collicular recess organ, and the area postrema (17,22,25). Figure 1 provides an overview of the distribution of estrogen target cells in the rat brain, including the midbrain, pons, and medulla oblongata. A similar distribution to that in the rat forebrain is observed in the other mammalian species studied thus far, including the squirrel monkey and tree shrew (3). A detailed topographical description for the different species is provided in *Anatomical Neuroendocrinology* (18). Examples of the topography of estrogen target neuron distribution in the region of the pons-caudal colliculus and medulla oblongata are shown here for the mouse (Fig. 2) and in the preoptic-central hypothalamic region for the squirrel monkey (3) (Fig. 3) and the guinea pig (11) (Fig. 4).

Estrogen-concentrating cells can be demonstrated in the 2-day neonatal rat brain (12) (Fig. 6) and 10-day fetal brain of the chick embryo (6) (Fig. 7). This suggests that steroid hormone action on nervous tissues exists at those early stages of life. Most likely, the early organizational effects of steroids that result in permanent alterations of gonadotropin secretion and behavior in mature life are exerted through genomic action on these target cells.

³H-PROGESTERONE

Thus far only one successful study on the cellular distribution of ³H-progesterone or its metabolites in the brain has been published (8). Metabolism and receptor variability may account for the difficulties in localizing this type of hormone. Progestin-concentrating neurons in the guinea pig were described in the preoptic-periventricular region and the central hypothalamus (Fig. 5). This distribution appears to correspond to the sites of ³H-estradiol uptake (11) (Fig.

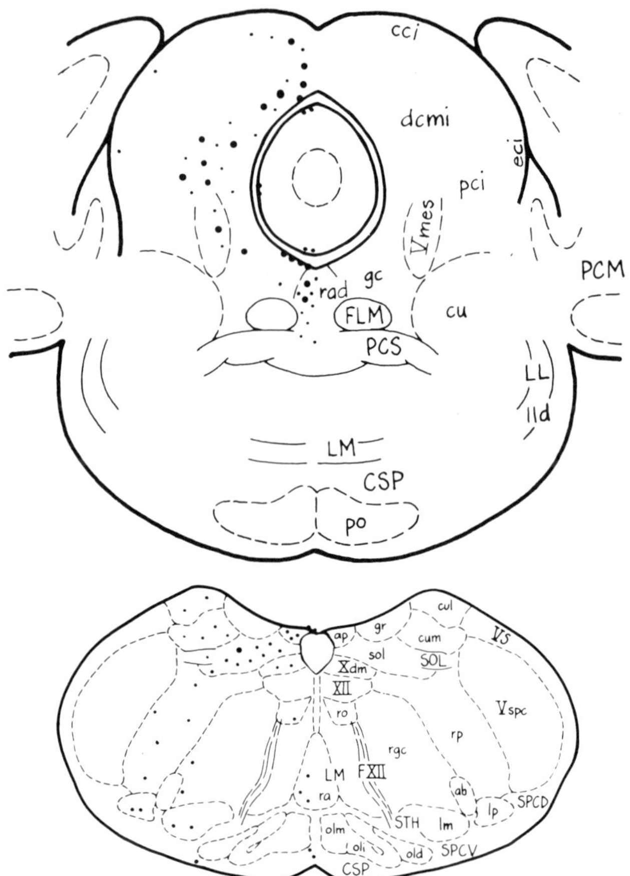

FIG. 2. Drawings of cross sections of the colliculus caudalis and pons region **(top)** and the medulla oblongata at the level of the area postrema **(bottom),** prepared after autoradiograms of mouse brain, 1 hr after ^{3}H-estradiol injection. The dots *(left half)* represent intensity of labeling and density of distribution of estrogen target neurons. **Top:** Strong labeling exists in such structures as the extensive central gray of the organum recessus colliculi caudalis and the nucleus raphes dorsalis (rad). Also labeled are certain ependymal cells. **Bottom:** Labeled cells are observed, for instance, in the area postrema (ap), nucleus tractus solitarii (sol), nucleus dorsalis motorius nervi vagi (Xdm), nucleus cuneatus (cul and cum), nucleus reticularis parvocellularis (rp), and nucleus raphes magnus (ra). (From Stumpf and Sar, ref. 22.)

4); however, it seems less extensive. The data currently available for progestins cover only the guinea pig hypothalamus. Further experiments with different species and under different hormonal conditions must be performed to establish the mechanism of action of progestins in the central nervous system.

Figure 8 shows typical autoradiograms of the guinea pig hypothalamic arcuate nucleus after injection of ^{3}H-estradiol or ^{3}H-progesterone. Since estrogen pretreatment enhances nuclear uptake of radioactivity after ^{3}H-progesterone injec-

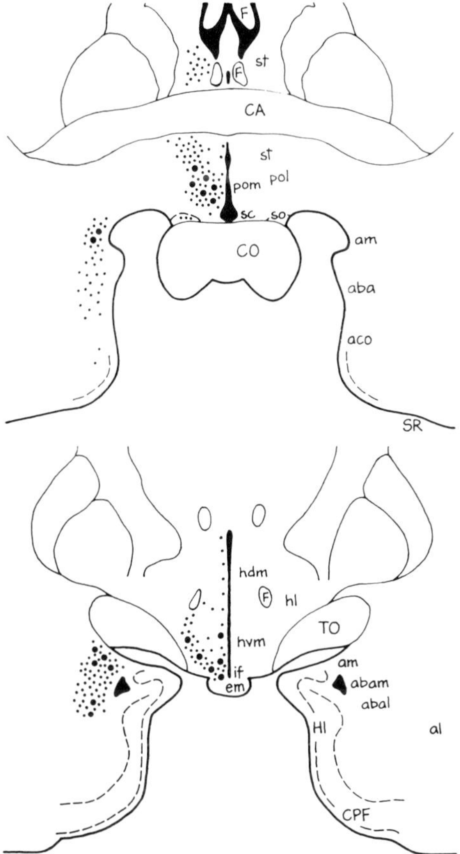

FIG. 3. Drawings of the preoptic **(top)** and central hypothalamic **(bottom)** region of squirrel monkey brain (frontal plane) showing the distribution of estrogen-concentrating neurons (black dots on left half) as seen in autoradiograms 1 hr after injection of ^{3}H-estradiol. High concentration of labeled hormone exists in the nucleus preopticus medialis (pom) and the bed nucleus of the stria terminalis (st), the pars ventrolateralis of the nucleus ventromedialis hypothalami (hvm), and certain nuclei of the amygdala (am, abam, and abal). (After Keefer and Stumpf, ref. 3.)

tion (8,11), and target neurons for both types of hormones appear in identical regions, it is likely that estrogens and progestins act on the same neurons.

The evidence available to date on estrogen and progestin target cell distribution as reviewed here and on the androgen target cell distribution as reviewed elsewhere (9,10) suggests widespread action of the components of steroidal contraceptives on central nervous structures. Contrary to earlier concepts, not only are the "hypophyseotrophic area" and the hypothalamus involved but also rather extensive regions including the "limbic system," the rhinencephalon, and the

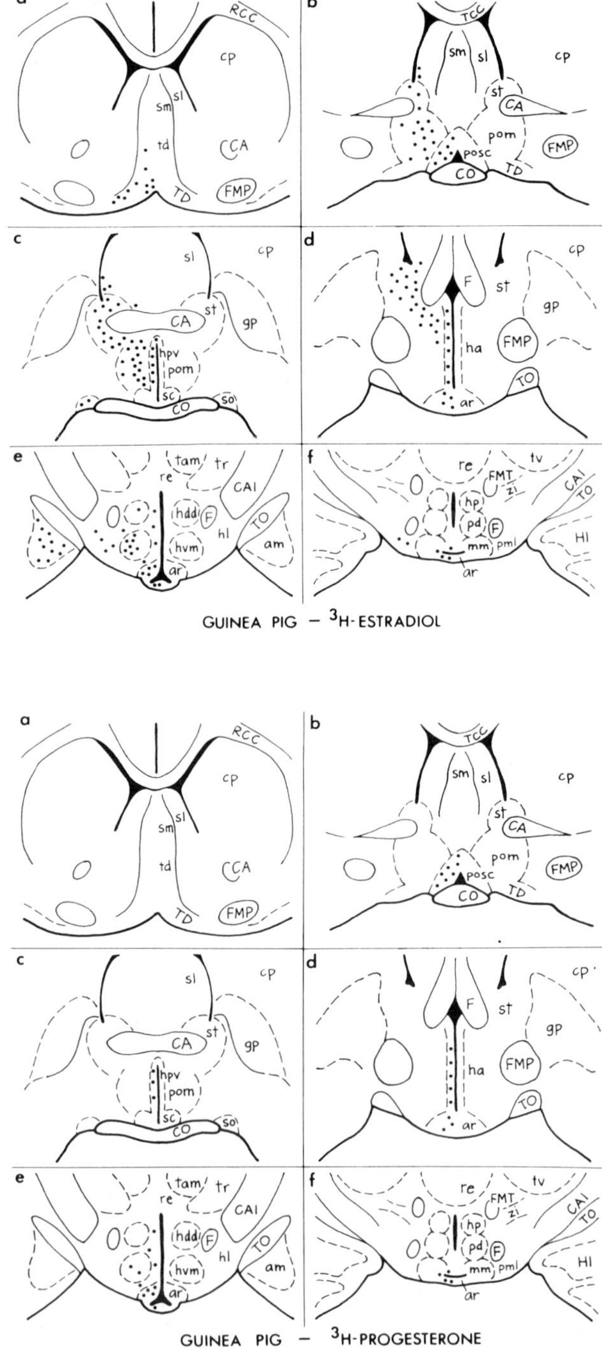

FIGS. 4 and 5. Distribution of estrogen-concentrating neurons (Fig. 4) and progestin-concentrating neurons (Fig. 5) in guinea pig hypothalamus. The dots (left half) indicate the intensity of labeling and frequency of occurrence of labeled neurons as obtained in autoradiograms. **a–f** represent frontal sections in rostrocaudal sequence. (From Sar and Stumpf, ref. 11.)

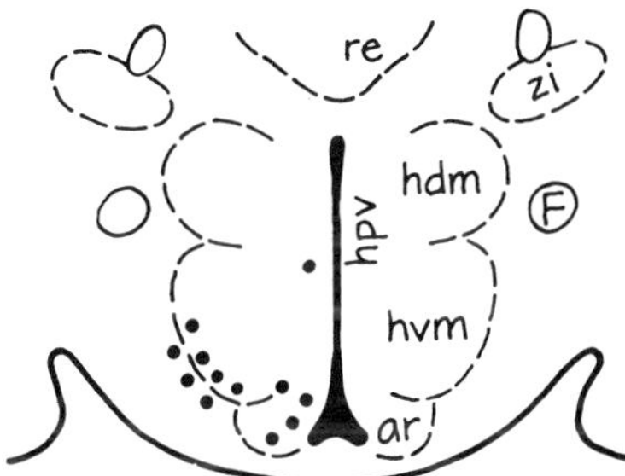

FIG. 6. Distribution of estrogen-concentrating neurons in the central hypothalamus of a 2-day neonatal rat. (From Sheridan et al., ref. 12.)

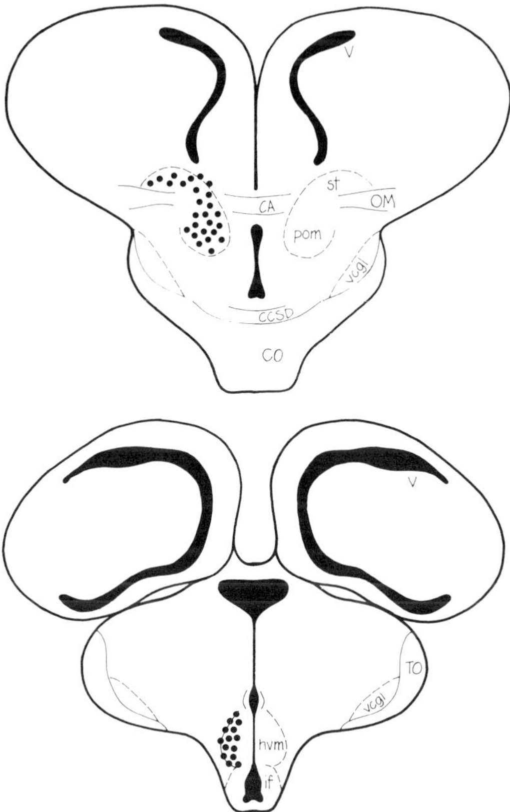

FIG. 7. Distribution of estrogen-concentrating cells in the hypothalamus of a 10-day chick embryo. Estrogen-concentrating cells are accumulated in the nucleus preopticus medialis (pom) and the nucleus interstitialis striae terminalis (st) as shown at the top and in the nucleus ventromedialis hypothalami (hvm) at bottom. At this stage no labeling is observed in the nucleus infundibularis (if); labeling of this nucleus appears later in the neonate. (After Martinez-Vargas et al., ref. 6.)

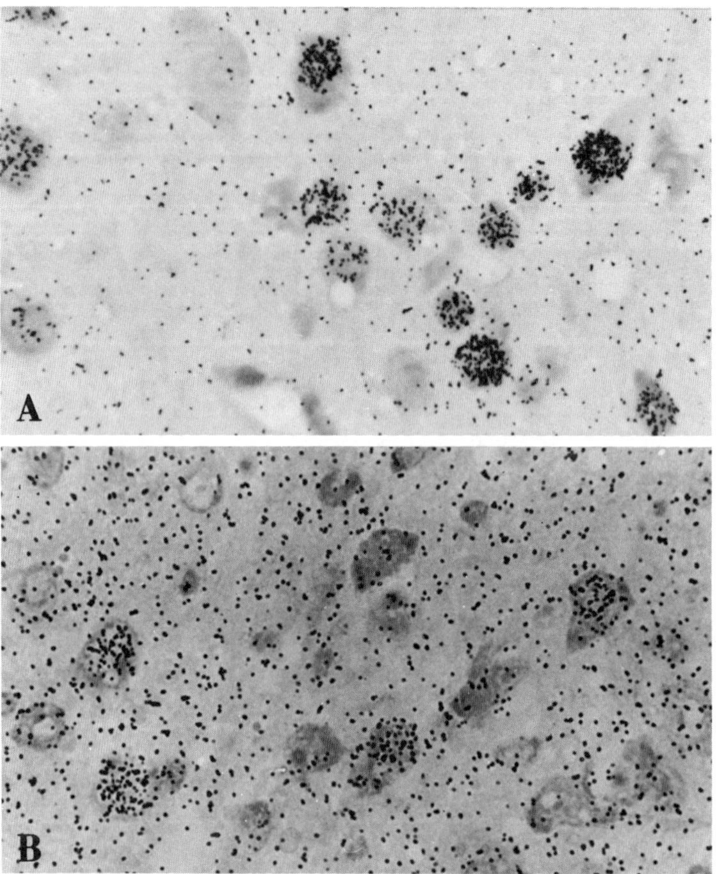

FIG. 8. Autoradiograms of nucleus arcuatus hypothalami of guinea pig obtained 1 hr after injection of ^{3}H-estradiol-17β **(A)** and 15 min after injection of ^{3}H-progesterone **(B).** Nuclear concentration of radioactivity exists in certain neurons with both estrogen and progestin. Priming with estradiol enhances nuclear uptake of radioactivity after ^{3}H-progesterone injection, whereas pretreatment with unlabeled progesterone reduces or abolishes the nuclear concentration. **(A,** from Sar and Stumpf, ref. 11. **B,** from Sar and Stumpf, ref. 8.)

lower brainstem (22), as well as the spinal cord (4,25) and sensory ganglia (26). Moreover, target cells have been identified in the pituitary (13,23).

It is likely that some or all of the central nervous structures can be activated by components of the contraceptive pill, depending on dose. This may account, more or less, for the many actions and the positive and negative side effects, e.g., changes in blood pressure, alterations of behavior and libido, and modifications of eating and metabolism. Thus in addition to the well-known direct actions of contraceptive steroids on peripheral target tissues, direct central effects and indirect peripheral effects mediated through the central nervous system and pituitary must be considered.

ACKNOWLEDGMENTS

Supported by USPHS grants 2 R01 NS09914 and AE021.

REFERENCES

1. Appelgren, L-E., and Karlsson, R. (1971): The distribution of ^{14}C-4-mestranol in mice. *Acta Pharmacol. Toxicol. (Kbh.),* 29:65–74.
2. Eisenfeld, A. (1974): Oral contraceptives: Ethinyl estradiol binds with higher affinity than mestranol to macromolecules from the sites of anti-fertility action. *Endocrinology,* 94:803–814.
3. Keefer, D. A., and Stumpf, W. E. (1975): Estrogen localization in the primate brain. In: *Anatomical Neuroendocrinology,* edited by W. E. Stumpf and L. D. Grant, pp. 153–165. Karger, Basel.
4. Keefer, D. A., Stumpf, W. E., and Sar, M. (1973): Topographical localization of estrogen-concentrating cells in the rat spinal cord following ^{3}H-estradiol administration. *Proc. Soc. Exp. Biol. Med.,* 143:414–417.
5. Laumas, V., Malkani, P. K., and Laumas, K. R. (1971): Distribution and uptake of radioactivity in rat tissues after a single injection and constant infusion of ^{3}H-norethynodrel. *Am. J. Obstet. Gynecol.,* 109:457–462.
6. Martinez-Vargas, M. C., Gibson, D. B., Sar, M., and Stumpf, W. E. (1975): Estrogen target cells in brain of the chick embryo. *Science,* 190:1307–1308.
7. Martinez-Vargas, M. C., Stumpf, W. E., and Sar, M. (1975): Estrogen distribution in dove brain: phylogenetic considerations and implications for nomenclature. In: *Anatomical Neuroendocrinology,* edited by W. E. Stumpf and L. D. Grant, pp. 166–175. Karger, Basel.
8. Sar, M., and Stumpf, W. E. (1973): Neurons of the hypothalamus concentrate ^{3}H progesterone or metabolites of it. *Science,* 182:1266–1268.
9. Sar, M., and Stumpf, W. E. (1973): Autoradiographic localization of radioactivity in the rat brain after the injection of 1,2-^{3}H testosterone. *Endocrinology,* 92:251–256.
10. Sar, M., and Stumpf, W. E. (1975): Distribution of androgen-concentrating neurons in rat brain. In: *Anatomical Neuroendocrinology,* edited by W. E. Stumpf and L. D. Grant, pp. 120–133. Karger, Basel.
11. Sar, M., and Stumpf, W. E. (1975): Cellular localization of progestin and estrogen in guinea pig hypothalamus by autoradiography. In: *Anatomical Neuroendocrinology,* edited by W. E. Stumpf and L. D. Grant, pp. 142-152. Karger, Basel.
12. Sheridan, P. J., Sar, M., and Stumpf, W. E. (1974): Autoradiographic localization of ^{3}H estradiol or its metabolites in the central nervous systems of the developing rat. *Endocrinology,* 94: 1386–1390.
13. Stumpf, W. E. (1968): Cellular and subcellular ^{3}H estradiol localization in the pituitary by autoradiography. *Z. Zellforsch.,* 92:23–33.
14. Stumpf, W. E. (1968): Estradiol concentrating neurons: Topography in the hypothalamus by dry-mount autoradiography. *Science,* 162:1001–1003.
15. Stumpf, W. E. (1970): Estrogen-neurons and estrogen-neuron systems in the periventricular brain. *Am. J. Anat.,* 129:207–218.
16. Stumpf, W. E. (1971): Probable sites for estrogen receptors in brain and pituitary. *J. Neurovisc. Relations (Suppl.),* 10:102–106.
17. Stumpf, W. E. (1975): The brain, an endocrine gland and hormone target. In: *Anatomical Neuroendocrinology,* edited by W. E. Stumpf and L. D. Grant, pp. 2–8. Karger, Basel.
18. Stumpf, W. E., and Grant, L. D., (editors) (1975): *Anatomical Neuroendocrinology.* Karger, Basel.
19. Stumpf, W. E., and Sar, M. (1971): Estradiol concentrating neurons in the amygdala. *Proc. Soc. Exp. Biol. Med.,* 136:102–106.
20. Stumpf, W. E., and Sar, M. (1973): Hormonal inputs to releasing factor cells, feedback sites. *Prog. Brain Res.,* 39:53–71.
21. Stumpf, W. E., and Sar, M. (1975): Autoradiographic techniques for localizing steroid hormones. *Methods Enzymol.,* 36:135–156.
22. Stumpf, W. E., and Sar, M. (1975): Hormone architecture of the mouse brain with ^{3}H estradiol. In: *Anatomical Neuroendocrinology,* edited by W. E. Stumpf and L. D. Grant, pp. 82–103. Karger, Basel.
23. Stumpf, W. E., Sar, M., and Keefer, D. A. (1975): Localization of hormones in pituitary cells:

receptor sites for hormones from hypophyseal target glands and the brain. In: *Pituitary: Ultrastructure in Biological Systems,* edited by A. Tixier-Vidal and M. Farquhar, pp. 63–82. Academic Press, New York.

24. Stumpf, W. E., Sar, M., and Keefer, D. A. (1975): Anatomical distribution of estrogen in the central nervous system of mouse, rat, tree shrew and squirrel monkey. *Adv. Biosci.,* 15:77–88.

25. Stumpf, W. E., Sar, M., and Keefer, D. A. (1975): Atlas of estrogen target cells in rat brain. In: *Anatomical Neuroendocrinology,* edited by W. E. Stumpf and L. D. Grant, pp. 104–119. Karger, Basel.

26. Stumpf, W. E., Sar, M., Keefer, D. A., and Martinez-Vargas, M. C. (1976): The anatomical substrate of neuroendocrine regulation as defined by autoradiography with ^{3}H estradiol, ^{3}H testosterone, ^{3}H dihydrotestosterone and ^{3}H progesterone. In: *Neuroendocrine Regulation of Fertility,* edited by T. C. Anand-Kumar, pp. 46–56. Karger, Basel.

27. Watanabe, H., Saha, N. N., and Layne, D. S. (1968): Distribution of radioactivity in rat tissues after administration of tritiated 17α-ethynyl-19-norsteroids. *Steroids,* 11:97–101.

28. Zaldivar, A., and Gallegos, A. J. (1971): Metabolism and tissue localization of [14–15^{3}H] d-norgestrel in the human. *Contraception,* 4:169–182.

Pharmacology of Steroid Contraceptive Drugs
edited by S. Garattini and H. W. Berendes.
Raven Press, New York © 1977.

Biochemical Effects of Steroid Contraceptive Drugs on Some Neurotransmitters in the Central Nervous System

S. Algeri, M. Bonati, M. Curcio, A. Jori, H. Ladinsky,
F. Ponzio, and S. Garattini

Istituto di Ricerche Farmacologiche "Mario Negri," 20157 Milan, Italy

The secretion of hypothalamic releasing factors is controlled by neuronal circuits of the hypothalamus and adjacent parts. The intersynaptic chemical mediators of these neurons seem to be represented by monoamines. In fact, it has been shown that some putative neurotransmitters (e.g., dopamine, norepinephrine, and acetylcholine) or drugs active on these mediators may influence the secretion of the hypophyseal hormones that regulate gonadal function (6,14,17,20,22,27). On the other hand there is a great deal of experimental evidence indicating that changes in the normal balance of gonadal hormones which occur during the estrous cycle, pregnancy, and castration alter the metabolism of monoaminergic neurotransmitters (12,40).

These findings point out the possibility that steroid hormones interact in a complex way with biogenic monoamines. Steroid contraceptive drugs (SCD) are structurally related to natural steroid sexual hormones, and so it is reasonable to imagine that they may influence the neuronal activity in a similar manner. Relative to this, Fuxe et al. (9) reported that estrogens and contraceptive drugs stimulate dopamine turnover in the median eminence of the hypothalamus. There is the possibility—although the problem awaits clarification—that these effects may be related in some way to the contraceptive action. On the other hand, it is possible that the effects of SCDs on the neuronal system may not be limited to the neuroendocrine circuits but may influence other regions of the brain as well.

In view of the evidence relating changes in neuronal monoamine metabolism with emotional and neurological disorders (30) and the controversial problem of behavioral side effects that are sometimes reported in women using oral contraceptives (7,10,11,15,21), we thought it of interest to study the effect of these drugs on the metabolism of some neurotransmitters in the brain. Therefore we studied specifically the effect of SCD treatment on dopamine (DA), norepinephrine (NE), and serotonin (5-HT) turnover, as well as its effect on the acetylcholine level and the activity of tyrosine hydroxylase and choline acetyltransferase in several brain regions of the rat and guinea pig.

MODALITY OF ANIMAL TREATMENT

As the SCD we chose Lyndiol (Organon Oss Holland), a combination of lynestrenol (17α-ethinyl-17β-hydroxy-estr-4en) and mestranol [17α-ethinyl-17β-hydroxy-3-methoxy-1,3,5 (10)-estratrien]. These compounds were administered in a fixed ratio (1:0.06) at doses in the range of the minimal doses producing 100% antifertility. These doses were 5–0.3 mg/kg for the rat and 1.25–0.075 mg/kg for the guinea pig. The drugs were dissolved in corn oil and administered orally by gavage. Control animals received the vehicle only. In the rat the "acute" treatment consisted of the drugs being administered daily for 4 days, which is the duration of one estrous cycle; they were given for 30 days in the "chronic" treatment. The "chronic" treatment of guinea pigs was prolonged to 3 months since the estrous cycle of this animal is much longer (16 days). At the end of treatment the estrous phase was checked by cytological examination. After chronic treatment most of the animals were in the diestrous phase. The exceptions, which were more numerous with the shorter treatment, were discarded. To avoid any effect due to the difference in the estrous phase, control animals were also selected in the diestrous phase. The last administration was given 24 hr before sacrifice except where indicated in Tables 10 and 11.

EFFECTS OF SCD ADMINISTRATION ON THE CATECHOLAMINERGIC SYSTEM IN SOME RAT BRAIN REGIONS

The noradrenergic system, which utilizes NE, and the dopaminergic system, which utilizes DA, have been implicated to various extents in the neuroendocrine mechanisms or in affective disorders. Both mediators originate from tyrosine, which is hydroxylated in position 3 by the enzyme tyrosine hydroxylase. This enzyme catalyzes a three-substrate reaction (tyrosine, oxygen, and a reduced pteridine cofactor) and represents the rate-limiting step in catecholamine synthesis.

The degree of nerve activity does not modify the levels of neurotransmitters, which are maintained relatively constant by a balance between synthesis and release. For this reason determination of the synthesis or turnover rate of a neurotransmitter is a better index of the functional status of a neuronal population.

In the experiments described we determined the effect of SCDs on the turnover of DA and NE in some brain regions with different methodological approaches. The first method consists in measuring the rate of radioactivity incorporation into catecholamines after administration of ^{3}H-tyrosine (50 Ci/mmole). This radioactive amino acid may be administered intravenously (1 mCi/kg) or directly into the brain lateral ventricles (14 μCi/animal) through two permanently implanted polyethylene cannulas (34).

The amount of synthesis is approximated by calculating the conversion index (C.I.) according to Sedvall et al. (31). This index corrects for the radioactivity incorporated into a catecholamine in a given brain area by the specific activity of tyrosine in the same area, and is expressed in millimicromoles per gram of tissue per time interval considered:

$$C.I. = (dpm\ catecholamine/g) \div \left(\frac{dpm\ tyrosine}{m\mu moles\ tyrosine/g} \right)$$

The second method consists in calculating the decline rate of catecholamine concentration in a given brain region after blocking its synthesis by specific inhibitors of tyrosine hydroxylase activity, as described by Brodie et al. (3).

In an initial experiment we determined the effect of chronic SCD treatment on the incorporation of ^{3}H-tyrosine into DA and NE in the neurons of the forebrain regions (limbic, striatum, and cortex). The C.I. was determined 10 and 25 min after an intravenous injection of ^{3}H-tyrosine. The treatment significantly decreased endogenous tyrosine concentration as well as the accumulation of ^{3}H-tyrosine. However, the specific activity of this amino acid was never affected by the treatment (Table 1). The incorporation of radioactivity into DA was significantly enhanced in the treated group at both time intervals (Table 2). This significance was maintained when we calculated the DA C.I. In contrast, NE metabolism was not modified by SCD treatment (Table 2).

Similar results were obtained in more restricted brain areas after an injection of ^{3}H-tyrosine directly into the brain lateral ventricles. In the striatum, an area rich in DA nerve terminals, the conversion of tyrosine into DA was increased in the chronically treated group (Table 3). It should be noted that in this area the treatment also decreased the concentration of endogenous and radioactive tyrosine. Nevertheless, the specific activity of the precursor was similar in the two experimental groups (Table 3). In the diencephalon or in the lower brainstem (pons, medulla, and mesencephalon)—areas containing, respectively, noradrenergic nerve terminals or noradrenergic cell bodies (Table 4)—NE was not affected by the treatment.

The rate of DA decline, after block of its synthesis by the administration of α-methyltyrosine, was faster in the striata of SCD chronically treated rats than in the corresponding brain area of normal animals (Fig. 1), indicating an increased turnover rate. Therefore the effect of steroid contraceptives on DA metabolism was confirmed by this methodological approach.

In the second experiment endogenous DA levels were significantly lower in the treated group. This finding may be taken as further indication of increased utilization of this neurotransmitter. When the SCD was administered to rats "acutely," no effect on catecholamine turnover was evident in any of the brain areas (striatum, diencephalon, and brainstem) examined (Table 5). In fact, the only significant modification was the accumulation of ^{3}H-NE in the brainstem. Nevertheless, when this value is corrected by the corresponding specific activity of tyrosine (C.I.), the difference disappeared, indicating that it is simply due to the increase in specific activity of the precursor (Table 5). In turn, the latter was due to the decrease of brainstem endogenous tyrosine (Table 5). A parallel

TABLE 1. *Tyrosine content and ³H-tyrosine levels in the forebrain of SCD chronically treated rats*

Treatment	Tyrosine (mµmole/g)	^{3}H-Tyrosine (dpm $\times 10^{-3}$/g)		Tyrosine specific activity (dmp/mµmole)	
		10 min	25 min	10 min	25 min
Vehicle	60.9 ± 3.1 (8)	330.3 ± 13.5 (3)	139.2 ± 3.6 (5)	5,450 ± 468 (3)	2,342 ± 99 (5)
Lynestrenol + mestranol	46.5 ± 5 N (8)[a]	265.1 ± 32.7 (3)	115.9 ± 7.5 (5)[b]	6,168 ± 183 (3)	2,476 ± 157 (5)

Animals were treated for 30 days with daily lynestrenol-mestranol (5:0.3 mg/kg p.o.) and were sacrificed 10 and 25 min after an injection of ³H-tyrosine (1 mCi/kg i.v.). All animals were sacrificed in the diestrous phase.
The number of animals are in parentheses.
Data are presented as the mean ± SE and were analyzed by the *t*-test.
[a] $p < 0.01$.
[b] $p < 0.05$.

TABLE 2. *DA and NE content, and ^{3}H-DA and ^{3}H-NE accumulation in forebrain of normal and SCD chronically treated rats*

Treatment	DA (mμmole/g)	^{3}H-DA formed in forebrain (dpm/g)		DA C.I.[a]	NE (mμmole/g)	^{3}H-NE formed in forebrain (dpm/g)		NE C.I.[a]
		10 min	25 min			10 min	25 min	
Vehicle	4.6 ± 0.2 (8)	5,780 ± 579 (3)	9,500 ± 531 (5)	0.15 ± 0.014 (8)	2.05 ± 0.09 (9)	2,397 ± 614 (3)	3,457 ± 255 (5)	0.057 ± 0.006 (8)
Lynestrenol + mestranol	5.2 ± 0.3 (8)	8,790 ± 192[b]	11,760 ± 823[c] (5)	0.20 ± 0.08[c] (8)	1.99 ± 0.09 (8)	2,760 ± 314 (3)	4,730 ± 600 (5)	0.068 ± 0.008 (8)

Animals were treated for 30 days with daily lynestrenol-mestranol (5:0.3 mg/kg p.o.) and were sacrificed 10 and 25 min after an injection of ^{3}H-tyrosine (1 mCi/kg i.v.). All animals were sacrificed in the diestrous phase.

The number of animals are in parentheses.

Data are presented as mean ± SE and were analyzed by the *t*-test.

[a] C.I. = conversion index = monoamine (dpm/g tissue)/tyrosine specific activity.

[b] $p < 0.05$.

[c] $p < 0.01$.

TABLE 3. *Conversion of tyrosine into DA in the striatum of normal and SCD chronically treated rats*

Measurement	Vehicle	Lynestrenol + mestranol
Tyrosine (mμmole/g)	136 ± 3.5 (18)	112 ± 4.2 (23)[a]
^{3}H-tyrosine (dpm × 10^{-3}/g)	2,480 ± 165 (18)	1,770 ± 103 (23)[a]
Tyrosine specific activity (dmp × 10^{-2}/mμmole)	175.6 ± 11 (18)	169.4 ± 15.4 (23)
DA (mμmole/g)	53.7 ± 1.7 (18)	57.41 ± 1.6 (23)
^{3}H-DA (dpm × 10^{-3}/g)	172.2 ± 15 (18)	187.5 ± 10 (23)
DA C.I.[b]	9.3 ± 0.9 (18)	12.4 ± 0.6 (23)[c]

Animals were treated for 30 days with lynestrenol-mestranol (15:0.9 mg/kg p.o.) and were sacrificed 25 min after intraventricular administration of ^{3}H-tyrosine (14 μCi/animal). All animals wore sacrificed in the dicstrous phase.

The number of observations are in parentheses.

Data are presented as mean ± SE and were analyzed by the *t*-test.

[a] $p < 0.001$.

[b] C.I. = conversion index = monoamine (dpm/g tissue)/tyrosine specific activity.

[c] $p < 0.05$.

TABLE 4. *Conversion of tyrosine into NE in the diencephalon and brainstem of normal and SCD chronically treated rats*

	Diencephalon		Brainstem	
Measurement	Vehicle	Lynestrenol-mestranol	Vehicle	Lynestrenol-mestranol
Tyrosine (mμmole/g)	100.9 ± 3.9 (7)	89.1 ± 7.8 (8)	106 ± 10 (9)	87 ± 8 (7)
Tyrosine specific activity (dpm × 10^{-2} mμmole)	244 ± 32 (7)	292 ± 40 (8)	486 ± 45 (9)	530 ± 48 (7)
NE (mμmole/g)	2.3 ± 0.28 (7)	2.4 ± 0.2 (8)	1.8 ± 0.05 (9)	2.5 ± 0.16 (7)
^{3}H-NE (dpm × 10^{-2}/g)	312 ± 52 (7)	411 ± 53 (8)	498 ± 64 (9)	477 ± 42 (7)
NE C.I.[a]	1.10 ± 0.1 (7)	1.34 ± 0.2 (8)	1.024 ± 0.1 (9)	0.90 ± 0.04 (7)

Animals were treated for 30 days with lynestrenol-mestranol (15:0.9 mg/kg p.o.) and were sacrificed 25 min after an intraventricular administration of ^{3}H-L-tyrosine (14 μCi/animal). All animals were sacrificed in the diestrous phase.

The number of observations are in parentheses.

Data are presented as mean ± SE and were analyzed by the *t*-test.

[a] C.I. = conversion index = monoamine (dpm/g tissue)/tyrosine specific activity.

decrease of endogenous and injected amino acid was present in the striatum of the treated animals; therefore its specific activity was not modified.

EFFECT OF CHRONIC SCD TREATMENT ON CATECHOLAMINE METABOLISM IN SOME BRAIN AREAS OF THE GUINEA PIG

The study of the effects of SCD on the rate of incorporation of ^{3}H-tyrosine was extended to another animal species, the guinea pig. Female guinea pigs were treated for 90 days, the time interval equivalent to approximately six estrous

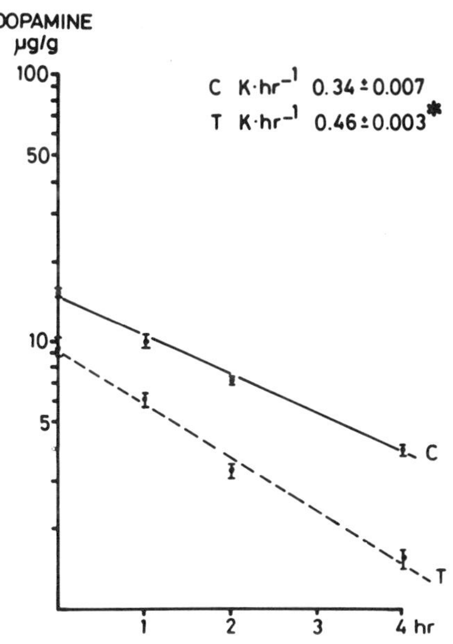

FIG. 1. Decline of striatal DA concentration after its synthesis inhibition by α-methyltyrosine (200 mg/kg i.v.) in female rats treated chronically with a combination of lynestrenol-mestranol (5:0.3 mg/kg p.o.) (- - - - -) or with the vehicle (———). Animals were treated with the inhibitor 24 hr after the last SCD administration. Each point is the average ± SE of four animals. The asterisk indicates the statistical significance ($p < 0.01$) of the difference between TK hr⁻¹ and CK hr⁻¹ according to student's t-test.

cycles. The brain areas examined were the striatum for DA, the lower brainstem (pons, medulla, and midbrain) for NE, and the hypothalamus for both catecholamines.

The results obtained were similar to those observed in the female rat after chronic treatment with the same drugs (Table 6). DA synthesis was enhanced in the striatum and hypothalamus of the treated group. The treatment did not affect NE synthesis. In fact, the increased concentration of ³H-NE in the lower brainstem was not due to an enhanced synthesis but to the higher specific activity reached by the amino acid in this brain area (Table 6).

"IN VITRO" EFFECT OF SCD CHRONIC TREATMENT ON TYROSINE HYDROXYLASE CHARACTERISTICS

The effects of SCD on the metabolism reported above could be due to the interaction of these steroids with some of the mechanisms which control DA synthesis in the neurons. The mechanisms involved in this control are: modification of tyrosine hydroxylase concentration (28), product inhibition of this enzyme (25,33), inhibition of neuronal activity by the polysynaptic neuronal loop (4), and activation of the specific receptors located in the membrane of the nerve terminals (16). The hypothesis of an action exerted by the contraceptive steroids on tyrosine hydroxylase, the enzyme controlling the rate-limiting step of catecholamine biosynthesis, was particularly appealing. In fact, specific binding sites for these steroids exist in the brain (24,36), and they selectively bind to the nuclei of the neurons (2,30); for this reason they may influence the synthesis of some specific

TABLE 5. *Conversion of tyrosine into NE and DA in the striatum, diencephalon, and brainstem of normal and short-term SCD-treated rats*

Measurement	Striatum		Diencephalon		Brainstem	
	Vehicle	Lynestrenol + mestranol	Vehicle	Lynestrenol + mestranol	Vehicle	Lynestrenol + mestranol
Tyrosine (mμmole/g)	74.5 ± 3.1 (9)	58.8 ± 2.8[a] (8)	76.1 ± 6.1 (8)	71.9 ± 4.5 (8)	77.1 ± 2.7 (9)	46.9 ± 3.9[a] (8)
Tyrosine specific activity (dpm × 10^{-2}/mμmole)	150 ± 15 (7)	170 ± 26 (6)	102.6 ± 10 (8)	92.9 ± 8.2 (8)		
DA (mμmole/g)	64.6 ± 2.2 (8)	67.9 ± 3 (8)	ND	ND	ND	ND
^{3}H-DA (dpm × 10^{-3}/g)	219 ± 32 (8)	240 ± 21.4 (8)	ND	ND	ND	ND
DA C.I.	13.8 ± 1.3 (8)	15 ± 1.3 (8)	ND	ND	ND	ND
NE (mμmole/g)	ND	ND	2.2 ± 0.1 (10)	1.9 ± 0.2 (8)	2.4 ± 0.4 (8)	2.3 ± 0.5 (8)
^{3}H-NE (dpm × 10^{-3}/g)	ND	ND	127.4 ± 15.5 (10)	143.9 ± 22.6 (8)	100.1 ± 10.6 (7)	147.4 ± 13[b] (8)$_2$
NE C.I.[c]	ND	ND	1.37 ± 0.14 (8)	1.52 ± 0.16 (7)	1.0 ± 0.08 (8)	0.9 ± 0.14 (8)

Animals were treated for 4 days with lynestrenol-mestranol (15:0.9 mg/kg p.o.) and were sacrificed 10 and 25 min after an injection of ^{3}H-tyrosine (1 mCi/kg i.v.). All animals were sacrificed in the diestrous phase.

The number of animals are in parentheses.

Data are presented as mean ± SE and were analyzed by *t*-test. ND, not determined.

[a] $p < 0.01$.

[b] $p < 0.05$.

[c] C.I. = conversion index = monoamine (dpm/g tissue)/tyrosine specific activity.

TABLE 6. *Conversion of tyrosine into DA and NE in the striatum, lower brainstem, and hypothalamus of normal and SCD chronically treated guinea pigs*

Measurement	Striatum		Lower brainstem		Hypothalamus	
	Vehicle	Lynestrenol-mestranol	Vehicle	Lynestrenol-mestranol	Vehicle	Lynestrenol-mestranol
Tyrosine (mμmole/g)	70 ± 3	68 ± 2	71 ± 1	68 ± 1	62 ± 2	63 ± 3
Tyrosine specific activity (dpm/mμmole)	41,985 ± 2,310	38,608 ± 3,479	4,234 ± 387	8,710 ± 800[a]	6,072 ± 716	7,310 ± 1,262
DA (mμmole/g)	40 ± 1.5	43 ± 1.7	ND	ND	ND	ND
^{3}H-DA (dpm/g)	220,822 ± 19,420	266,584 ± 14,689	ND	ND	4,521 ± 697	7,252 ± 919[b]
DA C.I.[c]	5.4 ± 0.6	7.2 ± 0.5[b]	ND	ND	0.7 ± 0.1	1.1 ± 0.1
NE (mμmole/g)	ND	ND	2.6 ± 0.1	2.7 ± 0.1	10.3 ± 0.4	11.5 ± 0.5
NE (dpm/g)	ND	ND	5,201 ± 617	12,720 ± 1,321[a]	17,430 ± 2,999	17,871 ± 2,300
NE C.I.[c]	ND	ND	1.3 ± 0.1	1.4 ± 0.1	2.9 ± 0.1	2.9 ± 0.2

Animals were treated for 3 months with daily lynestrenol-mestranol (1.25:0.075 mg/kg p.o.) and were sacrificed 15 min after intraventricular administration of ^{3}H-tyrosine (14 μCi/animal).

Data are presented as means ± SE of eight determinations, each made on a pool of two samples. The data are analyzed by *t*-test. ND, not determined.

[a] $p < 0.01$.

[b] $p < 0.05$.

[c] C.I. = conversion index = monoamine (dpm/g tissue)/tyrosine specific activity.

TABLE 7. *Specific activity and kinetic parameters of tyrosine hydroxylase enzyme from striatum of rats and guinea pigs treated chronically with lynestrenol-mestranol*

Condition	Specific activity (nmole CO_2/min/mg protein)	Km (DMPH$_4$) (mM)
Rat		
Vehicle	0.10 ± 0.008	0.31 ± 0.4
Lynestrenol-mestranol	0.10 ± 0.008	0.29 ± 0.1
Guinea pig		
Vehicle	0.20 ± 0.024	2.39 ± 0.39
Lynestrenol-mestranol	0.22 ± 0.025	0.95 ± 0.09[a]

Rats were treated with lynestrenol 15 mg/kg + mestranol 0.9 mg/kg for 30 days; guinea pigs were treated with lynestrenol 1.25 mg/kg + mestranol 0.075 mg/kg. Tyrosine hydroxylase activity was measured using 1.6 M MDMPH$_4$ with the standard assay system according to the method of Waymire et al. (38).

The K_m DMPH$_4$ was determined using DMPH$_4$ concentration 0.32–3.2 mM and the standard assay system.

[a] $p < 0.05$.

proteins. This kind of action has been shown to be exerted by corticosterone on the synthesis of brain serotonin (1).

To test this hypothesis, we studied *in vitro* the activity of tyrosine hydroxylase prepared from striata of female rats or guinea pigs. The animals were treated with SCD at the same dose that enhanced DA synthesis in the *in vivo* studies.

Two parameters were taken into consideration: the specific activity of the enzyme, which is related to the concentration of tyrosine hydroxylase in the sample, and the K_m for the reduced pteridine cofactor (DMPH$_4$), which is involved in the regulation of the product inhibition mechanism. Catecholamines inhibit tyrosine hydroxylase by competing for the reduced pterine cofactor; therefore a change in the affinity constant for the cofactor may reflect a change in the catecholamine competition for the binding site. Table 7 summarizes the results of this investigation. In the rat striatum tyrosine hydroxylase was not modified in either its activity or its K_m for the cofactor.

The results are different in the guinea pig because the treatment with SCD in this species does not change the activity of this enzyme, whereas its affinity constant for DMPH$_4$ is significantly decreased. This indicates a higher affinity for the cofactor by the striatal enzyme of the treated animals.

These results suggest that the action of SCD on DA biosynthesis is probably different in the various animal species, although the final effect is the same. In fact, although in the guinea pig the increased DA synthesis may be explained at least in part by modification of the enzyme K_m, the mechanism that increases DA synthesis, observed in the rat, has to be different.

EFFECT OF SCD ON SEROTONIN METABOLISM IN THE RAT BRAIN

Serotonin is another important putative neurotransmitter in the central nervous system (CNS). Abnormalities in its metabolism are sometimes correlated with affective disorders (30). Therefore it is important to elucidate the problem of the behavioral side effects of SCDs and to establish if these drugs affect this system. It has been reported that sexual steroids cause an increased 5-HT turnover in rat brain (19). In this way we studied the effect of lynestrenol and mestranol on serotonin metabolism of two brain areas of female rats: the lower brainstem, where most of the serotonergic cell bodies are located, and the limbic area (olfactory tubercles, olfactory bulbs, nucleus accumbens, and nucleus amygdaloideus inferioris), which is rich in serotonergic nerve terminals.

The animals were treated acutely or chronically as previously described. The effect of the different treatments on 5-HT turnover rate and on the concentrations of 5-HT, its catabolite 5-hydroxyindoleacetic acid (5-HIAA), and its amino acid precursor tryptophan (TP) were determined. 5-HT turnover was calculated, according to the method of Tozer et al. (37), from the product of the rate constant of 5-HIAA decline after inhibition of its formation by pargyline (75 mg/kg i.p.), a monoamine oxidase (MAO) inhibitor. The levels of TP in the brain were also determined. In fact, a change in the concentration of this amino acid may influence the rate of 5-HT synthesis (8).

Chronic treatment with SCDs (a combination of lynestrenol-mestranol) did not change the concentration of 5-HT, 5-HIAA, or TP, or the 5-HT turnover rate in either of the two brain areas considered (Table 8). However, during the acute treatment the effect on 5-HT metabolism was clearly evident (Table 8) in the brainstem and the limbic area. In the brainstem, in fact, the 5-HT and 5-HIAA concentrations were significantly increased in the treated group. When pargyline is administered to the two experimental groups, the slope of 5-HIAA decline is similar, indicating that the fractional rate constant (K) is equal in the two groups (Fig. 2). Nevertheless, the 5-HIAA steady-state level in the brainstem of rats receiving SCD is higher, indicating that neurotransmitter turnover is increased. In fact, the value of the turnover rate, calculated from the product of the rate constant of 5-HIAA decline and the steady-state level of this catabolite, was significantly higher in the treated group (Table 8). This enhancement in 5-HT turnover is not dependent on an increased concentration of the amino acid precursor in the tissue because TP was, on the contrary, significantly decreased (Table 8). In the limbic area no change in the concentrations of 5-HT, 5-HIAA, or TP is evident (Table 8); but when the formation of 5-HIAA is blocked by pargyline, the slope of its decline is faster in the treated group (Fig. 3), indicating an increased turnover rate. These experiments show that SCD affect the serotonergic system by increasing utilization of the neurotransmitter. However, this effect seems of short duration because prolonged treatment failed to produce the same effects.

At this point we studied if the effect of the treatment was due to the lynestrenol-mestranol combination or to only one component. We treated the animals acutely with lynestrenol (the progestinic component) or mestranol (the estrogenic component). The results of the experiment (Table 9) indicate that the effects on the serotonergic system are due to the progestinic component of the tested combination. In fact, when the two steroids are administered separately (Table 9), 5-HT

TABLE 8. *Effect of short-term and chronic treatment with SCD combinations on the concentrations and turnover rate of various substances in two areas of rat brain*

	Brainstem				Limbic area			
Treatment	TP (μg/g)	5-HT (μg/g)	5-HIAA (μg/g)	5-HT turnover rate (μg/g/hr)	TP (μg/g)	5-HT (μg/g)	5-HIAA (μg/g)	5-HT turnover rate (μg/g/hr)
Thirty-day treatment								
Lynestrenol-mestranol	6.2 ± 0.5	0.83 ± 0.15	1.18 ± 0.16	0.52 ± 0.06	5.07 ± 0.3	1.3 ± 0.06	0.89 ± 0.06	0.97 ± 0.10
Vehicle								
Four-day treatment	4.4 ± 0.4	0.70 ± 0.07	1.05 ± 0.14	0.41 ± 0.04	5.30 ± 0.5	1.3 ± 0.04	0.89 ± 0.06	0.85 ± 0.06
Lynestrenol-mestranol	3.4 ± 0.2[a]	1.01 ± 0.03[b]	1.00 ± 0.05[b]	0.52 ± 0.02[b]	3.50 ± 0.1	0.93 ± 0.04	0.61 ± 0.03	0.61 ± 0.05[b]
Vehicle	5.3 ± 0.1	0.76 ± 0.06	0.70 ± 0.07	0.40 ± 0.03	3.70 ± 0.1	0.90 ± 0.03	0.60 ± 0.03	0.41 ± 0.02

The results are the mean ± SE of eight samples.

5-HT turnover rate is calculated from the product of the rate constant of 5-HIAA decline after its formation blockade by the administration of the MAO inhibitor pargyline. The animals were sacrificed 0, 50, and 100 min after pargyline administration.

SCDs (lynestrenol 15 mg/kg, mestranol 0.9 mg/kg) were administered orally, dissolved in corn oil.

[a] $p < 0.001$.

[b] $p < 0.01$.

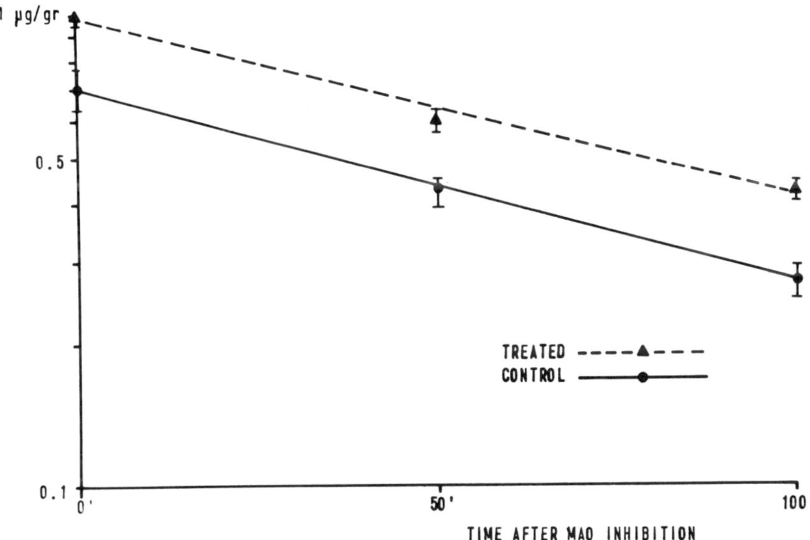

FIG. 2. Decline of 5-HIAA concentration in brainstem of vehicle or SCD (lynestrenol-mestranol 15:0.9 mg/kg p.o.) treated rats after inhibition of MAO by pargyline administration (75 mg/kg i.p.). The animals were treated daily for 4 days. The last SCD administration was given 2 hr before MAO inhibition. Each point is the average ± SE of eight animals.

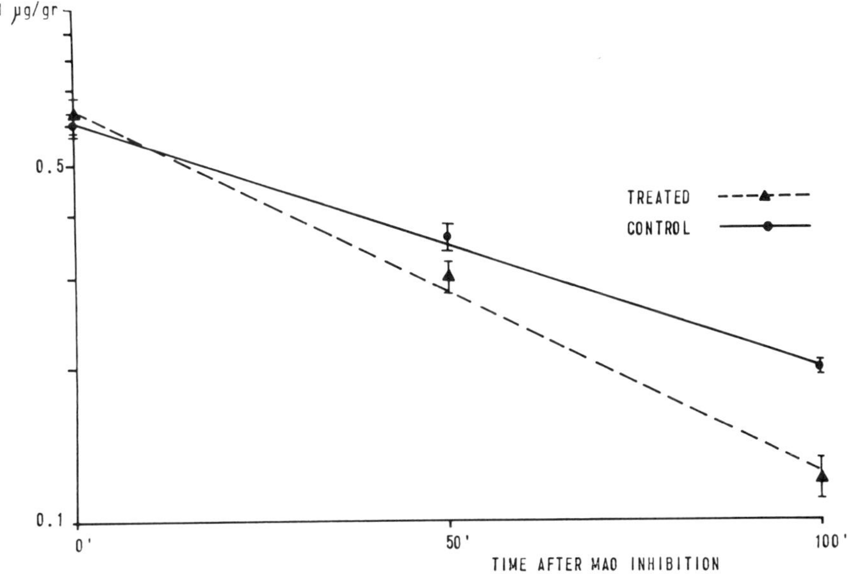

FIG. 3. Decline of 5-HIAA concentration in limbic areas of vehicle or SCD (lynestrenol-mestranol 15:0.9 mg/kg p.o.) treated rats after inhibition of MAO by pargyline administration (75 mg/kg i.p.). The animals were treated daily for 4 days. The last SCD administration was given 2 hr before MAO inhibition. Each point is the average ± SE of eight animals.

TABLE 9. *Effect of short-term treatment with lynestrenol or mestranol on the concentrations and turnover rate of various substances in two areas of rat brain*

Treatment	Brainstem				Limbic area			
	TP (μg/g)	5-HT (μg/g)	5-HIAA (μg/g)	5-HT turnover rate (μg/g/hr)	TP (μg/g)	5-HT (μg/g)	5-HIAA (μg/g)	5-HT turnover rate (μg/g/hr)
Lynestrenol	4.4 ± 0.3	0.88 ± 0.05	0.77 ± 0.08	0.38 ± 0.07[a]	6.3 ± 0.3	1.14 ± 0.07	0.67 ± 0.03	0.49 ± 0.02[b]
Vehicle	5.2 ± 0.3	0.87 ± 0.04	0.76 ± 0.03	0.26 ± 0.04	5.9 ± 0.2	1.15 ± 0.06	0.73 ± 0.04	0.33 ± 0.02
Mestranol	5.3 ± 0.3	0.81 ± 0.04	0.95 ± 0.06	0.57 ± 0.03	4.5 ± 0.3	0.98 ± 0.04	0.74 ± 0.05	0.44 ± 0.03
Vehicle	5.9 ± 0.3	0.78 ± 0.04	0.94 ± 0.03	0.66 ± 0.02	4.0 ± 0.2	0.94 ± 0.07	0.79 ± 0.04	0.48 ± 0.02

The results are the average of eight samples.

5-HT turnover rate is calculated from the product of the rate constant of 5-HIAA decline after its formation blockade by administration of the MAO inhibitor pargyline. The animals were sacrificed at 0, 50, and 100 min after pargyline administration.

Lynestrenol (15 mg/kg) or mestranol (0.9 mg/kg) was administered orally, dissolved in corn oil.

[a] $p < 0.05$.
[b] $p < 0.01$.

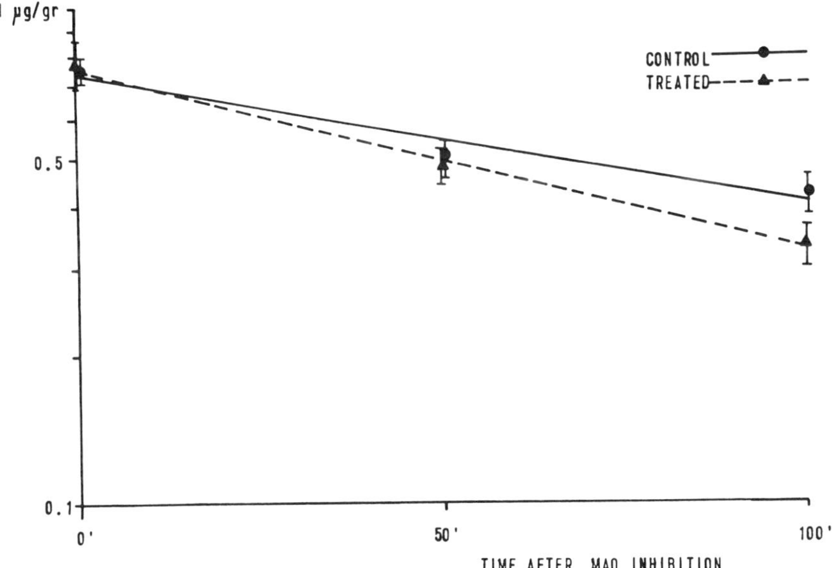

FIG. 4. Decline of 5-HIAA concentration in brainstem of vehicle or lynestrenol (15 mg/kg p.o.) treated rats after inhibition of MAO by pargyline (75 mg/kg i.p.). The animals were treated daily for 4 days. The last lynestrenol administration was 2 hr before MAO inhibition. Each point is the average ± SE of eight animals.

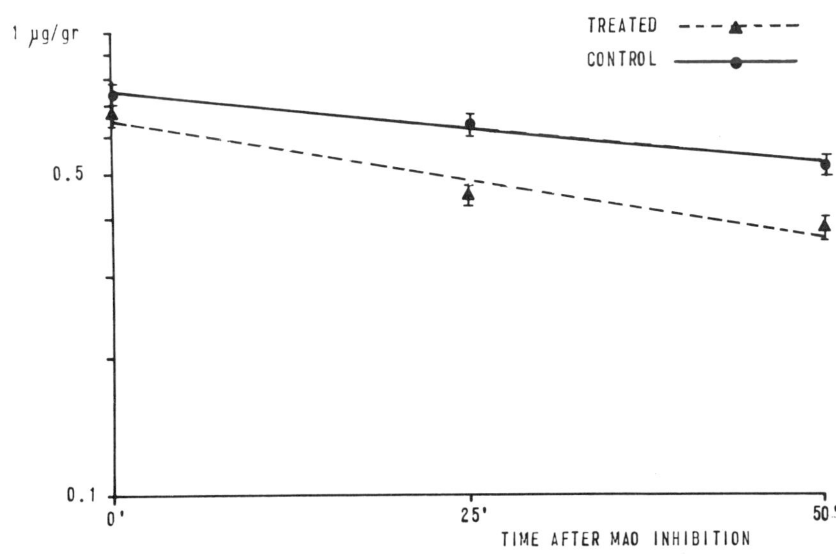

FIG. 5. Decline of 5-HIAA concentration in limbic areas of vehicle or lynestrenol (15 mg/kg p.o.) treated rats after inhibition of MAO by pargyline (75 mg/kg i.p.). The animals were treated daily for 4 days. The last lynestrenol administration was 2 hr before MAO inhibition. Each point is the average ± SE of eight animals.

turnover was enhanced only in the group treated with lynestrenol (Figs. 4 and 5), whereas mestranol was ineffective.

EFFECT OF SCD ON ACETYLCHOLINE LEVEL AND CHOLINE-O-ACETYLTRANSFERASE ACTIVITY IN MESENCEPHALON, DIENCEPHALON, AND CEREBRAL HEMISPHERES OF FEMALE RATS

There are no data on the effect of short-term or chronic treatment with SCDs on the acetylcholine level or choline-O-acetyltransferase activity of rat brain areas, although the provocative findings of Simonovic et al. (32) and Justo et al. (13) that acetylcholine stimulated the release of follicle-stimulating hormone-releasing hormone and lutenizing hormone-releasing hormone *in vivo* and *in vitro* imply a role for the cholinergic system in the regulation of ovulatory function in the rat (see also ref. 22). It was thus of interest to determine if short-term or chronic treatment with SCD can affect the acetylcholine level or the activity of its synthesizing enzyme choline-O-acetyltransferase (parameters indicative of the presence of cholinergic neurons) in the cerebral hemispheres, diencephalon, and

TABLE 10. *Effect of short-term and chronic SCD on acetylcholine in some rat brain areas*

Treatment (mg/kg p.o.)	Acetylcholine (nmoles/g wet wt $\pm$ SE)		
	Hemispheres	Diencephalon	Mesencephalon
Five-day treatment			
Vehicle[a]	14.3 $\pm$ 0.7 (6)	23.9 $\pm$ 1.3 (6)	17.8 $\pm$ 1.3 (6)
Lynestrenol (5 mg/kg) + mestranol (0.3 mg/kg)	13.7 $\pm$ 0.7 (7)	24.6 $\pm$ 1.3 (6)	17.8 $\pm$ 0.7 (6)
Thirty-day treatment			
Vehicle[a]	13.7 $\pm$ 0.7 (6)	23.3 $\pm$ 0.7 (5)	18.5 $\pm$ 1.3 (6)
Lynestrenol (5 mg/kg) + mestranol (0.3 mg/kg)	15.1 $\pm$ 1.3 (4)	25.3 $\pm$ 0.7[b] (5)	17.1 $\pm$ 0.7 (6)

Number of animals is in parentheses.
Acetylcholine was measured by the radiochemical method of Saelens et al. (29) as modified by Ladinsky et al. (18).
The last dose of SCD was administered 2 hr before sacrifice.
[a] Vehicle-treated animals in diestrus were selected for these controls.
[b] $p < 0.05$ (Student's *t*-test).

mesencephalon of the rat. Except for a small increase—approximately 10% ($p < 0.05$)—in the acetylcholine level in the diencephalon (Table 10), Lyndiol had no effect on these cholinergic parameters in the brain areas considered after 5 or 30 days' treatment (Tables 10 and 11).

TABLE 11. *Effect of short-term and chronic SCD on in vitro choline acetyltransferase from various rat brain areas*

	Choline acetyltransferase (μmoles ACh formed/g protein/hr ± SE)		
Treatment (mg/kg p.o.)	Hemispheres	Diencephalon	Mesencephalon
Five-day treatment			
Vehicle	68.4 ± 0.0 (5)	44.7 ± 1.6 (7)	61.6 ± 1.9 (7)
Lynestrenol (5 mg/kg) + mestranol (0.3 mg/kg)	66.9 ± 3.8 (5)	41.8 ± 1.3 (5)	61.5 ± 2.1 (5)
Thirty-day treatment			
Vehicle	48.4 ± 2.1 (4)	48.2 ± 3.3 (4)	73.7 ± 4.0 (4)
Lynestrenol (5 mg/kg) + mestranol (0.3 mg/kg)	53.2 ± 2.2 (6)	48.5 ± 1.7 (6)	65.5 ± 3.4 (6)

Choline-O-acetyltransferase was measured by the radiochemical method of McCaman and Hunt (23) as modified by Consolo et al. (5).
The last dose of SCD was administered 2 hr before sacrifice.
The number of animals is in parentheses.

CONCLUSION

The results of our experiments indicate that SCDs administered at the minimal doses that give 100% antifertility modify the metabolism of some monoamines, and so also modify the functionality of the neurons which utilize these neurotransmitters. The monoamines affected are DA and serotonin, which present an increased turnover, whereas the turnover and the NE and acetylcholine levels were not modified. The mechanism of interaction between steroidal sexual hormones and these two monoaminergic systems remains to be clarified. These hormones could act directly in the neurons or indirectly through their actions on gonadotropin release. It has been demonstrated that sexual steroids are specifically bound in the neurons in certain brain areas, especially the hypophysis and hypothalamus (35), and to a minor extent in other brain regions (24,26,35,36). Moreover, there is evidence indicating that these binding sites are located at least partly in the neuronal cell nuclei (2,39). This suggests the possibility that the specific binding may alter some of the processes connected with the synthesis of proteins involved in dopaminergic or serotonergic synthesis.

It is interesting to note in this respect that in the guinea pig it has been possible to demonstrate a change in the kinetic characteristics of tyrosine hydroxylase (Table 7). Although the modifications determined by the SCD treatment are significant, the extent of this effect is limited to approximately 25–30% for the increase in DA and the serotonin turnover.

The meaning of this effect in terms of behavioral modification is therefore questionable, and it is particularly difficult to assess if these findings are related to the side effects, such as the mental depression observed in women taking the pill. Nevertheless, it should be kept in mind that the small changes we have seen in relatively larger brain areas may be much more pronounced at the level of some specific neuronal population.

ACKNOWLEDGMENT

The research on which this publication is based was performed pursuant to Contract No. NIH-NICHD-72–2733 with the National Institutes of Health; Department of Health, Education and Welfare.

REFERENCES

1. Azmitia, E. C., Jr., and McEwen, B. S. (1969): Corticosterone regulation of tryptophan hydroxylase in midbrain of the rat. *Science,* 166:1274–1276.
2. Baulieu, E-E. (1977): This volume.
3. Brodie, B. B., Costa, E., Dlabac, A., Neff, N. H., and Smookler, H. H. (1966): Application of steady state kinetics to the estimation of synthesis rate and turnover time of tissue catecholamines. *J. Pharmacol. Exp. Ther.,* 154:493–498.
4. Carlsson, A., and Lindqvist, M. (1963): Effect of chlorpromazine or haloperidol on formation of 3-methoxytyramine and normetanephrine in mouse brain. *Acta Pharmacol. Toxicol. (Kbh.),* 20:140–144.
5. Consolo, S., Garattini, S., Ladinsky, H., and Thoenen, H. (1972): Effect of chemical sympathectomy on the content of acetylcholine, choline and choline acetyltransferase activity in the cat spleen and iris. *J. Physiol. (Lond.),* 220:639–646.
6. Donoso, A. O., Bishop, W., Fawcett, C. P., Krulich, L., and McCann, S. M. (1971): Effects of drugs that modify brain monoamine concentrations on plasma gonadotropin and prolactin levels in the rat. *Endocrinology,* 89:774–784.
7. F.D.A. statement on oral contraceptives. *F.D.C. Reports,* August 15, 1966.
8. Fernstrom, J. D., and Wurtman, R. J. (1971): Brain serotonin content: Physiological dependence on plasma tryptophan levels. *Science,* 173:149–152.
9. Fuxe, K., Hökfelt, T., Jonsson, G., and Löfström, A. (1973): Recent morphological and functional studies on hypothalamic dopaminergic and noradrenergic mechanisms. In: *Frontiers in Catecholamine Research,* edited by E. Usdin and S. H. Snyder, pp. 787–794. Pergamon Press, New York.
10. Grounds, D., Davies, B., and Mowbray, R. (1970): The contraceptive pill, side effects and personality: Report of a controlled double blind trial. *Br. J. Psychiatry,* 116:169–172.
11. Huffer, V., Levin, L., and Aronson, H. (1970): Oral contraceptives: Depression and frigidity. *J. Nerv. Ment. Dis.,* 151:35–41.
12. Jori, A., and Cecchetti, G. (1973): Homovanillic acid levels in rat striatum during the oestrous cycle. *J. Endocrinol.,* 58:341–342.
13. Justo, G., Motta, M., and Martini, L. (1975): In vivo effects of acetylcholine on LH secretion. *Experientia,* 31:598–600.
14. Kamberi, I. A., Mical, R. S., and Porter, J. C. (1970): Effect of anterior pituitary perfusion and intraventricular injection of catecholamines and indoleamines on LH release. *Endocrinology,* 87:1–12.
15. Kay, C. R. (1977): This volume.
16. Kehr, W., Carlsson, A., Lindqvist, M., Magnusson, T., and Atack, C. (1972): Evidence for a receptor-mediated feedback control of striatal tyrosine hydroxylase activity. *J. Pharm. Pharmacol.,* 24:744–747.
17. Kordon, C., and Glowinski, J. (1972): Role of hypothalamic monoaminergic neurones in the gonadotrophin release-regulating mechanisms. *Neuropharmacology,* 11:153–162.
18. Ladinsky, H., Consolo, S., Bianchi, S., and Jori, A. (1976): Increase in striatal acetylcholine by picrotoxin in the rat: Evidence for a gabergic-dopaminergic-cholinergic link. *Brain Res.,* 108: 351–361.
19. Ladisich, W. (1974): Effect of progesterone on regional 5-hydroxytryptamine metabolism in the rat brain. *Neuropharmacology,* 13:877–883.

20. Lichtensteiger, W. (1973): Catecholamines in sexual hormone regulation: forebrain influence on tubero-infundibular dopamine neurones and interaction with cholinergic systems. In: *Frontiers in Catecholamine Research,* edited by E. Usdin and S. H. Snyder, pp. 803–809. Pergamon Press, New York.

21. Marcotte, D. B., Kane, F. J., Obrist, P., and Lipton, M. A. (1970): Psychophysiologic changes accompanying oral contraceptive use. *Br. J. Psychiatry,* 116:165–167.

22. Martini, L. (1977): This volume.

23. McCaman, R. E., and Hunt, J. M. (1965): Microdetermination of choline acetylase in nervous tissue. *J. Neurochem.,* 12:253–259.

24. McEwen, B. S., Zigmond, R. E., and Gerlach, J. L. (1972): Sites of steroid binding and action in the brain. In: *The Structure and Function of Nervous System,* Vol. 5, edited by G. H. Bourne, pp. 205–291. Academic Press, New York.

25. Neff, N. H., and Costa, E. (1968): Application of steady-state kinetics to the study of catecholamine turnover after monoamine oxidase inhibition or reserpine administration. *J. Pharmacol. Exp. Ther.,* 160:40–47.

26. Pfaff, D. W., and Keiner, M. (1973): Altas of estradiol-concentrating cells in the central nervous system of the female rat. *J. Comp. Neurol.,* 151:121–158.

27. Piva, F., Sterescu, N., Zanisi, M., and Martini, L. (1969): Non-steroidal antifertility agents affecting brain mechanisms. *Bull. WHO,* 41:275–288.

28. Pletscher, A. (1972): Regulation of catecholamine turnover by variations of enzyme levels. *Pharmacol. Rev.,* 24:225–232.

29. Saelens, J. K., Allen, M. P., and Simke, J. P. (1970): Determination of acetylcholine and choline by an enzymatic assay. *Arch. Int. Pharmacodyn. Ther.,* 186:279–286.

30. Schildkraut, J. J. (1973): Neuropharmacology of the affective disorders. *Annu. Rev. Pharmacol.,* 13:427–454.

31. Sedvall, G. C., Weise, V. K., and Kopin, I. J. (1968): The rate of norepinephrine synthesis measured "in vivo" during short intervals: Influence of adrenergic nerve impulse activity. *J. Pharmacol. Exp. Ther.,* 159:274–282.

32. Simonovic, I., Motta, M., and Martini, L. (1974): Acetylcholine and the release of the follicle-stimulating hormone-releasing factor. *Endocrinology,* 95:1373–1379.

33. Spector, S., Gordon, R., Sjoerdsma, A., and Udenfriend, S. (1967): End-product inhibition of tyrosine hydroxylase as a possible mechanism for regulation of norepinephrine synthesis. *Mol. Pharmacol.,* 3:549–555.

34. Strada, S. J., Sanders-Bush, E., and Sulser, F. (1970): p-Chloramphetamine temporal relationship between psychomotor stimulation and metabolism of brain norepinephrine. *Biochem. Pharmacol.,* 19:2621–2629.

35. Stumpf, W. E. (1968): Estradiol-concentrating neurons: Topography in the hypothalamus by dry-mount autoradiography. *Science,* 162:1001–1003.

36. Stumpf, W. E., and Madhabananda, S. (1977): This volume.

37. Tozer, T. N., Neff, N. H., and Brodie, B. B. (1966): Application of steady state kinetics to the synthesis rate and turnover time of serotonin in the brain of normal and reserpine-treated rats. *J. Pharmacol. Exp. Ther.,* 153:177–182.

38. Waymire, J. C., Bjur, R., and Weiner, N. (1971): Assay of tyrosine hydroxylase by coupled decarboxylation of dopa formed from 1-^{14}C-L-tyrosine. *Anal. Biochem.,* 43:588–600.

39. Zigmond, R. E., and McEwen, B. S. (1970): Selective retention of oestradiol by cell nuclei in specific brain regions of the ovariectomized rat. *J. Neurochem.,* 17:889–899.

40. Zschaeck, L. L., and Wurtman, R. J. (1973): Brain ^{3}H-catechol synthesis and the vaginal estrous cycle. *Neuroendocrinology,* 11:144–149.

Pharmacology of Steroid Contraceptive Drugs
edited by S. Garattini and H. W. Berendes.
Raven Press, New York © 1977.

Metabolic Pathways of Steroid Contraceptive Drugs

Heinz Breuer

*Institut für Klinische Biochemie, Universität Bonn, D 5300 Bonn-Venusberg,
F. R. Germany*

Synthetic progestational and estrogenic steroids have been in use for more than
15 years as oral contraceptive drugs. Much effort has been devoted to the study
of their metabolism, and these investigations have revealed various specific metabolic pathways, including ring A reductions, hydroxylations, and conjugations.
The most widely used contraceptive steroids are shown in Fig. 1. Norethister-

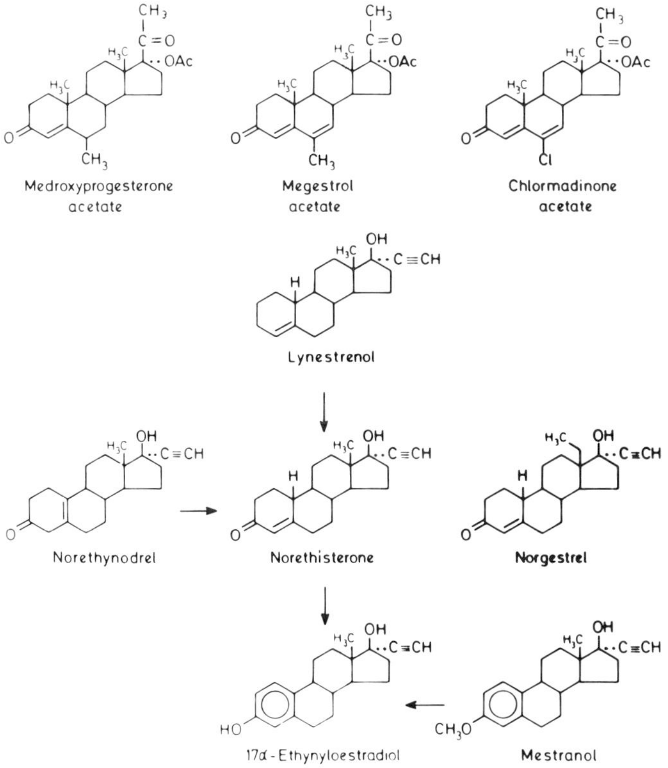

FIG. 1. Chemical structure and relationship of the most widely used contraceptive steroids.

one, lynestrenol, norethynodrel, and norgestrel belong to the group of C_{19}-nor-steroids which are derived from 19-nortestosterone. As indicated by the arrows, there is a close chemical relationship between lynestrenol, norethynodrel, and norethisterone. A second group of progestational compounds comprises the C-6-substituted C_{21}-steroids medroxyprogresterone acetate, megestrol acetate, and chlormadinone acetate. The only estrogenic contraceptive agents so far developed are 17α-ethynylestradiol and its 3-methyl ether. The main features of the metabolic pathways of the compounds in Fig. 1 are discussed in this chapter, with special reference to qualitative aspects; in addition, some metabolic interactions are dealt with.

NORETHISTERONE

Norethisterone, which has been in use for more than 15 years, is a progestational compound commonly found in both sequential- and combination-type birth control pills. Quantitative and qualitative aspects of its metabolism have been studied in numerous laboratories. It is well established that metabolic attacks occur at several points in norethisterone. These include reduction of ring A, hydroxylations, and, probably only to a small extent, reactions at the ethynyl side chain (5). The major metabolities in urine and plasma result from reduction of the Δ^4-3-oxo group to give a mixture of 5α- and 5β-reduced 3-hydroxy compounds (Fig. 2). 17α-Ethynyl-5β-estrene-3α,17β-diol was identified as the main metabolite of norethisterone in the glucuronide fraction of the urine (19); this metabolite accounted for 25–28% of compounds that could be extracted from the urine after glucuronide cleavage. In addition, the 5α-H-3α-hydroxysteroid

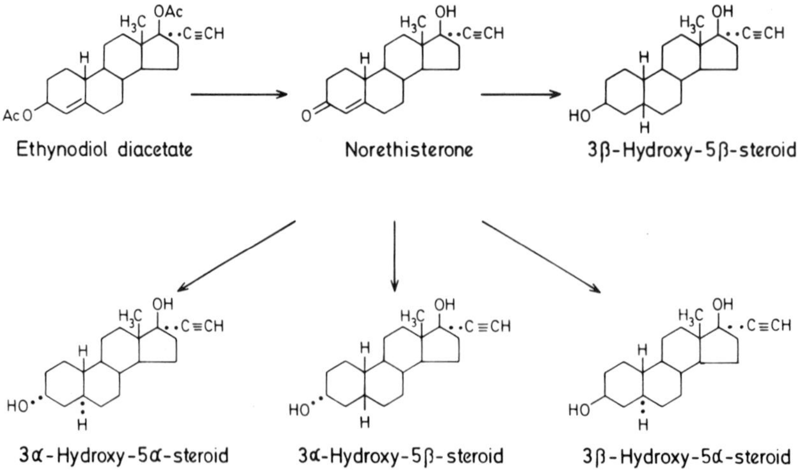

FIG. 2. Reductive metabolism of norethisterone.

was identified in the glucuronide fraction. The 3β-hydroxy compound (5α-H and 5β-H) occurred only in small amounts (19).

For many years considerable interest has been focused on the question to what extent norethisterone may be aromatized to 17α-ethynylestradiol under physiological conditions. When we first studied the metabolic fate of norethisterone in man (8), we noted a marked increase in the urinary excretion of 17α-ethynylestradiol. This finding was confirmed by Brown and Blair (11), who came to the conclusion that a dose of 12–30 mg norethisterone is converted in the human body to approximately 1 mg 17α-ethynylestradiol. Similar findings were reported by Langecker (26), Okada et al. (36), and later by Kamyab et al. (22). However, none of these investigators could demonstrate an increase in the urinary estriol fraction. This negative finding suggested that the 17α-ethynylestradiol found in the urine of subjects treated with norethisterone may have been formed as an artifact during analysis of the urine specimens (6).

To find out if norethisterone is in fact converted to 17α-ethynylestradiol by human tissue, a number of C_{19}-steroids were incubated with the human placental aromatizing enzyme system (38) and were also perfused through fresh human placenta (42). Whereas testosterone, 19-nortestosterone, and the 17α-methyl derivative were aromatized to the corresponding phenolic compounds in a yield of 35–53%, neither 17α-ethynyltestosterone nor 17α-ethynyl-19-nortestosterone (norethisterone) were converted to 17α-ethynylestradiol to any measurable extent. These results strongly suggested that the 17α-ethynyl side chain prevents aromatization of C_{19}- or C_{18}-steroids to estrogenic compounds.

At this stage the question arises of how to explain the discrepancy between the *in vitro* and perfusion experiments on the one hand and the *in vivo* findings on the other. Townsley et al. (45) discovered in 1966 that 19-norandrostenedione is converted by placental preparations to 1β-hydroxy-19-norandrostenedione; similar findings were obtained with minced human ovary (44). Treatment of 1β-hydroxy-19-norandrostenedione with either acid or base results in the formation of estrone (43). Since in all reported studies in which the metabolism of norethisterone has been investigated the isolation and estimation procedures involved acid hydrolysis and partition between aqueous base and organic solvent, the presence of 1β-hydroxylated derivatives of 19-norsteroids would have artificially inflated the value for estrogens. Thus on the basis of the *in vitro* findings, it seemed reasonable to conclude that the various phenolic compounds arose as artifacts during the analysis of urine from subjects treated with norethisterone.

In this connection it should be pointed out that Sinsenwine et al. (41) recently isolated 1β-hydroxynorgestrel from the urine of women treated with *dl*-norgestrel; they demonstrated that this metabolite is aromatized to 18-homoethynylestradiol under acidic or mildly alkaline conditions (Fig. 3). They devised a method by which 1-hydroxylated metabolites are eliminated prior to fractionation and analysis. This method is based on the reduction by sodium borohydride of the 1-hydroxy-4-en-3-one grouping in ring A, thereby excluding the possibility of aromatization. When the method was applied to urine from women who had

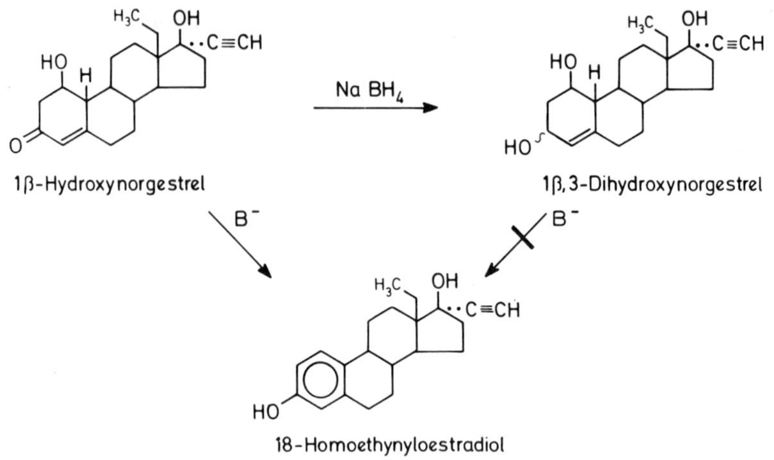

FIG. 3. Spontaneous aromatization of 1β-hydroxynorgestrel to 18-homoethynylestradiol and prevention of this reaction by reduction of 1β-hydroxynorgestrel with NaBH$_4$. (From Sinsenwine et al., ref. 41.)

received norethisterone, only trace amounts, if any, of 17α-ethynylestradiol were found (H Breuer, *unpublished experiments*). The extremely small amounts persisting after sodium borohydride reduction could be artifacts from 1β-hydroxylated metabolites in urine formed during the time between excretion and analysis.

NORETHISTERONE ENANTHATE

Recently norethisterone enanthate has been used increasingly as an injectable formulation which produces a long-lasting antifertility effect. *In vivo* and *in vitro* studies indicate that the metabolism of the enanthate does not differ qualitatively from that of the free compound (21). However, the cleavage rates of norethisterone enanthate and norethisterone acetate (tertiary 17β-esters) are significantly slower than those of the corresponding testosterone esters (secondary 17β-esters) (3).

NORETHYNODREL

Norethynodrel belongs to the most frequently prescribed progestational compounds in oral contraceptives. A study of the uptake of tritiated norethynodrel after a single injection and constant infusion showed that the steroid was selectively taken up by the uterus and other tissues of the reproductive tract of the rat (28,39). Norethynodrel is also known to modify the uptake of tritiated estradiol-17β in the uterus (27). Moreover, a study of the fate of tritiated norethynodrel in women revealed that the steroid had a relatively long half-life and showed retention in the endometrium (29). These findings led Laumas and his colleagues to investigate the metabolism of norethynodrel in the human endometrium and myometrium (34). As summarized in Fig. 4, the major metabolite identified after incubation of norethynodrel with minced uterine tissue was norethisterone. The shift of the double bond from the 5(10) to the 4(5) position of the steroid nucleus requires the enzyme $\Delta^{5(10)}$-3-oxosteroid isomerase. Under the experimental conditions used, the spontaneous conversion of norethynodrel to norethisterone accounted for only 1–2% of the substrate, whereas in the presence of the uterine tissue the conversion of norethynodrel to norethisterone was approximately 50% on the average. This suggests that the conversion of norethynodrel was an enzymatic process. The myometrial 105,000 g supernatant converted norethynodrel to norethisterone more than the mitochondrial and microsomal fractions did. This implies that the highest total activity of the enzyme $\Delta^{5(10)}$-3-oxosteroid isomerase is localized in the supernatant fraction.

The conversion of norethynodrel to the 3α-hydroxy compound (Fig. 4) was two times greater in the proliferative endometrium than in the secretory phase, suggesting that the enzyme 3α-hydroxysteroid oxidoreductase (3-oxosteroid reductase) is present in greater quantities in the proliferative endometrium. In the subcellular fractions of the myometrium, the conversion of norethynodrel to the 3α-hydroxy compound was found mainly in the 105,000 g supernatant fraction.

Chen and Lee (12) investigated the steroid-protein binding complex of norethynodrel and liver microsomes. The formation of this metabolite proceeded rapidly in the complete oxygenase system. It started at a linear rate and reached a plateau within 10 min with an apparent K_m value of 3.33 × 10^{-5} moles/liter. The reaction required oxygen as well as NADPH. Norethynodrel is probably metabolized to a reactive intermediate that is able to bind covalently to the

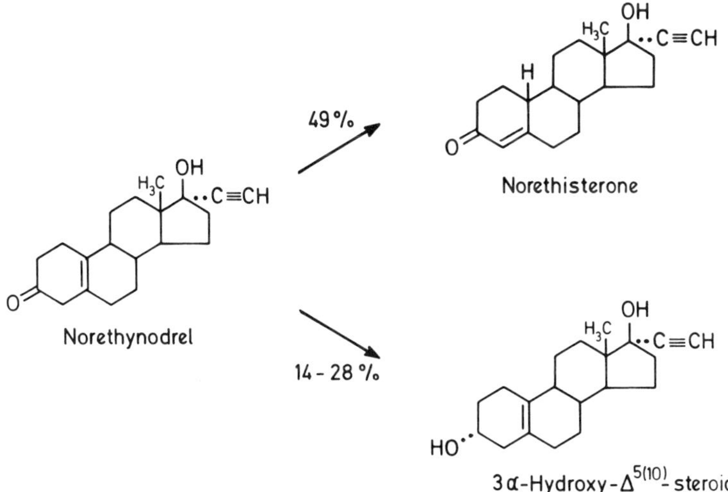

Fig. 4. Metabolism of norethynodrel in minced uterine tissue. (From Murugesan et al., ref. 34.)

proteins present in the incubation mixture. It may be speculated that the active steroid intermediate is either a hydroperoxide derivative (17α-ethynyl-10β-hydroperoxy-19-nortestosterone) or an epoxide intermediate (17α-ethynyl-5α, 10α-oxidoestron-17β-ol-3-one). Hydroperoxides and epoxides form during steroid metabolism.

LYNESTRENOL

Although lynestrenol is closely related chemically to norethisterone, the two compounds show differences in biological activities. On the other hand, Kamyab et al. (23) reported that there are similarities between the *in vivo* metabolism of ^{14}C-labeled norethisterone and lynestrenol in man. This led to an investigation which revealed that under *in vitro* conditions lynestrenol is converted to norethisterone (32). As indicated in Fig. 5, norethisterone formation in these experiments may be due to direct hydroxylation of lynestrenol at carbon atom C3, followed by dehydrogenation. It is well known that steroids containing the 3-hydroxy-4-ene group (allylic alcohols) are easily oxidized by liver tissue to the Δ^4-3-ketone. The 3α-hydroxylated 5α-reduced metabolite of lynestrenol (13,32) could arise by reduction of either the 3-hydroxy-Δ^4-steroid or norethisterone. It is interesting to note that these experiments demonstrate for the first time direct hydroxylation of a steroid at carbon atom C3.

A comparative study of the metabolism of lynestrenol acetate and lynestrenol showed that the two compounds are, at least to some extent, metabolized via different pathways (13). After intravenous administration to rats, lynestrenol

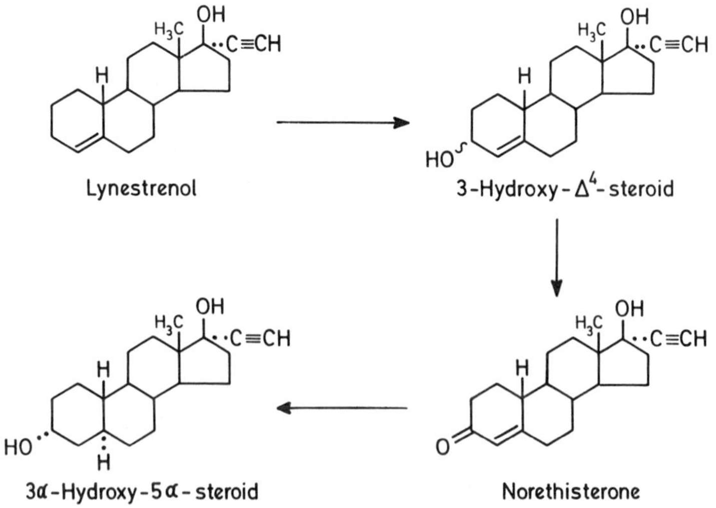

Lynestrenol   3-Hydroxy-Δ^4-steroid

3α-Hydroxy-5α-steroid   Norethisterone

FIG. 5. Metabolic pathways leading to 3-oxygenated metabolites of lynestrenol. (From Mazaheri et al., ref. 32.)

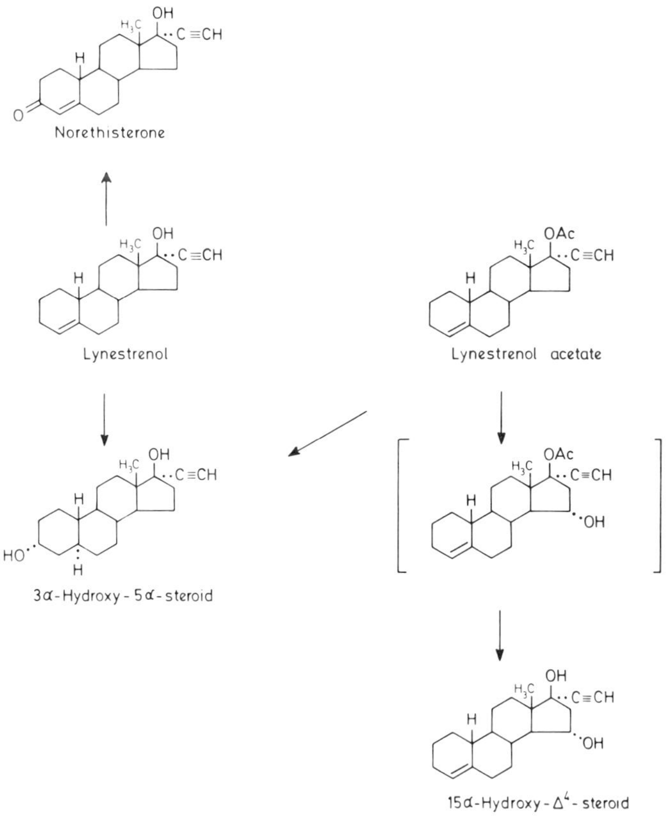

Fig. 6. Metabolism of lynestrenol and lynestrenol acetate. (From Coert et al., ref. 13.)

acetate was altered in the nucleus in the presence of the acetate group. The acetate group itself was removed, either when the alteration took place or after it had been completed. The results of IR, NMR, and mass spectrometry analysis indicated the introduction of a 15α-hydroxyl group (Fig. 6). The 15α-hydroxy metabolite was formed only from lynestrenol acetate, not from lynestrenol. In contrast, the 3α-hydroxy-5α-steroid was an important metabolite of both lynestrenol and lynestrenol acetate. These results indicate that esterification of a steroid can lead to deviation from the metabolic pathway of the original free steroid.

NORGESTREL

Before turning to the qualitative aspects of the metabolism of *dl*-norgestrel, it should be noted that its A-ring reduction proceeds more slowly than that of norethisterone (19); the inhibition of ring A reduction is probably due to the methyl group at carbon atom C18. It may be assumed that the higher biological activity of norgestrel—as compared with norethisterone—can be attributed to this inhibition of ring A reduction, as a result of which the unchanged compound remains longer in the organism.

Sinsenwine et al. (40) studied in detail the qualitative metabolism of *dl*-norgestrel in woman (Fig. 7). The major metabolite (approximately 30% of the urinary activity) was found to be 16β-hydroxynorgestrel sulfate. The conjugated as well as the free fractions comprised at least 23 metabolites. Among them were biological transformation products resulting from hydroxylation at the 16α, 16β, 1β, 2α-, and 6-positions; *d*-homoannulation; and ring-A reduction (3α,5β-tetrahydronorgestrel and its 3β,5β- and 3α,5α-isomers, and a 16-hydroxylated tetrahydronorgestrel). The 16β-hydroxylated and the 3α-hydroxy-5β-reduced metabolites are quantitatively the most important ones. On the basis of the results of Sinsenwine et al. (40), it is evident that the norgestrel molecule is intensively hydroxylated, whereas reduction of ring A is less prominent. This agrees with the kinetic studies mentioned previously (19).

The identification of 1β-hydroxynorgestrel among the urinary metabolites of *dl*-norgestrel and the easy transformation of this compound under mild alkaline conditions to a potentially estrogenic phenol (Fig. 3) suggested that the estrogens present in the urine of subjects treated with synthetic progestational steroids are artifacts formed during analytical workup. As already pointed out, Sinsenwine

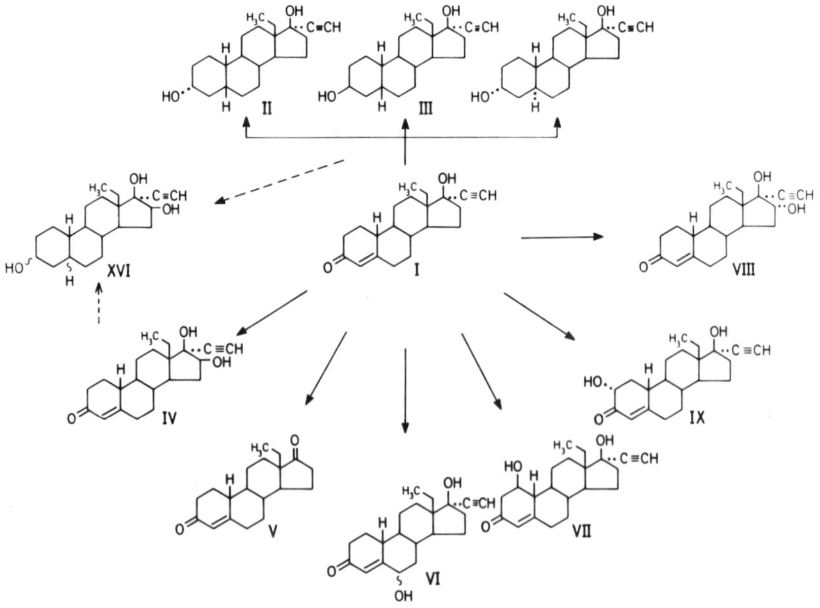

FIG. 7. Urinary metabolites of *dl*-norgestrel in women. (From Sinsenwine et al., ref. 40.)

et al. (41) worked out a method which eliminates 1-hydroxylated metabolites as potential sources of phenolic artifacts. After reduction of the 1-hydroxy-4-en-3-one grouping in ring A with sodium borohydride, the urine of women treated with [14]C-*dl*-norgestrel contained only 0.17–0.27% of the dose as phenolic material. Thus it remains to be shown whether norgestrel and norethisterone are truly metabolized to estrogenic compounds.

CHLORMADINONE ACETATE

The metabolism of chlormadinone acetate, a highly active synthetic progestational steroid derived from progesterone, is influenced to a great extent by barbiturate induction (20). Under noninduced conditions (Fig. 8), the microsomal

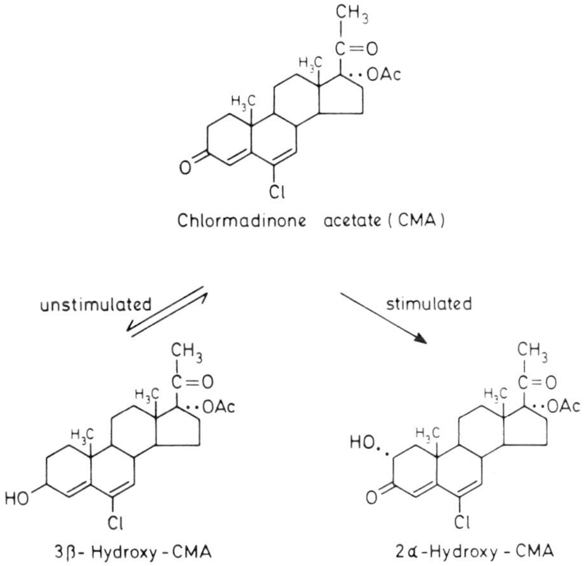

FIG. 8. Metabolism of chlormadinone acetate under various conditions. (From Handy et al., ref. 20.)

enzyme system from male rats and humans formed predominantly 3β-hydroxychlormadinone acetate (17β-acetoxy-6-chloro-3β-hydroxypregna-4,6-dien-2-one). After barbiturate induction (Fig. 8), 2α-hydroxychlormadinone acetate was the major metabolite formed in rat and rabbit liver homogenates (20). From these results it may be concluded that microsomal hydroxylation, dominant in the metabolism of megesterol and medroxyprogesterone, is not a significant initial pathway in the noninduced *in vitro* metabolism of chlormadinone acetate.

MEGESTROL ACETATE

When radioactively labeled megestrol acetate was administered orally to women, three metabolites, excreted as glucuronide conjugates, were identified (14). Hydroxylation had occurred at C2, at the 6-methyl, and at both positions (Fig. 9). It should be noted that the metabolic attack at carbon atom C6 opens

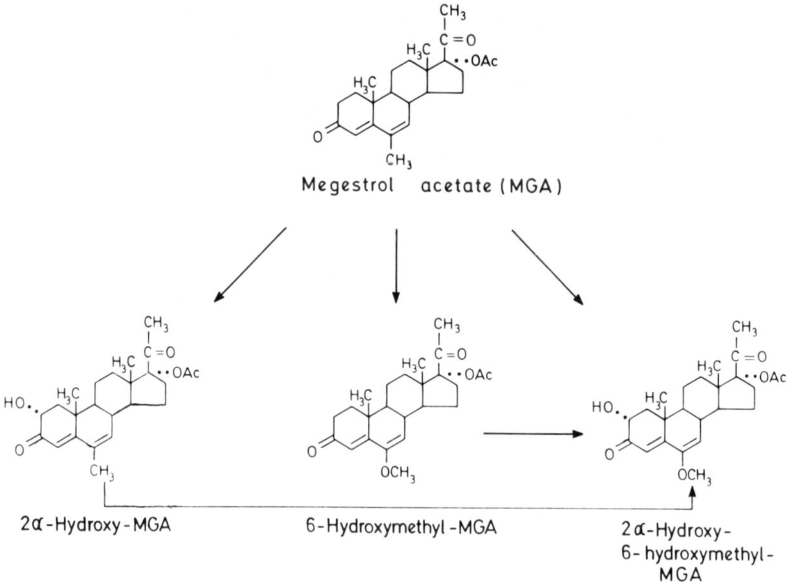

FIG. 9. Metabolism of megestrol acetate in women. (From Cooper and Kellie, ref. 14.)

a possible route for the removal of the 6-methyl group by further oxidation. For comparison, progesterone is metabolized by reduction and hydroxylation to less lipophilic compounds; the metabolites of progesterone also become more hydrophilic by conjugation. Megestrol acetate is resistant to this type of metabolism and, in addition, is less hydrophilic than progesterone. This difference in metabolism indicates that the temporary storage of megestrol acetate in body fat may be greater than that of progesterone.

ETHYNYLESTRADIOL

The metabolism of 17α-ethynylestradiol and its 3-methyl ether (mestranol) has been the subject of intensive study during the last decade. In 1969 Fotherby and his colleagues (24) stated that 17α-ethynylestradiol undergoes a considerable metabolism in women. After oral or intravenous administration of ^{14}C-labeled 17α-ethynylestradiol, only small amounts of radioactivity were detected in the fraction which would have contained any 17α-ethynylestradiol present in the

urine. Later the same group (37) reported that up to 16.5% of the administered
17α-ethynylestradiol was excreted unchanged in urine, whereas excretion via
feces accounted for up to 30% of the administered dose.

Since it has been shown that women who take 17α-ethynylestradiol have an
abnormal metabolism of endogenous estradiol (31), it appeared reasonable to
study the effects which 17α-ethynylestradiol might have on its own metabolism.
Surprisingly, it was found that the mean metabolic clearance rates of 17α-
ethynylestradiol of the two groups—normals and 17α-ethynylestradiol users
—are not significantly different. Thus ingestion of 17α-ethynylestradiol does not
appear to alter the metabolism of 17α-ethynylestradiol (30). It may be that
different enzymes are responsible for the metabolism of estradiol-17β as compared
to 17α-ethynylestradiol, and that 17α-ethynylestradiol induces the estradiol-
metabolizing enzyme system but not the 17α-ethynylestradiol-metabolizing system. It may also be that estradiol metabolism is more sensitive than 17α-
ethynylestradiol metabolism to the cholestatic effect of 17α-ethynylestradiol.

Qualitative aspects of the metabolic fate of 17α-ethynylestradiol and mestranol
have been investigated in detail by a number of laboratories. The main findings
are summarized in Fig. 10. Mestranol is demethylated to 17α-ethynylestradiol.
Demethylation of 3-methoxyestrogens is a well-known reaction which was documented many years ago (9,10). An interesting metabolite of mestranol is mestranol glucuronide (47). The only position available for conjugation of mestranol

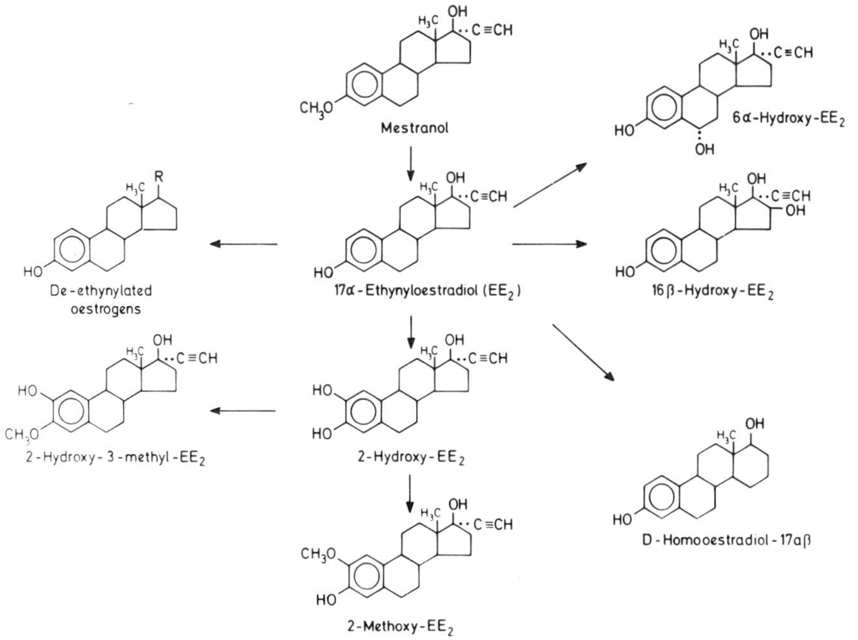

FIG. 10. Metabolic transformations of mestranol and 17α-ethynylestradiol.

is the sterically hindered tertiary 17β-hydroxyl group. This appears to be the only instance in which a steroid is conjugated *in vivo* by mammals at a tertiary hydroxyl group.

An important reaction in the metabolism of 17α-ethynylestradiol involves substitution at carbon atom C2. Thus 2-hydroxy-17α-ethynylestradiol and the corresponding 2- and 3-methyl ethers have been identified as major metabolites of 17α-ethynylestradiol in man (1,46,47). In addition, 16β-hydroxy- and 6α-hydroxy-17α-ethynylestradiol (46) and also *d*-homoestradiol-17β (1) were detected as minor metabolites in urine. The de-ethynylation of 17α-ethynylestradiol deserves special mention. Using nondestructive methodology for the separation and isolation of metabolic products of 17α-ethynylestradiol, Goldzieher and his colleagues (46) obtained evidence for the presence of the following four de-ethynylated estrogens in the urine of women treated with 17α-ethynylestradiol: estrone, estradiol-17β, estriol, and 2-methoxyestradiol-17β. Similar results were obtained by Williams and his colleagues (47), who also identified 2α-hydroxyestrone among the de-ethynylated metabolites of mestranol. They found that the extent of *in vivo* de-ethynylation of mestranol amounted to no more than 1–2% of the administered dose, as estimated by measurement of the derived urinary estrone, estradiol-17β, estriol, and 2-hydroxyestrone.

2-Hydroxylation, which was first described by Fishman and colleagues in 1960 (17), is an important pathway not only with natural estrogens but also with 17α-ethynylestradiol. There are two examples which indicate that 2-hydroxylated derivatives of 17α-ethynylestradiol may in fact become important in women taking 17α-ethynylestradiol.

Some years ago, we observed disturbances of the menstrual cycle in a high proportion of women with tuberculosis who were treated with rifampicin and who were also taking oral contraceptives (35). In spite of taking oral contraceptives, five patients became pregnant. Of 88 patients treated with rifampicin, 62 suffered spotting, intermenstrual bleeding, or failure of menstruation. In contrast, of 26 patients receiving streptomycin and oral contraceptives, only one had a menstrual disturbance. In all patients, variations in the urinary excretion of estrogens were observed. However, these changes could not be correlated to the various forms of cyclical disturbances. It was suggested that rifampicin may have an influence on the biogenesis or the metabolism of steroids, thus leading to the frequently observed disturbance of menstruation in patients taking oral contraceptives. In fact, Bolt et al. (4) observed that 2-hydroxylation of 17α-ethynylestradiol by human liver microsomes is increased approximately fourfold after only several days of rifampicin treatment. As already mentioned, aromatic hydroxylation is the only metabolic route of quantitative significance for the oxidative inactivation of 17α-ethynylestradiol. It can therefore be assumed that treatment with rifampicin leads to an increased breakdown of 17α-ethynylestradiol *in vivo*. This may explain the unexpected pregnancies which occurred during rifampicin treatment of patients with tuberculosis receiving oral contraceptives.

The second example that indicates a possible significance of 2-hydroxy-17α-ethynylestradiol is concerned with the interaction of 2-hydroxylated estrogens with catecholamines. In previous experiments from our laboratory, it was shown *in vitro* that enzymic methylation of catecholamines by S-adenosylmethionine catechol-O-methyltransferase (COMT) from the liver of various species is strongly inhibited by 2-hydroxylated estrogens (2,25). The report by Fishman (16) that 2-hydroxylation of estrogens takes place in certain areas of the brain and similar results obtained recently with 17α-ethynylestradiol (Breuer, *unpublished experiments*) prompted us to study the question whether 2-hydroxyestradiol and 2-hydroxy-17α-ethynylestradiol inhibit the enzymatic methylation

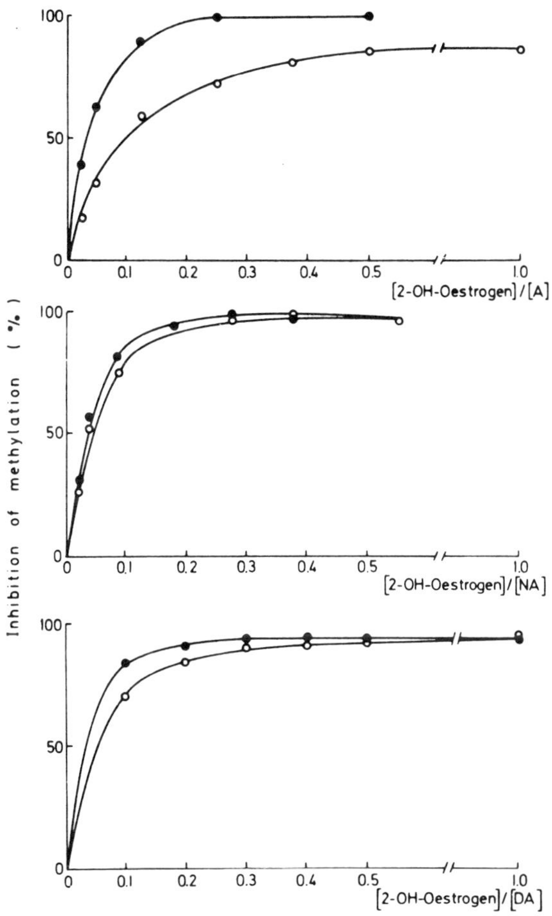

FIG. 11. Inhibition of the methylation of adrenaline (A), noradrenaline (NA), and dopamine (D), respectively, by increasing amounts of 2-hydroxyestradiol-17β (○) and 2-hydroxy-17α-ethynylestradiol-17β (●), respectively. Incubations were carried out with a catechol-O-methyltransferase preparation from rat brain. (From Breuer and Köster, ref. 7.)

of catecholamines by brain COMT (7). When epinephrine was incubated with the COMT preparation from rat brain in the presence of increasing amounts of 2-hydroxyestradiol, methylation of the catecholamine was increasingly inhibited (Fig. 11). At a molar ratio of 0.1 for inhibitor to substrate, methylation was inhibited by 50%; at a molar ratio of unity, inhibition was 85%. 2-Hydroxy-17α-ethynylestradiol was an even more potent inhibitor than 2-hydroxyestradiol; at a ratio of 0.25 (inhibitor to substrate), there was 100% inhibition of methylation of epinephrine. Similar results were obtained with norepinephrine and dopamine as substrates. Methylation of the catecholamines by catecholestrogens was inhibited competitively.

The biochemical findings reported here lead to speculation about the possible significance of these experiments. There can be no doubt that the actual amount of free norepinephrine accessible to enzymatic methylation by brain COMT must be extremely small. From experiments with peripheral nerve preparations (18), it has been calculated that only 0.002% of catecholamines present in nervous tissue is liberated during a single impulse. The concentration of norepinephrine in brain tissue of rats has been found to vary from 0.2 to 2μg/g wet weight (15), with an approximate mean of 0.5 μg/g wet weight. If approximately 99% is inactivated by reuptake, only 1% of norepinephrine can be methylated by COMT; this corresponds to 0.1 pg norepinephrine per gram wet weight. On the other hand, after intravenous injection of tritiated estradiol, its uptake by pituitary tissue is similar to that by uterine tissue; the uptake by hypothalamus is significantly lower, probably by a factor of 10 (33). The concentration of tritiated estradiol in hypothalamic tissue was approximately 2 pg/g wet weight. A similar figure can be expected after oral uptake of 50 μg 17α-ethynylestradiol per day. If the estrogens are converted to 2-hydroxylated estrogens at a rate of 1% in hypothalamus, a concentration of 0.02 pg catechol estrogen per gram wet weight would result. This figure is comparable to that calculated for the free norepinephrine methylated.

On the basis of these calculations, it may be concluded that an interaction between 2-hydroxy-17α-ethynylestradiol and catecholamines takes place at the hypothalamic level. It remains to be shown if some of the effects of 17α-ethynylestradiol are due to such an interaction.

REFERENCES

1. Abdel-Aziz, M. T., and Williams, K. I. H. (1970): Metabolism of radioactive 17α-ethynylestradiol by women. *Steroids,* 15:695–710.
2. Ball, P., Knuppen, R., Haupt, O., and Breuer, H. (1972): Interaction between estrogens and catechol amines. III. Studies on the methylation of catechol estrogens, catechol amines and other catechols by the catechol-O-methyltransferase of human liver. *J. Clin. Endocrinol.,* 34:736–746.
3. Bellmann, O., Duhme, H-J., and Gerhards, E. (1976): In vitro studies on enzymatic cleavage of steroid esters in the female organism. *Acta Endocrinol. (Kbh.),* 81:839–853.
4. Bolt, H. M., Kappus, H., and Bolt, M. (1975): Effect of rifampicin treatment on the metabolism of oestradiol and 17α-ethinyloestradiol by human liver microsomes. *Eur. J. Clin. Pharmacol.,* 8:301–307.

5. Breuer, H. (1964): Studies on the metabolism of 17α-ethyinyl-19-nortestosterone. *Int. J. Fertil.,* 9:181–187.
6. Breuer, H. (1970): Metabolism of progestagens. *Lancet,* 7673:615–616.
7. Breuer, H., and Köster, G. (1974): Interaction between oestrogens and neurotransmitters at the hypophysial-hypothalamic level. *J. Steroid. Biochem.,* 5:961–967.
8. Breuer, H., Dardenne, U., and Nocke, W. (1960): Ausscheidung von 17-Ketosteroiden, 17-ketogenen Steroiden und Östrogenen beim Menschen nach Gaben von 17α-Äthynyl-19-nortestosteron-estern. *Acta Endocrinol. (Kbh.),* 33:10–26.
9. Breuer, H., Knuppen, M., Gross, D., and Mittermayer, C. (1964): Demethylierung von Methoxyöstrogenen in vitro und in vivo. *Acta Endocrinol. (Kbh.),* 46:361–378.
10. Brown, J. B. (1962): Metabolic demethylation of oestrogen methyl ethers. *J. Endocrinol.,* 24: 251–252.
11. Brown, J. B., and Blair, H. A. F. (1960): *Proc. R. Soc. Med.,* 53:433.
12. Chen, C., and Lee, S-G. (1975): Covalent binding of norethynodrel to proteins and glutathione initiated by rat liver oxygenase. *Mol. Pharmacol.,* 11:409–420.
13. Coert, A., Geelen, J., and von der Vies, J. (1975): Metabolites of lynestrenol acetate in the bile of rats after intravenous administration: A comparison with lynestrenol. *Acta Endocrinol. (Kbh.),* 78:791–800.
14. Cooper, J. M., and Kellie, A. E. (1968): The metabolism of megestrol acetate (17α-acetoxy-6-methylpregna-4,6-diene-3,20-dione) in women. *Steroids,* 11:133–149.
15. Coyle, J. T., and Henry, D. (1973): Catechol amines in fetal and newborn rat brain. *J. Neurochem.,* 21:61–67.
16. Fishman, J. H. and Norton, B. (1975): Catechol estrogen formation in the central nervous system of the rat. *Endocrinology,* 96:1054–1059.
17. Fishman, J., Cox, R. J., and Gallagher, T. F. (1960): 2-Hydroxyestrone: The new metabolite of estradiol in men. *Arch. Biochem. Biophys.,* 90:318–319.
18. Folkow, B., Häggendal, J., and Linsander, B. (1967): Extent of release and elimination of noradrenaline and peripheral adrenergic nerve terminals. *Acta Physiol. Scand. [Suppl. 307],* 72:1–38.
19. Gerhards, E., Hecker, W., Hitze, H., Nienweboer, B., and Bellmann, O. (1971): Zum Stoffwechsel von Norethisteron (17α-Äthinyl-4-östren-17β-ol-3-on) und DL- sowie D-Norgestrel (18-Methyl-17α-äthinyl-4-östren-17β-ol-3-on) beim Menschen. *Acta Endocrinol. (Kbh.),* 68:219–248.
20. Hendy, R. W., Palmer, K. H., Wall, M. E., and Piantadosi, C. (1974): The metabolism of antifertility steroids: The in vitro metabolism of chlormadinone acetate. *Drug Metab. Dispos.,* 2:214–220.
21. Howard, G., Khan, F. S., Warren, R. J., and Fotherby, K. (1975): Metabolism of norethisterone oenanthate in vivo and in vitro. *J. Endocrinol.,* 65:20P–21P.
22. Kamyab, S., Fotherby, K., and Klopper, A. I. (1968): Metabolism of [4-^{14}C] norethisterone in women. *J. Endocrinol.,* 41:263–272.
23. Kamyab, S., Fotherby, K., and Klopper, A. I. (1968): Metabolism of [4-^{14}C] lynestrenol in man. *J. Endocrinol.,* 42:337–343.
24. Kamyab, S., Fotherby, K., and Steele, S. J. (1969): Metabolism of 4-^{14}C-ethynyl oestradiol in women. *Nature (Lond.),* 221:360–361.
25. Knuppen, R., Lubrich, W., Haupt, O., Ammerlahn, U., and Breuer, H. (1969): Wechselwirkung zwischen Östrogenen und Catecholaminen. I. Beeinflussung der enzymatischen Methylierung von Catecholaminen durch Östrogene und vice versa. *Hoppe Seylers Z. Physiol. Chem.,* 350:1067–1075.
26. Langecker, H. (1961): Die Metabolite in menschlichen Harn nach Verabreichung von 17α-Aethinyl-19-Nortestosteron (Noraethisteron). *Acta Endocrinol. (Kbh.),* 37:14–18.
27. Laumas, V., Farooq, A., and Laumas, K. R. (1972): Priming effect of norethynodrel on the uptake of [6,7-^{3}H] estradiol in the mouse uterus. *J. Steroid Biochem.,* 3:871–876.
28. Laumas, V., Malkani, P. K., and Laumas, K. R. (1971): Distribution and uptake of radioactivity in rat tissue after a single injection and constant infusion of ^{3}H-norethynodrel. *Am. J. Obstet. Gynecol.,* 109:457–462.
29. Laumas, K. R., Murugesan, K., and Hingorani, V. (1971): Disappearance in plasma and tissue uptake of radioactivity after an intravenous injection of [6,7-^{3}H] norethynodrel in women. *Acta Endocrinol. (Kbh.),* 66:385–400.
30. Longcope, C., and Williams, K. I. H. (1975): The metabolism of synethetic estrogens in non-users and users of oral contraceptives. *Steroids,* 25:121–129.
31. Longcope, C., Watson, D., and Williams, K. I. H. (1974): The effect of synthetic estrogens on the metabolic clearance and production rates of estrone and estradiol. *Steroids,* 24:15–30.

32. Mazaheri, A., Fotherby, K., and Chapman, J. R. (1970): Metabolism of lynestrenol to norethisterone by liver homogenate. *J. Endocrinol.,* 47:251–252.
33. McGuire, J. L., and Lisk, R. D. (1968): Estrogen receptors in the intact rat. *Proc. Natl. Acad. Sci. USA,* 61:497–503.
34. Murugesan, K., Hingorani, V., and Laumas, K. R. (1973): In vitro metabolism of [6,7-^{3}H]norethynodrel in the human endometrium and the myometrium. *Acta Endocrinol., (Kbh.),* 74:576–591.
35. Nocke-Finck, L., Breuer, H., and Reimers, D. (1973): Wirkung von Rifampicin auf den Menstruationszyklus und die Östrogen-ausscheidung bei Einnahme oraler Kontrazeptiva. *Dtsch. Med. Wochenschr.,* 98:1521–1523.
36. Okada, H., Amatsu, M., Ishihara, S., and Tokuda, G. (1964): Conversion of some synthetic progestins to oestrogens. *Acta Endocrinol. (Kbh.),* 46:31–36.
37. Reed, M. J., Fotherby, K., and Steele, S. J. (1972): Metabolism of ethynyloestradiol in man. *J. Endocrinol.,* 55:351–361.
38. Ryan, K. J. (1959): Biological aromatization of steroids. *J. Biol. Chem.,* 234:268–272.
39. Saucier, R., Banerjee, R. C., Brazean, P., Jr., and Husain, S. M. (1970): Effect of norethynodrel on the tissue distribution of H^3-estradiol-17β in ovariectomized rats. *Steroids,* 16:463–470.
40. Sinsenwine, S. F., Kimmel, H. B., Lin, A. L., and Ruelius, H. W. (1973): Urinary metabolites of dl-norgestrel in women. *Acta Endocrinol. (Kbh.),* 73:91–104.
41. Sinsenwine, S. F., Lin, A. L., Kimmel, H. B., and Ruelius, H. W. (1974): Phenolic metabolites of dl-norgestrel: A method for the removal of 1-hydroxylated metabolites, potential sources of phenolic artifacts. *Acta Endocrinol. (Kbh.),* 76:789–800.
42. Stárka, L., Breuer, H., and Cedard, L. (1966): Biosynthesis of equilin and related ring B unsaturated oestrogens in perfused human placenta. *J. Endocrinol.,* 34:447–456.
43. Townsley, J. D., and Brodie, H. J. (1966): A new placental metabolite of oestr-4-ene-3,17-dione: A possible source of error in oestrogen estimation. *Biochem. J.,* 101:25c–27c.
44. Townsley, J. D., and Brodie, H. J. (1967): Mechanism of estrogen biosynthesis. IV. Ovarian metabolism of estr-4-ene-3,17-dione. *Biochim. Biophys. Acta,* 144:440–445.
45. Townsley, J. D., Possanza, G., and Brodie, H. J. (1966): Stereochemical studies on estrogen biosynthesis. *Fed. Proc.,* 25:282.
46. Williams, M. C., Helton, E. D., and Goldzieher, J. W. (1975): The urinary metabolites of 17α-ethynylestradiol-9α, 11ξ-^{3}H in women: Chromatographic profiling and identification of ethynyl and non-ethynyl compounds. *Steroids,* 25:229–246.
47. Williams, J. G., Longcope, Ch., and Williams, K. I. H. (1975): Metabolism of 4-^{3}H- and 4-^{14}C-17α-ethynylestradiol 3-methyl ether (mestranol) by women. *Steroids,* 25:343–354.

Pharmacology of Steroid Contraceptive Drugs
edited by S. Garattini and H. W. Berendes.
Raven Press, New York © 1977.

Ethynylestradiol and Mestranol: Their Pharmacodynamics and Effects on Natural Estrogens

C. Longcope and K. I. H. Williams

Worcester Foundation for Experimental Biology, Shrewsbury, Massachusetts 01545

Characterizing the metabolism of steroids has generally been done by analyses carried out on the blood or urine pool of the steroid and/or its metabolites following administration of the steroid labeled with a radioactive isotope. These analyses provide useful information (1), but a far more complete picture of the metabolism of a steroid can be obtained using both types than either one alone (1,2). We studied the metabolism of the synthetic estrogens ethynylestradiol (EE) and its 3-methyl ether (ME) using both analyses. In addition, since the usual mode of entry of these compounds into the body is by oral ingestion, we studied their metabolism following oral and intravenous administration. In this chapter we review our earlier findings (3–9) and discuss these as well as some newer findings.

METHODOLOGY

The intravenous administration of ^{3}H-EE or ^{3}H-ME was by pulse injection or constant infusion. Blood samples were obtained at increasing time intervals after the pulse injection and during the constant infusions. These samples were analyzed as described for radioactivity as free ^{3}H-ME, ^{3}H-EE, or both (7).

For oral administration, either ^{3}H-EE or ^{3}H-ME was dissolved in a small quantity of ethanol and then placed on a sugar cube or added to a carbonated drink. The subject then chewed and swallowed the sugar or swallowed the carbonated drink as rapidly as possible to prevent buccal absorption. Blood samples were drawn at increasing time intervals and analyzed for ^{3}H-ME and/or ^{3}H-EE.

The data from the pulse injections were analyzed as described to obtain volumes of distribution, fractional conversion rates, and metabolic clearance rates (7). For pulse injections of ^{3}H-ME, the data for radioactive concentrations of ^{3}H-ME and ^{3}H-EE were analyzed arithmetically and the conversion ratio calculated (7). The data from the oral administrations were analyzed arithmetically to obtain the conversion ratio (7). Data from the constant infusions were analyzed to obtain metabolic clearance rates, conversion ratios, and $[\rho]_{BB}$ values (5,7).

Plasma levels of EE and ME were measured following ether extraction and paper chromatographic separation by radioimmunoassay using an antibody generated in rabbits to an ethynylestradiol-Keyhole limpet hemocyanin (KLH) complex prepared by covalent linkage of 3-O-carboxymethylethynylestradiol to KLH. A 3,000 : 1 dilution of the antiserum gave 50% binding of radioactive ethynylestradiol; a 2,000 : 1 dilution gave a working curve sensitive at 10–200 pg ethynylestradiol.

Following the administration of ³H-EE or ³H-ME by any of the above methods, the subject collected all urine for the next 96 hr, each specimen being placed in a separate container. Urines were analyzed for radioactivity as free and conjugated steroids or as radioactivity in the urine water (3,4,6,8,9).

ETHYNYLESTRADIOL METABOLISM

Following the pulse injection of ³H-EE, the disappearance of radioactivity as EE can best be described as a function that is the sum of three exponentials (Fig. 1). The last exponential is suggestive of a slowly turning-over compartment compatible with the ethynylestradiol compartment noted by Reed et al. (10) and Bird and Clark (11). The initial volumes of distribution range from 12.2 to 67.5 liters, the highest value being found in a subject who had been a regular user of EE-containing medication. These volumes are larger than the plasma volume, indicating rapid transfer out of the vascular bed. The plasma protein binding of ethynylestradiol does not seem to affect this transfer to any great degree. Generally for steroids the initial volume of distribution correlates with the metabolic clearance rate (1); but for EE, although the initial volume of distribution is large, the metabolic clearance rate is relatively small. The mean ± SE in 9 subjects was

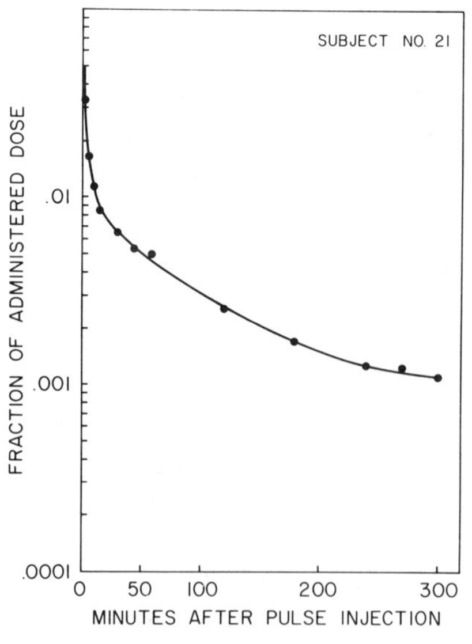

FIG. 1. Concentration of radioactivity expressed as fraction of administered dose for EE following pulse injection of ³H-EE. (From ref. 7, courtesy of *Steroids.*)

630 ± 30 liter/day/meter^2, which is lower than the value we found (790 ± 20 liter/day/meter^2 for estradiol-17β in 23 normal women. Therefore the 17α-ethynyl grouping in some manner impedes metabolism but does not interfere with the binding to the cellular receptors necessary for hormonal activity.

When ^{3}H-EE is taken by mouth there is rapid entry of ^{3}H-EE into the blood, and significant quantities of radioactivity as ^{3}H-EE are measurable within 6–10 min (Fig. 2). By 60–100 min peak levels are reached, and radioactivity then begins to decline at a slow rate such that measurable radioactivity as ^{3}H-EE is still present in the blood after 24 hr. The metabolic clearance rate calculated following the oral ingestion is similar to that after pulse injection. This suggests that there is excellent absorption from the gastrointestinal (GI) tract and little hepatic metabolism, so most of the oral dose enters the circulation unchanged.

Following oral ingestion of ^{3}H-EE, there is very slow elimination of radioactivity such that after 120 hr only 30–45% of the administered radioactivity has appeared in the urine (4). Following oral ingestion the $t_{1/2}$ of the ^{3}H-EE in the blood pool calculated from the last exponential is approximately 16 hr. These findings suggest that ^{3}H-EE when cleared from the blood remains in the body in a different form, which is more slowly cleared from the body. In addition, since less than 50% of the radioactivity appears in the urine in any form, it is probable that some degree of fecal excretion occurs as well (12).

Approximately 5–10% of the administered radioactivity was excreted in the urine as EE-"glucuronide." This amounts to approximately 50% of the urinary radioactivity, and lesser amounts of the urinary radioactivity (approximately 8–10%) appear as EE-"sulfate." In addition, small amounts of 2-methoxy-17α-EE and 2-hydroxy-17α-EE-3 methyl ether were also identified (4).

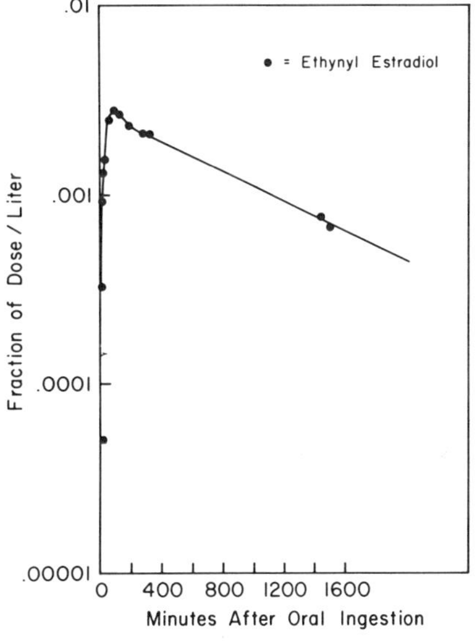

FIG. 2. Concentration of radioactivity expressed as fraction of administered dose for EE following oral ingestion of ^{3}H-EE.

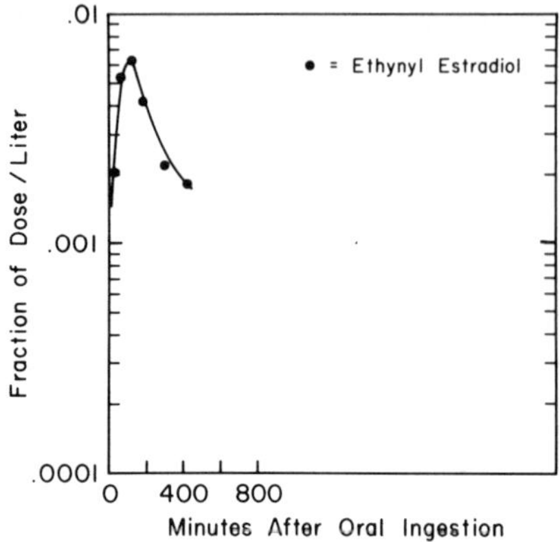

FIG. 3. Concentration of EE in plasma expressed as fraction of administered dose following ingestion of an oral contraceptive containing 50 μg EE.

The previous studies were carried out using ^{3}H-EE; when EE was measured by radioimmunoassay following the ingestion of an EE-containing oral contraceptive, the pattern of EE concentration in the plasma (Fig. 3) was similar to that noted for radioactivity in the previous experiments. These results are also similar to those reported earlier by Warren and Fotherby using a receptor assay (13). In one subject who used an EE-containing oral contraceptive, blood samples were drawn frequently during one cycle of EE use and analyzed for EE concentration. These results are shown in Fig. 4. EE levels gradually increased from being undetectable to a relative steady-state concentration on day 5, with a rapid fall-off following cessation of therapy on day 20. It should be noted that the blood samples were obtained 10–12 hr after pill ingestion, so peak levels were probably somewhat higher than shown here. Thus EE appears to be readily absorbed from the GI tract, with most of the dose entering the peripheral circulation. From there

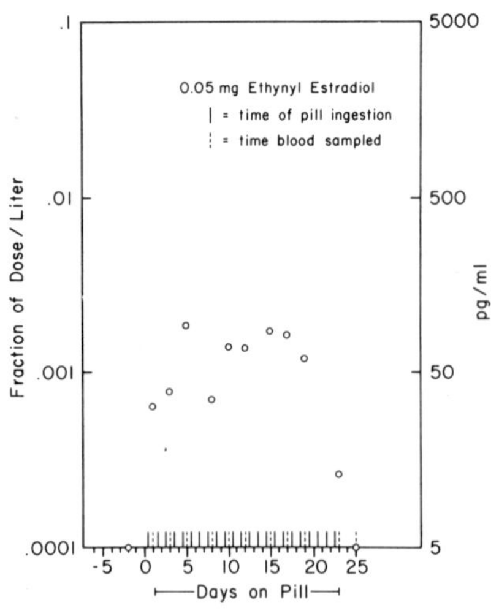

FIG. 4. Concentrations of EE in plasma expressed as fraction of administered dose and in picograms per milliliter following ingestion of an oral contraceptive containing 50 μg EE daily for 21 days. EE concentration (○).

it is cleared largely irreversibly into body pools from which it is excreted relatively slowly in the urine and feces.

MESTRANOL METABOLISM

Following the pulse injection of ^{3}H-ME, the disappearance of radioactivity as ME could be described as a function that was the sum of two exponentials (Fig. 5). This finding suggests that for the time interval of our studies (5 hr) there is no slowly turning-over pool such as we noted for EE. The initial volumes of distribution were 24–46 liters, which is in the same range as for EE, in spite of the greater plasma protein binding of EE. In 12 women the mean metabolic clearance rate was 690 ± 45 liters/day/meter^2, which is similar to the mean value of 630 liters/day/meter^2 for EE. There is an initial rapid appearance of EE in the plasma, reflecting rapid demethylation of ME and transport of the newly formed EE back into the blood compartment. The decline in radioactivity of EE, however, was slower than that of ME. Since the metabolic clearance rates of the two substances are similar, this finding suggests that either a portion of ME is sequestered outside the blood compartment and is returned somewhat slowly as EE, or that EE itself is sequestered outside the blood compartment, perhaps as EE-sulfate and slowly enters the blood pool of EE. In all 5 subjects the concentration of ^{3}H-ME remained above that of ^{3}H-EE for the time interval that samples were obtained. Approximately 15–23% of the ME injected re-entered the blood as EE.

Following oral ingestion of ^{3}H-ME, there was an initial rapid rise in the concentration of ^{3}H-ME in the blood, reaching a peak within 60–120 min (Fig.

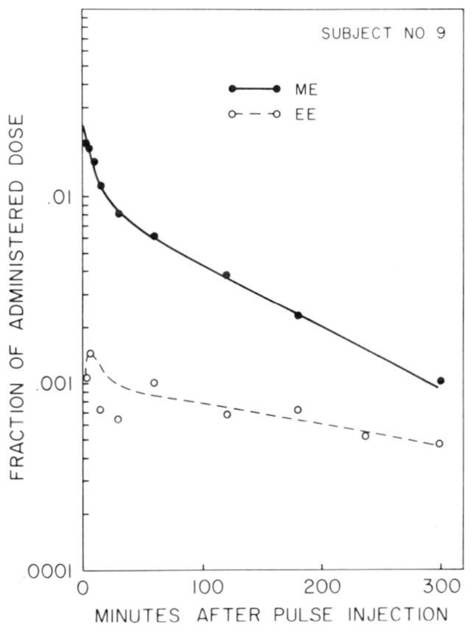

FIG. 5. Concentration of radioactivity expressed as fraction of administered dose for ME and EE following pulse injection of ^{3}H-ME. (From ref. 7, courtesy of *Steroids.*)

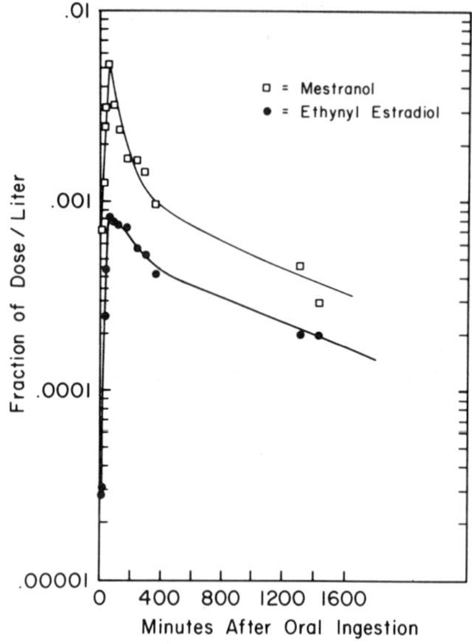

FIG. 6. Concentration of radioactivity expressed as fraction of administered dose of ME and EE following oral ingestion of ^{3}H-ME.

6). There was a gradual decline thereafter, with measurable quantities of radioactivity persisting in the blood 24 hr after ingestion of the ^{3}H-ME.

Similar to the ^{3}H-ME, the concentrations of ^{3}H-EE also rose rapidly, peaking 80–120 min after ingestion of the ^{3}H-ME. A gradual decline in the concentrations of ^{3}H-EE followed, with measurable quantities still present after 24 hr. Interestingly, the slopes of the concentrations of ^{3}H-ME and ^{3}H-EE were roughly parallel from 4 to 24 hr after ingestion of ^{3}H-ME, with the concentrations of ^{3}H-ME being above those of ^{3}H-EE at all time intervals.

The fractional conversion of ^{3}H-ME to ^{3}H-EE when measured in the blood following oral ingestion ranged from 0.36 to 0.59, with a mean $\pm$ SE of 0.44 $\pm$ 0.05. This mean is considerably greater than the mean values of 0.18 and 0.19 reported by Bird and Clark (11) and ourselves (7) following intravenous administration, but is close to the value of 0.54 reported by Bolt and Bolt (14), who used somewhat different methodology. The disparity between the values we obtained following intravenous and oral administration is perhaps due to the different time span over which the experiments were carried out, i.e. 24 versus 5 hr. It is unlikely that immediate metabolism by the liver is responsible for these differences since the metabolic clearance rates of EE and ME were similar following either method of administration. This suggests that hepatic extraction is considerably less than 100%.

The appearance of radioactivity in the urine following the ingestion of ^{3}H-ME was slow, with only 30–45% appearing after 8 days. As for ^{3}H-EE, this suggests a large pool of ^{3}H which does not re-enter the blood as ^{3}H-ME but is only slowly excreted.

The major excretory product was EE-"glucuronide," accounting for 7–11%

of the administered dose. Since 5–10% of the administered dose of ^{3}H-EE appeared in the urine as EE-"glucuronide," and if one assumes that all the ^{3}H-ME excreted as ^{3}H-EE-"glucuronide" was demethylated prior to conjugation, then most of the orally administered ^{3}H-ME would be converted to ^{3}H-EE in the body. It should be realized that we are combining data from different subjects; but since we calculated that only 40–50% of orally ingested ^{3}H-ME passed through the blood pool of ^{3}H-EE, these urinary data indicate that a major part of the conversion to EE occurs in a compartment not freely communicating with the blood pool of EE. Minimal amounts of mestranol conjugates and de-ethynylated compounds were found in the urine. De-ethynylation was also reported by Williams et al. (15), who noted significant quantities of de-ethynylated metabolites in the urine after intravenous and oral administration of ^{3}H-EE. We were unable to find ^{3}H-estrone or ^{3}H-estradiol in the blood in our studies, so it is unlikely that de-ethynylation contributes significantly to circulating estrone or estradiol levels.

Radioimmunoassay measurements of ME and EE in the plasma of women following the ingestion of ME-containing oral contraceptives revealed a pattern (Fig. 7) that was not dissimilar from that noted for radioactivity. In one subject taking an ME-containing oral contraceptive, blood samples were obtained frequently over the course of one pill-taking cycle. As noted in Fig. 8, ME levels were relatively stable over the latter part of the cycle. EE levels rose rapidly and were relatively stable after day 2. It should be noted that blood samples were drawn only 2–3 hr after ingestion of a pill so that the levels measured are somewhat higher than those noted in Fig. 4. Although levels of ME are higher than those of EE in acute studies using either labeled or unlabeled steroids, in this chronic study EE attains levels equal to or higher than ME. Thus ME also is almost completely absorbed after oral ingestion, and at least 50% of the

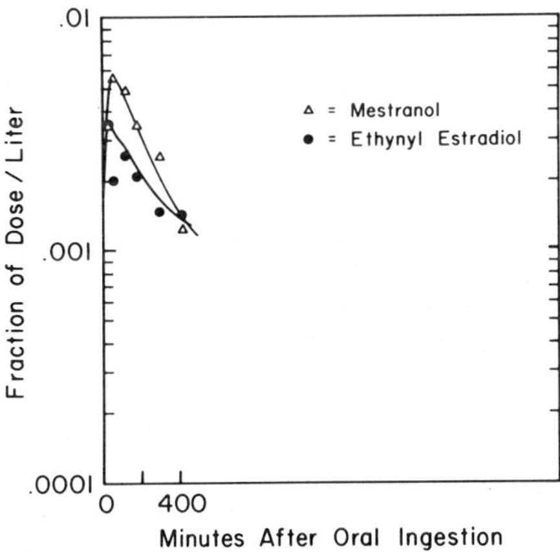

FIG. 7. Concentration of ME and EE in plasma expressed as fraction of administered dose per liter following ingestion of an oral contraceptive tablet containing 50 μg ME.

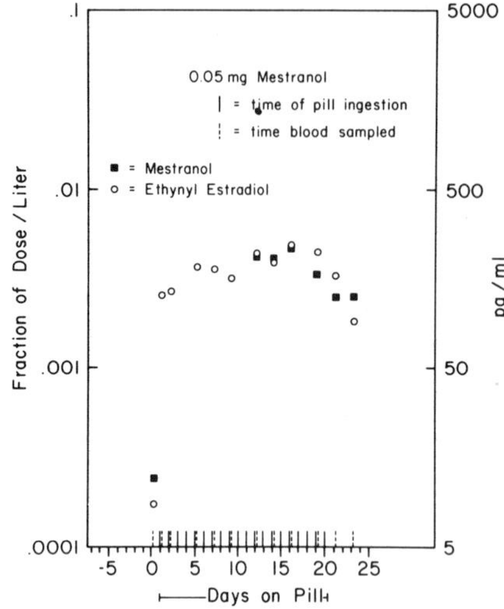

FIG. 8. Concentration of ME and EE in plasma expressed as fraction of administered dose per liter and picograms per milliliter following daily ingestion (for 21 days) of an oral contraceptive containing 50 μg ME.

ingested ME passes through the blood pool of EE. It is this EE which in large part is responsible for the biologic activity of ME.

EFFECTS OF EE AND ME ON THE METABOLISM OF ESTRONE AND ESTRADIOL

Metabolic clearance rates (MCR) and urinary metabolite excretion patterns of estrone and estradiol were obtained in nonusers and users of ME- and EE-containing oral contraceptives (5). Although mestranol did not appear to alter the MCR for estradiol, the MCR of estradiol in users of EE-containing compounds was increased significantly (Fig. 9). It is not likely that this increase is due to an alteration in the binding of estradiol to the sex-steroid binding globulin. An increase in the binding globulin would tend to decrease the MCR of estradiol. The concentration of ethynylestradiol present in the blood of users is not sufficient to displace estradiol from the binding globulin (16) and thus increase its metabolic clearance. We suggested that this alteration is probably secondary to changes occurring outside the vascular space (5). EE has no effect on the MCR of estrone, but the mean value for the MCR of estrone in ME users is slightly decreased compared to that of normals.

This alteration in the MCR, however, is not mirrored by the urinary excretion data (6). Somewhat paradoxically perhaps, the excretion of ^{3}H in the urine after ^{3}H-estradiol is administered to users of EE-containing oral contraceptives is significantly slower than in nonusers. Therefore, although estradiol is cleared more rapidly from the blood pool, it remains in the body for a longer time.

Along with the delayed urinary excretion of ^{3}H-estradiol metabolites, there appears to be a decrease in the excretion of ^{3}H as estriol following the administration of ^{3}H-estradiol, and a consequent shift in the ratio of the 2-oxygenated to

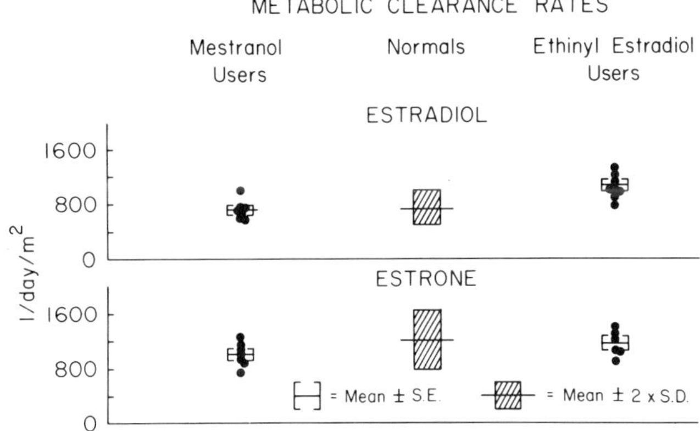

FIG. 9. Metabolic clearance rates of estradiol and estrone calculated in women who used ME-containing oral contraceptives, in normal nonusers, and in women who used EE-containing oral contraceptives.

16-oxygenated metabolites (6). We were not, however, able to show that use of oral contraceptives had any effect on the dynamic metabolism of EE or ME.

Thus the dynamic metabolism of ME and EE differ somewhat from the metabolism of estradiol, and EE at least appears to alter the metabolism of estradiol itself. That this change is related in some manner to any of the side effects of EE is conjectural at best.

ACKNOWLEDGMENTS

We wish to thank Charles Flood for excellent technical assistance in these studies. This work was supported by NIH Contract NICHD-71–2294, NIH Grant HD-08034, and NIH Contract N01-HD-5-2858.

REFERENCES

1. Tait, J. F., and Burstein, S. (1964): In vivo studies of steroid dynamics in man. In: *The Hormones,* Vol. 5, edited by G. Pincus, K. V. Thimann, and E. B. Astwood, p. 441. Academic Press, New York.
2. Horton, R., and Tait, J. F. (1966): Androstenedione production and interconversion rates measured in peripheral blood and studies on the possible site of its conversion to testosterone. *J. Clin. Invest.,* 45:301–313.
3. Williams, K. I. H. (1969): The metabolism of radioactive 17α-ethynylestradiol 3-methyl ether (mestranol) by women. *Steroids,* 13:539–544.
4. Abdel-Aziz, M. T., and Williams, K. I. H. (1970): The metabolism of radioactive 17α-ethynylestradiol by women. *Steroids,* 15:695–710.
5. Longcope, C., Watson, D., and Williams, K. I. H. (1974): The effects of synthetic estrogens on the metabolic clearance and production rates of estrone and estradiol. *Steroids,* 24:15–30.
6. Femino, A. M., Longcope, C., Williams, J. G., and Williams, K. I. H. (1974): The effect of oral contraceptive steroid therapy on the urinary metabolites of radioactive estrone and estradiol-17β. *Steroids,* 24:849–859.

7. Longcope, C., and Williams, K. I. H. (1975): The metabolism of synthetic estrogens in non-users and users of oral contraceptives. *Steroids,* 25:121–133.
8. Williams, J. G., Longcope, C., and Williams, K. I. H. (1975): Metabolism of 4-^{3}H- and 4-^{14}C-17α-ethynylestradiol 3-methyl ether (mestranol) by women. *Steroids,* 25:343–354.
9. Williams, J. G., and Williams, K. I. H. (1975): Metabolism of 2-^{3}H- and 4-^{14}C-17α-ethynylestradiol 3-methyl ether (mestranol) by women. *Steroids,* 26:707–720.
10. Reed, M. J., Fotherby, K., and Steele, S. J. (1972): Metabolism of ethynyloestradiol in man. *J. Endocrinol.,* 55:351–361.
11. Bird, C. E., and Clark, A. F. (1973): Metabolic clearance rates and metabolism of mestranol and ethynylestradiol in normal young women. *J. Clin. Endocrinol. Metab.,* 36:296–302.
12. Bolt, H. M., and Remmer, H. (1972): Retention, metabolism and elimination of 17α-ethynylestradiol-3-methyl ether (mestranol). *Xenobiotica,* 2:77–88.
13. Warren, R. J., and Fotherby, K. (1973): *J. Endocrinol.,* 59:369–370.
14. Bolt, H. M., and Bolt, W. H. (1974): *Eur. J. Clin. Pharmacol.,* 7:295–305.
15. Williams, M. C., Helton, E. D., and Goldzieher, J. W. (1975). The urinary metabolites of 17α-ethynylestradiol-9α,11ξ-^{3}H in women: Chromatographic profiling and identification of ethynyl and non-ethynyl compounds. *Steroids,* 25:229–246.
16. Hembree, W. C., Bardin, C. W., and Lipsett, M. B. (1969): A study of estrogen metabolic clearance rates and transfer factors. *J. Clin. Invest.,* 48:1809–1819.

Pharmacology of Steroid Contraceptive Drugs
edited by S. Garattini and H. W. Berendes.
Raven Press, New York © 1977.

Aspects of Megestrol Acetate and Medroxyprogesterone Acetate Metabolism

**F. Martin and †H. Adlercreutz*

*†Department of Clinical Chemistry, University of Helsinki, Helsinki, Finland; and *Department of Biochemistry, Trinity College, Dublin 2, Ireland*

Megestrol acetate (17α-acetoxy-6-methyl-4,6-pregnadiene-3,20-dione) and medroxyprogesterone acetate (17α-acetoxy-6α-methyl-4-pregnene-3,20-dione) have long been known as potent inhibitors of ovulation and have found wide usage in contraceptive preparations. Both compounds have also been used extensively in the treatment of cancer of the uterus. It has been established that these C_6,C_{17}-substituted progesterone derivatives have greatly increased resistance to progesterone-metabolizing enzymes (1–3), and it is suggested that their greatly enhanced progestational activity is related to this factor. Although these compounds have been widely used, knowledge of their absorption, plasma levels, and further metabolism in humans and experimental animals is far from complete.

In this chapter studies carried out at our laboratory on the metabolism of these compounds are reviewed. The monitoring of plasma megestrol acetate and medroxyprogesterone acetate (MPA) levels in humans after oral administration, using radioimmunoassay procedures, is described. Plasma megestrol acetate levels were also determined by a specific mass fragmentographic technique, and the results obtained using the two procedures are compared. In addition, preliminary data on megestrol acetate metabolites in humans and beagles after oral administration, obtained using a gas chromatographic-mass spectrometric procedure, are presented.

RADIOIMMUNOASSAY FOR MEGESTROL ACETATE AND MPA IN PLASMA

The radioimmunoassay procedure is the same for the determination of both compounds except that the standard curve is prepared using megestrol acetate in the one case and MPA in the other. $1,2\text{-}^3\text{H-MPA}$ is utilized in both assay systems as no high specific activity-labeled megestrol acetate is available. The one antiserum preparation serves both assays.

Prior to extraction, 20 μl (ca. 2,000 cpm) $1,2\text{-}^3\text{H-MPA}$ (specific activity 58 Ci/mmole) in 1% ethanol is added as internal standard to 0.5–1.5 ml plasma in suitable extraction tubes. After mixing on a vortex shaker, the tubes are placed in a water bath at 37°C for 5 min. They are then mixed with the vortex shaker for 30 sec and left standing at room temperature for 5 min prior to extraction. The samples are then extracted twice with 5 volumes of petroleum ether (b.p. 40–60) using a horizontal shaker. The extracts are transferred with a pasteur pipette to graduated glass tubes and evaporated to dryness under a stream of nitrogen.

To the dry residues 1.0 ml borate buffer, pH 8.0, 0.133 mole/liter containing 0.02% gelatin is added and the tubes mixed on a Vortex shaker, warmed in a water bath at 37°C for 5 min, and mixed again on the vortex shaker for a further minute. They are then left standing on the bench until they have reattained room temperature.

For recovery determination 400 μl of the buffer solution from each tube is transferred by Finnpipette (Labsystems Oy, Helsinki, Finland) into a scintillation vial, and 7 ml of scintillation fluid (Instagel, Packard) is added. The same volume of buffer and scintillation fluid is also added to three samples of the internal standard solution to allow determination of percent recovery. The scintillation vials are shaken by hand and left in a refrigerator (4°C) for 1–2 hr or overnight before counting. Futher aliquots (50–250 μl) of the buffer solution are pipetted into Eppendorf microtubes as are 50-μl amounts of the appropriate standards (0–1,000 pg) in borate buffer containing 1% ethanol. Antiserum [100 μl, anti-MPA-3-(O-carboxymethyl) oxime serum (from goat 16), dilution 1 : 45,000, final dilution 1 : 315,000] is added to all tubes. Borate buffer is added to equalize their volume content. Finally, 0.0125 μCi 1,2-^{3}H-MPA in 50 μl 1% ethanol is added to each tube, the tubes shaken on an Eppendorf Rotamixer for 2 min at room temperature, and then incubated in a cold room (4°C) overnight.

The following day separation of bound from unbound steroid is achieved by adding 400 μl cold dextran-coated charcoal suspension to each tube, incubating the tubes for 15 min in an ice bath, and then centrifuging them for 2 min in an Eppendorf centrifuge. Thereafter 400 μl of the supernatant fluid is transferred into scintillation vials and 7 ml of scintillation fluid added. The vials are shaken and cooled, as described above, and counted in a Wallac Dec-em liquid scintillation counter.

MASS FRAGMENTOGRAPHIC DETERMINATION OF MEGESTROL ACETATE IN PLASMA

A detailed description and evaluation of this procedure was published previously (4,5). Briefly the method involves: addition of MPA to the plasma sample as internal standard; extraction with diethyl ether-chloroform; purification of the extract on a column of silica gel; formation of the 3-monomethoxime derivatives and mass fragmentographic analysis in an LKB 9000 gas chromatograph-mass spectrometer fitted with an accelerating voltage alternator. The stationary phase used is 1% SE-30, and the two very abundant base peaks of the 3-monomethoxime derivatives of megestrol acetate (m/e 310) and MPA (m/e 312) (Fig. 1) are monitored on separate single-pen electrical recorders. The method has been

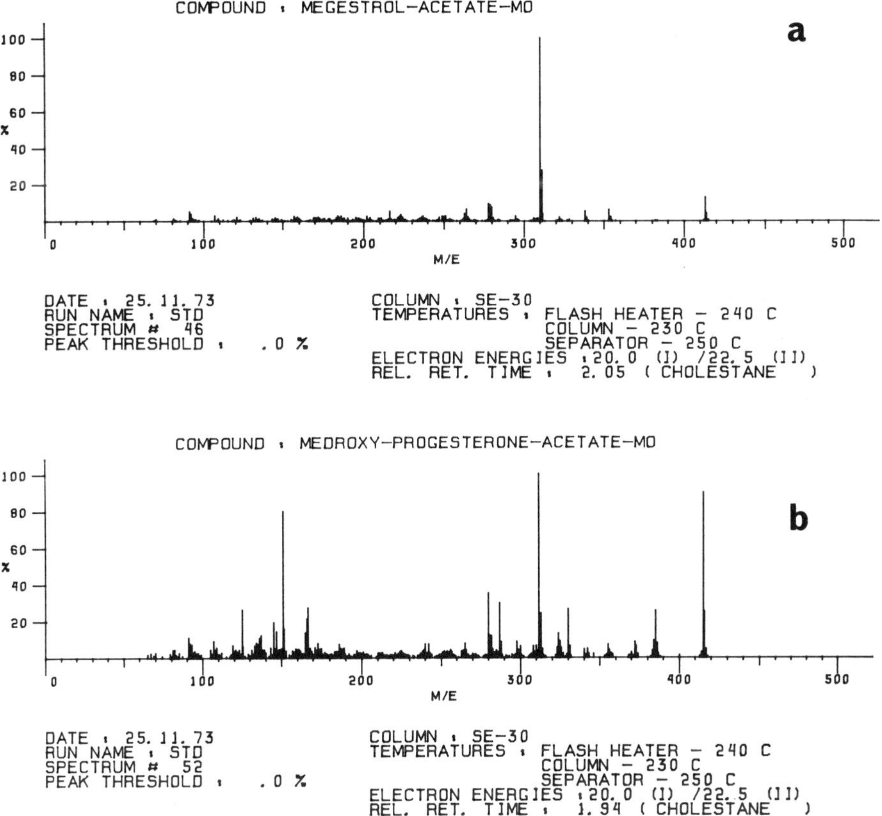

Fig. 1. Mass spectra of megestrol acetate 3-monomethoxime **(a)** and MPA 3-monomethoxime **(b)** taken with an LKB 9000 gas chromatograph-mass spectrometer linked to a Hewlett-Packard 2100A computer with an HP 7210A X/Y plotter. A 1% SE.30 stationary phase was used. The electron energy was 22.5 eV. The base peaks are at m/e 310 **(a)** and m/e 312 **(b)**.

shown to be specific for megestrol acetate measurement. The precision is very much dependent on the mass fragmentographic step, but repeated instrument calibration and injection of standards result in reasonable reproducibility. The practicable lower limit for quantitative megestrol acetate determination is of the order of 200 pg (4).

PROCEDURE FOR THE ISOLATION AND INVESTIGATION OF MEGESTROL ACETATE METABOLITES IN BIOLOGICAL FLUIDS AND TISSUES

The isolation of megestrol acetate metabolites is a direct adaptation of methods used in our (6) and other (7,8) laboratories for the isolation and investigation of endogenous neutral steroid metabolites in biological samples. The method was

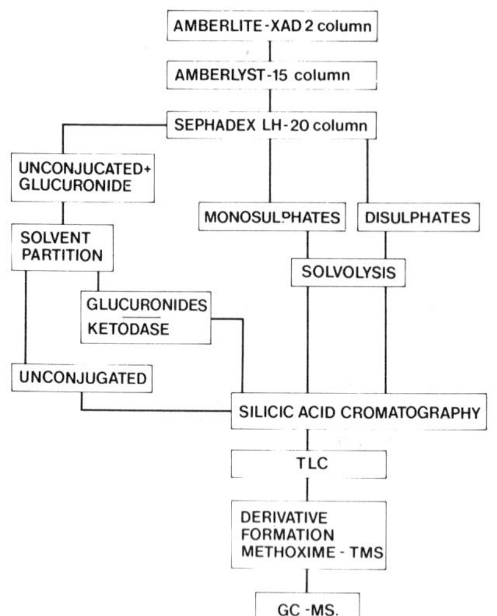

FIG. 2. Flow chart of the method used for isolation and identification of megestrol acetate and its metabolites in urine.

described by Adlercreutz et al. (5) and is summarized in Fig. 2. Urine samples are first subjected to Amberlite XAD-2 (9,10) and Amberlyst 15 (10) chromatography; bile samples are treated with an acetone-ethanol mixture overnight at 39°C; they are then filtered and evaporated (7). Liver samples are homogenized in an acetone-ethanol mixture and then processed as the bile samples. All extracts are subjected to Sephadex LH-20 chromatography (5,7), and fractions of unconjugated plus glucuronide-, monosulfate-, and disulfate-conjugated steroids are isolated. The unconjugated plus glucuronide fraction is partitioned between 8.4% (w/v) $NaHCO_3$ and ethyl acetate (11). The glucuronides are hydrolyzed with ketodase and the mono- and disulfates solvolyzed (12). All fractions are then fractionated by silicic acid column chromatography (7) and in some cases further purified by thin-layer chromatography (5). Methoxime trimethylsilyl ethers of all fractions are prepared and the fractions screened by gas chromatography-mass spectrometry on a 1% SE-30 stationary phase in an LKB 9000 gas chromatograph mass spectrometer. The mass spectra are recorded, normalized, stored, and printed by an on-line data processing system (HP 2100 A minicomputer, HP 7900 A disc drive, HP 7210 A digital plotter, and teletype printer; the programs were written by Mr. Esa Soini) (5).

MEGESTROL ACETATE AND MPA LEVELS IN HUMAN PLASMA AFTER ORAL ADMINISTRATION

The plasma levels of megestrol acetate after oral administration of 50-mg doses to a series of women under treatment for carcinoma corporis uteri were monitored using radioimmunoassay (RIA) and mass fragmentographic (MF) procedures. The plasma levels measured at intervals over the 25-hr period after megestrol acetate administration are compared in Table 1, and in Fig. 3 the levels attained in subject 1 are compared graphically. A similar comparison in another patient was described previously (5).

After oral administration of 50-mg doses, peak values of megestrol acetate, 25–100 ng/ml, were detected in plasma by either procedure within 2–5 hr. By 24–25 hr the levels had fallen to 2.6–26.3 ng/ml (radioimmunoassay) and 1.4–11.4 ng/ml (mass fragmentography) (Table 1; Fig. 3). Overall, but in particular after the peak values have been reached, higher plasma levels were obtained by radioimmunoassay. These higher levels may reflect cross reaction by plasma unconjugated megestrol acetate metabolites in the radioimmunoassay. It should be mentioned that no cross-reacting steroids were found in the plasma of untreated patients, and there is little likelihood of megestrol acetate metabolites interfering with the mass fragmentographic procedure.

To investigate if plasma from patients who had received megestrol acetate orally contained other immunoreactive compounds, the following experiment was carried out: a pool of plasma from such patients was subjected to extraction with diethyl ether/chloroform (3 : 1, v/v). The extract was then subjected to chromatography on a microcolumn of Lipidex 5000 (Packard Instrument Inter-

TABLE 1. *Plasma megestrol acetate levels after oral administration to female subjects: Comparison of values obtained by RIA and MF*

	Plasma megestrol acetate levels (ng/ml)							
	Subject 1		Subject 2		Subject 3		Subject 4	
Time (hr)	RIA[a]	MF[b]	RIA	MF	RIA	MF	RIA	MF
0[c]	0	0	0	0	0	0	0	0
1	19.4	19	16.4	11.6	18.5	10.8	6.1	3.0
2	63	—	30.2	21.5	—	23.3	9.7	5.8
2.5	86.5	91.0	39.8	30.0				
3	98.8	89.1	45.3	33.3	29.3	18.5	25.2	15.4
3.5	101.3	93.7	61.5	43.4				
4	82.9	80.3	71.9	43.4		12.5	11.0	6.7
5	75.3	71.5	32.9	19.4				
5.5					11.9	2.9	9.0	7.2
6	83.1	40.1	29.3	15.9				
7	52.6	29.8	20.9	9.1				
7.5					7.4	8.7	8.7	4.8
8	43.3	24.3	18.2	8.9				
9	38.8	23.3	18.5	8.1				
24					6.1	1.4	2.6	2.0
25	26.3	11.4	7.3	4.4				

[a] The intra-assay coefficient of variation for radioimmunoassay of megestrol acetate was 8.9% ($N = 13$; mean value of pool 15.8 ng/ml) and 9.9% ($N = 15$; mean value of pool 60.2 ng/ml). The interassay coefficient of variation was 10.6% ($N = 10$; mean value of duplicates analyzed 17.3 ng/ml).

[b] The values determined by mass fragmentography were reported elsewhere (4).

[c] At time 0, 50 mg megestrol acetate was administered to each subject.

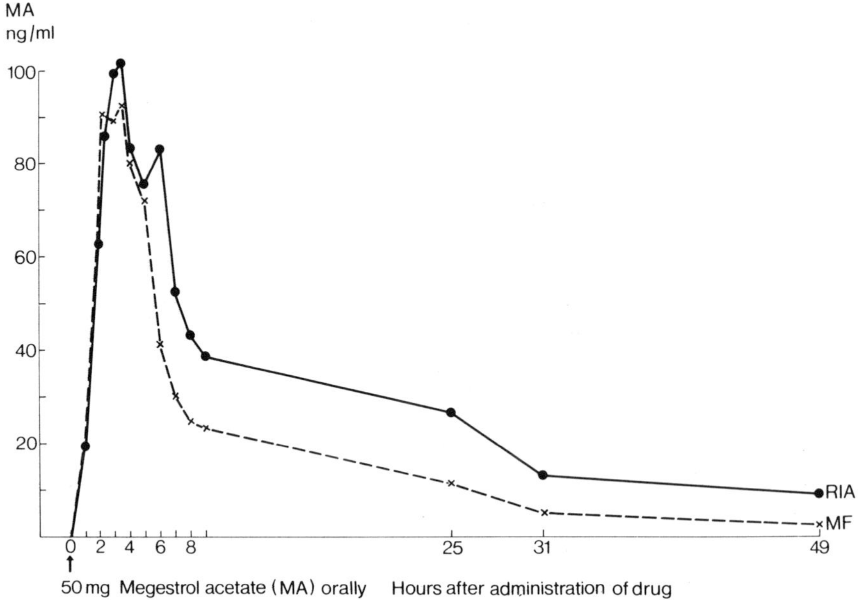

FIG. 3. Plasma concentration of megestrol acetate following a single oral dose of 50 mg of the steroid, measured by two methods: radioimmunoassay (RIA) and mass fragmentography (MF).

national S.A., Zurich, Switzerland) packed in petroleum ether (b.p. 40–60)/chloroform (95 : 5), and eluted first with 2.5 ml, then with 5 × 2-ml fractions of the same solvent, and finally with 2 ml methanol. A small amount of megestrol acetate reference standard was treated in the same way. The fractions of eluate were dried under nitrogen and subjected to radioimmunoassay. The results are presented in Table 2. It is apparent that all the megestrol acetate is eluted from the column in the first 10.5 ml of petroleum ether-chloroform. Thus the immunoreactivity detected in the methanolic eluate (6.9 ng, 25% of the total) strongly suggests the presence of cross-reacting megestrol acetate metabolites in the plasma extract. It must be emphasized, however, that the extraction solvent used was somewhat more polar than that used in the routine radioimmunoassay. It was also established that 6-hydroxymethylmegestrol acetate, a major urinary metabolite of megestrol acetate (13; see also below) elutes from these columns in the methanol fraction. Although unconjugated megestrol acetate metabolites have thus far not been identified in human plasma, significant amounts are found in human urine (13; see also below). Cooper and Kellie (13) detected a compound in the unconjugated fraction of human urine with a chromatographic mobility similar to that of 6-hydroxymethyl megestrol acetate. However, the principal unconjugated metabolite detected in our studies has its hydroxyl group linked to a secondarily substituted carbon atom, very likely C2 (13; see also below). If 2α-hydroxymegestrol acetate (13) were present in the plasma extracts, it could

TABLE 2. *Immunoreactivity spectrum of a plasma extract from subjects receiving megestrol acetate orally, after chromatography on Lipidex 5000*

Lipidex 5000 column elution regimen[a] (ml)	Plasma extract[b] (ng)	Megestrol acetate standard[c] (ng)
Petroleum ether/$CHCl_3$ (95 : 5)		
2.5	11.4	23.0
2.0	4.2	ND
2.0	1.8	ND
2.0	0.4	ND
2.0	0.04	ND
2.0	0	0
Methanol		
2.0	6.9	0

[a] Microcolumns of Lipidex 5000 were packed in petroleum ether/chloroform (95 : 5). The samples were applied in the same solvent and eluted as shown.

[b] A plasma pool from women who received megestrol acetate orally was extracted with diethyl ether/chloroform (3 : 1 v/v).

[c] ND, not determined.

be expected to cross react with antibodies raised against MPA-3-(carboxy) methyloxime-bovine serum albumin.

Plasma MPA levels were measured in a patient who received 3 × 10-mg oral doses of this drug at 24-hr intervals, and after an interval of 48 hr received 3 × 100-mg doses, also at 24-hr intervals; plasma levels were measured over 25-hr periods starting at the time of administration of the last dose of each regimen (Fig. 4). After the last 10-mg dose, the plasma level rose from a basal value of 0.15 ng/ml to a peak value of 1.13 ng/ml at 3 hr and fell to approximately the same basal level within 25 hr. After the last 100-mg dose, the plasma MPA concentration rose to a peak level of 7.3 ng/ml at 3 hr and thereafter fell gradually, the concentration being 1.2 ng/ml at 25 hr (Fig. 4).

Hiroi et al. (14), using the same antibody and a similar radioimmunoassay procedure, measured plasma MPA levels in serum of four women receiving 10-mg oral doses daily for 5 days. These patients showed peak plasma levels within the first 4 hr of 3.4–4.4 ng/ml, with the concentration falling to a basal level of 0.3–0.6 ng/ml by 24 hr. One of the subjects was exceptional in that her basal plasma level (plasma level 24 hr after each 10-mg dose, range 0.8–1.6 ng/ml) and peak plasma level (maximum 12.3 ng/ml) increased as the 5-day study progressed. Although the same antibody and very similar assay procedures were used, the peak plasma concentrations and the 24-hr plasma concentrations found by Hiroi et al. are threefold greater than those determined in our subject. However, both sets of values are much lower than earlier reports of plasma MPA levels in human subjects (15).

After the 100-mg dose a rapid but transient rise in plasma MPA levels to 7.3 ng/ml was apparent (Fig. 3). In contrast, Jeppsson and Johansson (16), using a similar radioimmunoassay procedure, showed that single intramuscular injec-

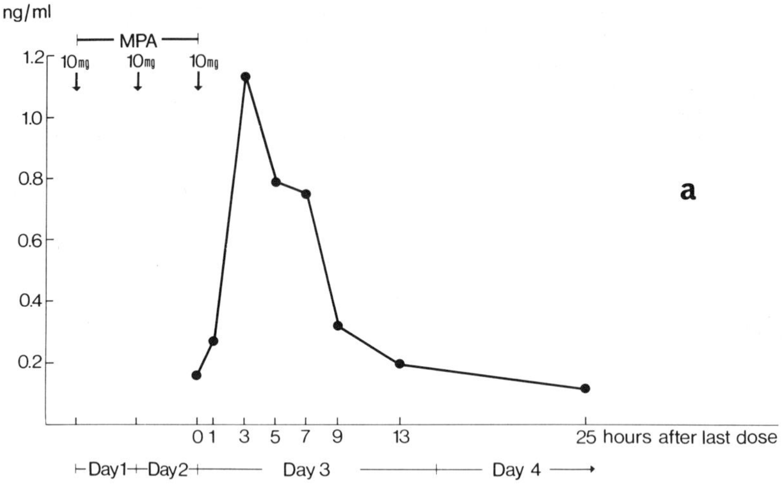

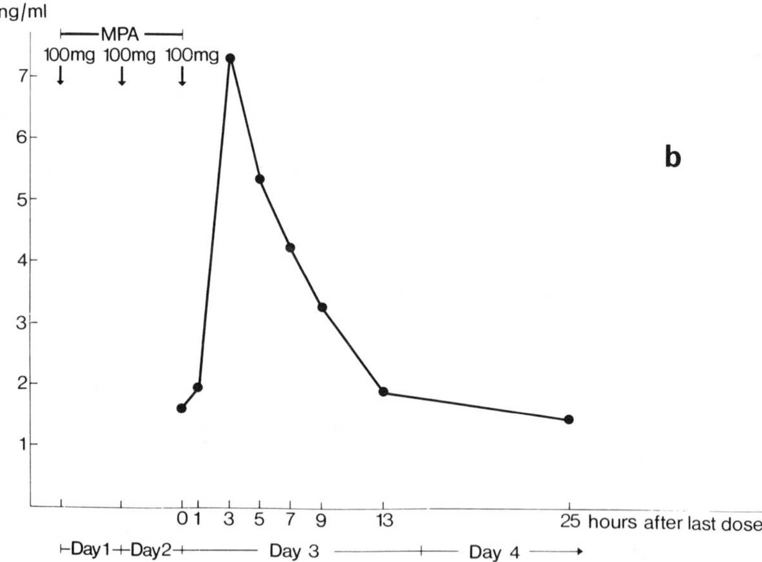

FIG. 4. Plasma concentration of MPA in a woman who received 3 × 10-mg oral doses of the drug at 24-hr intervals on days 1 and 2, and 3 ×100-mg doses at 24-hr intervals on days 5 and 6. The plasma measurements were made by radioimmunoassay on samples obtained over a 25-hr period after ingestion of the last 10-mg dose **(a)** and over a similar period after ingestion of the last 100-mg dose **(b)**. (From H. Adlercreutz, T. Laatikainen, and U. Nieminen, *unpublished.*)

tions of MPA (150 or 300 mg; Depo-Provera) for contraceptive purposes led to sustained maximal levels during the first week—of the order of 3–4 ng/ml (150 mg injection) or 10 ng/ml (300 mg injection); these fell gradually but still maintained values of 0.5–1.0 ng/ml after 80 days. Insertion of Silastic intravaginal rings impregnated with 100 or 200 mg MPA led to a rather rapid rise but relatively stable values (0.9–1.6 ng/ml) while the ring was in place; the values rapidly declined after removal (14).

On the basis of the differences in plasma megestrol acetate levels obtained by radioimmunoassay and mass fragmentography, the possibility of metabolite interference with the MPA radioimmunoassay must also be considered. Royer et al. (17) investigated the cross reactivities of steroids similar to MPA with antisera raised against MPA conjugated to albumin through C11 and C3 (as used here). Both antibodies showed considerable cross reactivity with steroid analogs, with alterations at C5 and C4. The anti-C3 conjugate serum showed very significant cross reactivity, but the anti-C11 conjugate serum showed little, with analogs containing C3 or C6 hydroxy groups. In addition, the anti-C11 conjugate serum gave consistently lower results when assays carried out with both antisera were used to monitor plasma MPA in dogs given doses of 30 mg/kg intramuscularly, but similar results were obtained when the two antisera were used to assay plasma levels in monkeys. It seems, therefore, that metabolite interference could also be significant in this assay system, with the extent depending on the nature of the metabolites present.

A comparison of Figs. 3 and 4 suggests great differences in the intestinal absorption characteristics of megestrol acetate and MPA. Although plasma levels of 50–100 ng/ml are seen in women after 50-mg oral doses of the former, a 100-mg dose of the latter results in plasma levels of only 7 ng/ml. It is possible that a large proportion of orally administered MPA is deactivated in the intestinal tract or becomes unavailable for absorption. When progesterone, which shows little biological activity on oral administration, is incubated with intestinal microorganisms, the 3-oxo-4-ene system is reduced (18). In addition, other bacterial enzymes attack progesterone with resultant opening of ring A (19,20). The cortisol side chain can be split off in the human intestinal tract (21). Thus the intestine and its contents play a major role in determining the biological effectiveness of orally administered steroids. One factor, however, favoring orally administered megestrol acetate over MPA is that 4,6-diene structures are more resistant to bacterial reduction than 4-ene structures (22,23), but it is not known if this has a significant bearing on their grossly different plasma levels.

GAS CHROMATOGRAPHIC-MASS SPECTROMETRIC PROPERTIES OF MEGESTROL ACETATE METABOLITES IN HUMAN URINE AND BILE

Gas chromatographic-mass spectrometric analysis of *urinary extracts* from two patients receiving 100-mg oral loads of megestrol acetate revealed the presence of the parent compound and several possible metabolites. In the unconjugated steroid fraction from one patient, unmetabolized megestrol acetate and two possible monohydroxylated metabolites, compounds I and II, were detected. In the glucuronide fraction these and two further possible monohydroxylated metabolites (compounds Ia and IIa) were found in addition to a dihydroxylated megestrol acetate derivative. No metabolites could be found in the sulfate conjugate fractions. Analysis of the combined unconjugated and conjugated urinary extracts from the second patient revealed the presence of dihydroxylated (compound III) and dihydrodihydroxylated (compound IV) megestrol acetate derivatives.

To achieve better overall gas chromatographic-mass spectrometric sensitivity all fractions were analyzed after O-methoxime trimethylsilyl (MO-TMS) ether formation. The mass spectra of the MO-TMS ethers of the megestrol acetate metabolites detected (Figs. 1a, 6a–c, 8–10) are dominated by fragments generated by the loss of the molecules' functional groups. The most characteristic of these fragmentations are summarized in Fig. 5 and include: loss of methyl group (M-15), scission of the N–O bond in the methoxime group (M-31), loss of the C-17α acetate group (M-60), loss of silanol (M-90), loss of the C-17$\alpha + \beta$ side chains (M-103), and loss of $-CH_2-O-Si(CH_3)_3$ (M-103) from steroids containing a primary substituted hydroxyl group (24,25), e.g., 6-hydroxymethyl megestrol acetate MO-TMS ether (Fig. 6a and b).

Megestrol acetate and each of the two groups of monohydroxy metabolites (compounds I, Ia and II, IIa) found in the urinary extracts were separated during chromatography on columns of silicic acid (7) prior to gas chromatography: Megestrol acetate was eluted with 27% ethyl acetate in toluene, compounds I and Ia with 35% ethyl acetate in toluene, and compounds II and IIa with ethyl acetate. The mass spectrum of compound II-MO-TMS ether (Fig. 5a) has a number of significant fragments [m/e 338 M-(103 + 60) and m/e 295 M-(2 × 103)], which suggest the presence of a primary substituted hydroxyl function. As Cooper and Kellie (13) had previously identified 6-hydroxymethyl megestrol acetate in human urine, partial synthesis of this compound from 17-acetoxy-6-methylene-4-pregnene-3,20-dione (kindly given to us by Dr. A. E. Kellie) using the method of Cooley et al. (26) was undertaken. The mass spectrum of the synthetic 6-hydroxymethyl megestrol acetate-MO-TMS ether was found to be

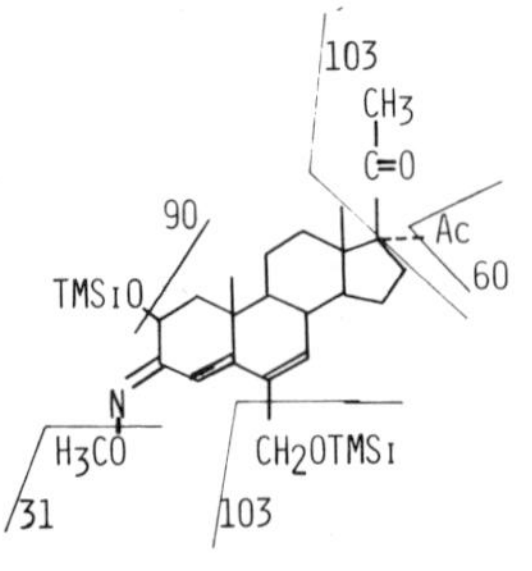

FIG. 5. Possible mass spectrometric fragmentation patterns of suspected megestrol acetate metabolites as methoxime-trimethylsilyl ethers.

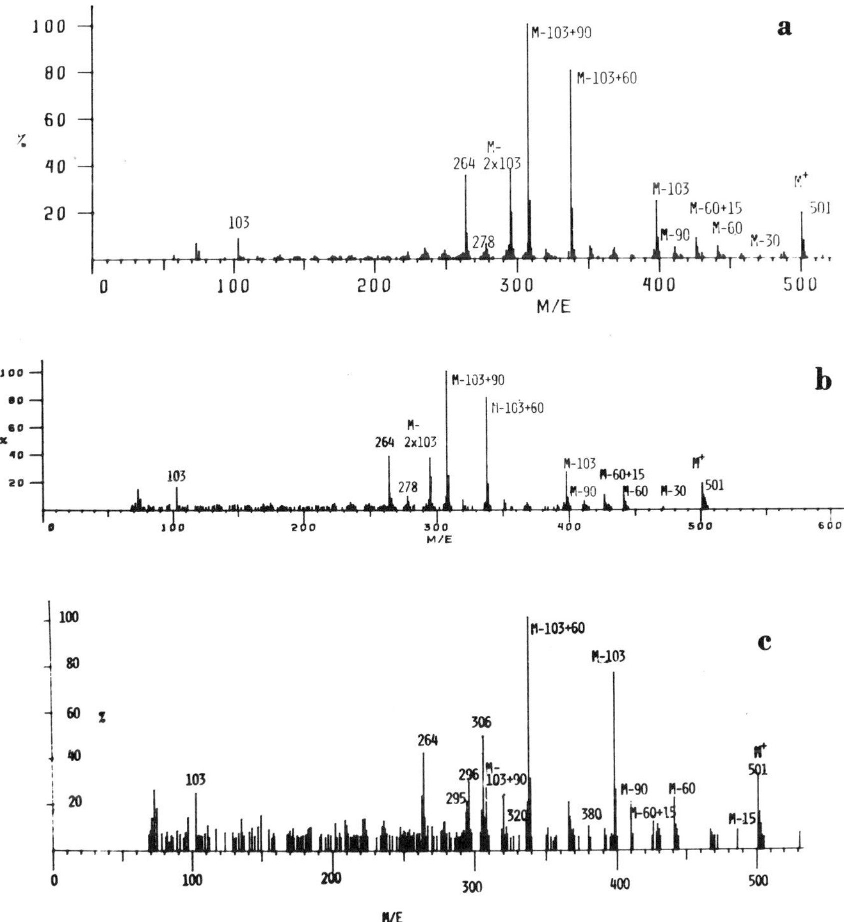

FIG. 6. Mass spectra of 6-hydroxymethylmegestrol acetate synthesized from 17-acetoxy-6-methylene-4-pregnene-3,20-dione-MO-TMS ether according to Cooley et al. (26) **(a)**, Compound II-MO-TMS ether **(b)**, and compound IIα-MO-TMS ether **(c)** detected in the glucuronide fraction of human urine after ingestion of megestrol acetate. The instrumentation and experimental conditions were as described in Fig. 1.

identical with that of compound II-MO-TMS ether (Fig. 6a and b). Compound IIa, which was found in the same silicic acid fraction of the urinary glucuronides as 6-hydroxymethyl megestrol acetate, has a mass spectrum qualitatively similar to the latter, but its base peak is at m/e 338 (Fig. 6c). It is very likely that compound IIa is also a monohydroxy megestrol acetate derivative with primary hydroxyl substitution, but as all mass spectra from this peak obtained to date seem to be contaminated the matter requires further investigation.

Compound I (unconjugated and glucuronide fractions), and compound Ia (glucuronide fraction) (Fig. 7) have almost identical mass spectra (Fig. 8). The

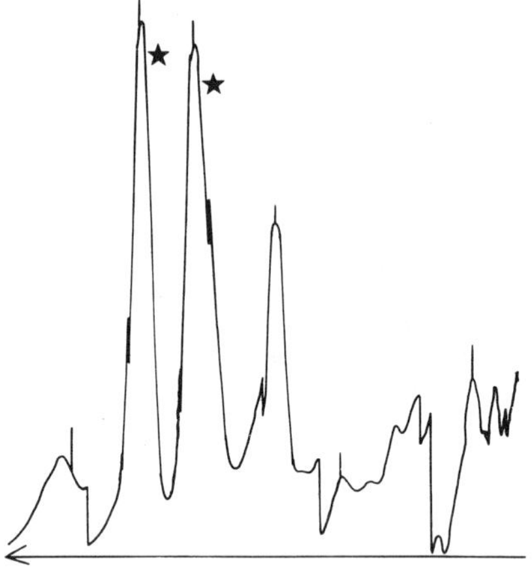

FIG. 7. Total ion current (TIC) chromatogram scan from 8 min after sample injection obtained for that fraction of steroid glucuronides, which, after hydrolysis, were eluted from the silicic acid column in 35% ethyl acetate in toluene. The analysis was made after methoxime-trimethylsilyl ether formation, and the scan runs from left to right. The vertical lines indicate the points at which mass spectra were recorded. Stars mark the peaks which gave spectra designated compound I *(left)* and compound Ia *(right)* in Fig. 8.

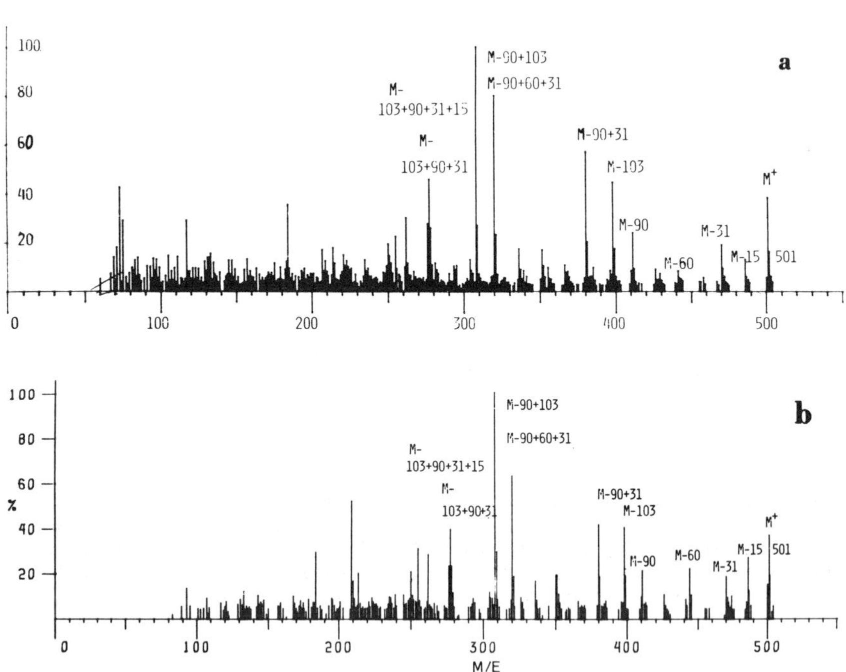

FIG. 8. Mass spectra of compound I-MO-TMS ether **(a)** and compound Ia-MO-TMS ether **(b)** detected in the glucuronide fraction of human urine after oral ingestion of megestrol acetate. Instrumentation and experimental conditions were as described in Fig. 1.

spectra seem to differ mainly in the intensity of the M-15 (m/e 386) and M-31 (m/e 370) fragments. They have the same molecular ion (m/e 501) and base peak [m/e 308 (M-(103 + 90)] as 6-hydroxymethylmegestrol acetate-MO-TMS ether. However, the spectra are otherwise dominated by fragments involving the loss of 31 mass units (scission of the N-O bond in the methoxime group): m/e 470 (M-31), 380 [M-(90 + 31)], 320 [M-(90 + 60 + 31)], 277 [M-(103 + 90 + 31)], and 262 [M-(103 + 90 + 31 + 15)] (Fig. 8), which are not seen in the spectrum of 6-hydroxymethylmegestrol acetate-MO-TMS ether (Fig. 6a and b); they do not show the fragments characteristic of the presence of a primary substituted hydroxyl function (see above) seen in the latter. The presence of 2α-hydroxymegestrol acetate in human urine has been reported (13), and it is at present being synthesized for comparison with compounds I and Ia.

The mass spectrum of compound III (Fig. 9a), a possible dihydroxylated metabolite, showed a molecular ion at m/e 589—that expected for dihydroxymegestrol acetate-MO-bis-TMS ether. The fragmentation pattern is a hybrid of those described above for the 6-hydroxymethyl metabolite and compound II. It is thought that it may be 6-hydroxymethyl-2α-hydroxymegestrol acetate, which has previously been described in both rabbit and human urine (13,27). The mass spectrum of compound IV in Fig. 9b shows a molecular ion at m/e 591, 2 mass units greater than compound III, which would be expected from a dihydrodihy-

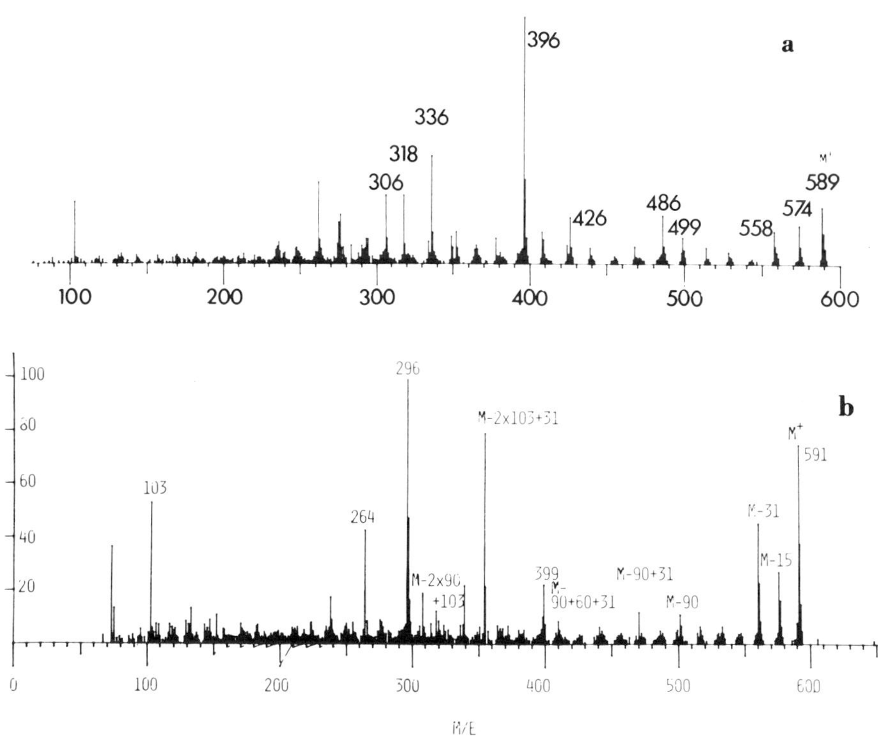

FIG. 9. Mass spectra of compound III-MO,bis-TMS ether **(a)** and compound IV MO-bis-TMS ether **(b)** detected in a combined unconjugated plus conjugated steroid extract of human urine after oral ingestion of megestrol acetate. Instrumentation and experimental conditions were as described in Fig. 1.

droxymegestrol acetate-MO-bis-TMS ether. The presence of this compound is evidence of the human organism's ability to reduce partially the 4,6-diene system in megestrol acetate.

In the *extracts* of *bile* from a postmenopausal woman with T-tube drainage of the main bile duct for therapeutic purposes, who received 2 X 50 mg megestrol acetate tablets, no unmetabolized megestrol acetate was detected nor any unconjugated metabolites. In the glucuronide fraction 6-hydroxymethylmegestrol acetate, compound IIa, and traces of compound I were found. No dihydroxy metabolites were detected. In the monosulfate fraction evidence of the presence of 6-hydroxymethylmegestrol acetate was obtained.

In their study of ^{14}C-megestrol acetate metabolism after its oral administration to women, Cooper and Kellie (13) recovered 56–78% of the dose in urine and 8–30% in the feces over a period of 7 days. They found approximately equal amounts of radioactivity in the unconjugated and glucuronide fractions of urine, with less in the sulfate fraction. In the glucuronide fraction they identified 2α-hydroxy-, 6-hydroxymethyl-, and 2α-hydroxy-6-hydroxymethylmegestrol acetate, and detected some more polar metabolites. They also detected 6-hydroxymethylmegestrol acetate in the unconjugated fraction. Our study thus far confirms the findings on 6-hydroxymethylmegestrol acetate in urine and extends its distribution to the glucuronide and monosulfate fractions of human bile. Our results also seem to indicate that megestrol acetate is hydroxylated in the human in positions other than the 6-methyl and 2α- positions, and that partial reduction, at least of the 4,6-diene system, takes place. In rat adrenals, 18- and 11-hydroxylation of megestrol acetate have been described (28). The possible formation of these metabolites in humans must now be investigated.

MEGESTROL ACETATE METABOLISM IN THE BEAGLE

Using the same procedure, urine, plasma, bile, and liver from a female and a male beagle who received 100 mg megestrol acetate orally for 10 days were studied. No unmetabolized megestrol acetate or megestrol acetate metabolites could be detected in plasma or urine from these animals using this method. However, in the unconjugated steroid fraction of the female beagle liver there was evidence of the presence of 6-hydroxymethylmegestrol acetate and compound I. More polar metabolites were not detected. The metabolites in female beagle bile are under investigation.

In the bile from the male beagle only one megestrol acetate metabolite (compound Ic) was detected, and this was in the glucuronide fraction. The mass spectrum of compound Ic (Fig. 10), like the other monohydroxylated metabolites, shows a molecular ion at m/e 501, but the base peak is at m/e 398. In fact, the spectrum resembles more that of megestrol acetate-MO (Fig. 1a) than that of any of the other monohydroxylated metabolites (Figs. 6 and 8). This metabolite seems unique to the male beagle, as there is no evidence of its presence in any of the other extracts studied. These preliminary experiments with beagles also suggest

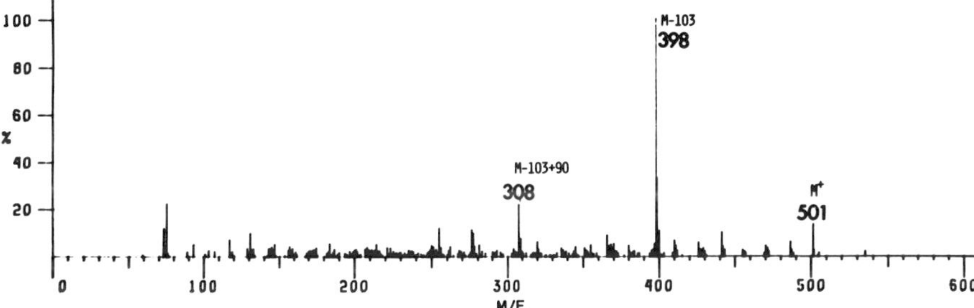

FIG. 10. Mass spectrum of compound Ic-MO-TMS ether detected in the glucuronide fraction from male beagle bile after oral administration of megestrol acetate. Instrumentation and experimental conditions were as described in Fig. 1.

that there may be considerable sex variation in megestrol acetate metabolism in this species.

Chainey et al. (29) investigated the metabolism of radioactively labeled megestrol acetate in the female beagle. They found that 79–92% of the administered dose was excreted in feces and only 8–10.5% in urine. Our findings also support the biliary-fecal axis as the main route of megestrol acetate excretion in the beagle. It is interesting to note that, although the routes of excretion in women and female beagles differ, the metabolites formed may be very similar. The biliary-fecal axis also seems to be the main route of excretion of endogenous androgen metabolites in the beagle: Studies in this laboratory (30–31) on endogenous androgens in plasma, urine, bile, and feces showed the presence of androgen metabolites (4,500 µg/liter) in bile (principally glucuronides) with androgen metabolites in urine at a concentration of only 76 µg/liter. In feces 177 µg androgen metabolites per 24 hr, mostly unconjugated, were detected.

SUMMARY

Radioimmunological and mass fragmentographic methods were used to monitor megestrol acetate and MPA levels in human plasma after oral administration of both drugs. The more-specific mass fragmentographic method for megestrol acetate gave lower plasma values than the radioimmunoassay. Evidence of megestrol acetate metabolite interference in the radioimmunoassay is presented. The specificity of the MPA radioimmunoassay is also discussed. The oral administration of megestrol acetate and MPA results in very much higher plasma levels of the former.

Megestrol acetate metabolites were detected in human urine and bile after oral administration using a gas chromatographic-mass spectrometric procedure. The metabolites in bile were almost exclusively glucuronide-conjugated, whereas in urine both unconjugated and glucuronide-conjugated metabolites were found. Mono- and dihydroxy metabolites predominated, although evidence of megestrol acetate reduction was also found. Metabolites in a female and male beagle were investigated by the same procedure. In the female beagle metabolites similar to those found in humans were detected in the liver. Only one metabolite was detected in the male, in the glucuronide fraction from bile; it was a monohydroxylated compound and seems to be unique to the male beagle.

ACKNOWLEDGMENTS

The excellent technical assistance of Mrs. Sirkka Tiainen, Anja Manner, Helena Lindgren, and Miss Inga Wiik is gratefully acknowledged. F.M. was in receipt of a fellowship from the World Health Organization from February 1973 to January 1975. This investigation was supported by grants from The Ford Foundation (to H.A.). The antiserum was kindly supplied by Dr. H. J. Rall, Upjohn International, Inc.

REFERENCES

1. Bush, I. E. (1962): Chemical and biological factors in the activity of adrenocortical steroids. *Pharmacol. Rev.,* 14:317–445.
2. Glenn, E. M., Richardson, S. L., and Bowman, B. I. (1959): Biologic activity of 6-alpha-methyl compounds corresponding to progesterone, 17-alpha-hydroxyprogesterone acetate and compound S. *Metabolism,* 8:265–285.
3. Cooke, B. A., and Vallance, D. K. (1965): Metabolism of megestrol acetate and related progesterone analogues by liver preparations in vitro. *Biochem. J.,* 97:672–677.
4. Adlercreutz, H., Nieminen, U., and Ervast, H-S. (1974): A mass fragmentographic method for the determination of megestrol acetate in plasma and its application to studies on the plasma levels after administration of the progestin to patients with carcinoma corporis uteri. *J. Steroid Biochem.,* 5:619–626.
5. Adlercreutz, H., Martin, F., Wahlroos, O., and Soini, E. (1975): Mass spectrometric and mass fragmentographic determination of natural and synthetic steroids in biological fluids. *J. Steroid Biochem.,* 6:247–259.
6. Martin, F., Peltonen, J., Laatikainen, T., Pulkkinen, M., and Adlercreutz, H. (1975): Excretion of progesterone metabolites and estriol in faeces from pregnant women during ampicillin administration. *J. Steroid Biochem.,* 6:1339–1346.
7. Laatikainen, T., and Vihko, R. (1969): Identification of $C_{19}O_2$ and $C_{21}O_2$ steroids in the glucuronide fraction of human bile. *Eur. J. Biochem.,* 10:165–171.
8. Janne, O. (1970): Quantitative determination of neutral steroid mono- and disulphates in human urine. *Clin. Chim. Acta,* 29:529–540.
9. Bradlow, H. L. (1968): Extraction of steroid conjugates with a neutral resin. *Steroids,* 11:265–272.
10. Viinikka, L., and Janne, O. (1973): Urinary excretion of neutral steroid glucuronides with reference to the menstrual cycle. *Clin. Chim. Acta,* 49:277–285.
11. Eriksson, H., and Gustafsson, J-A. (1970): Excretion of steroid hormones in adults: Steroids in urine from a pregnant woman. *Eur. J. Biochem.,* 16:268–277.
12. Janne, O., Vihko, R., Sjovall, J., and Sjovall, K. (1969): Determination of steroid mono- and disulphates in human plasma. *Clin. Chim. Acta,* 23:405–412.
13. Cooper, J. M., and Kellie, A. E. (1968): The metabolism of megestrol acetate (17α-acetoxy-6-methylpregna-4,6-diene-3,20-dione) in women. *Steroids,* 11:133–149.
14. Hiroi, M., Stanezyk, F. Z., Goebelsmann, U., Brenner, P. F., Lumkin, M. E., and Mishell, D. R., Jr. (1975): Radioimmunossay of serum medroxyprogesterone acetate (Provera[R]) in women following oral and intravaginal administration. *Steroids,* 26:373–386.
15. Cornette, J. C., Kirton, K. T., and Duncan, G. W. (1971): Measurement of medroxyprogesterone acetate (Provera[R]) by radioimmunoassay. *J. Clin. Endocrinol.,* 33:459–466.

16. Jeppsson, S., and Johansson, E. D. B. (1976): Medroxyprogesterone acetate, estradiol, FSH and LH in peripheral blood after intramuscular administration of Depo-Provera[R] to women. *Contraception (in press)*.

17. Royer, M. E., Ko, H., Campbell, J. A., Murray, H. C., Evans, J. S., and Kaiser, D. G. (1974): Radioimmunoassay of medroxyprogesterone acetate (Provera[R]) using the 11α-hydroxysuccinyl conjugate. *Steroids*, 23:713–730.

18. Schubert, K., Schlegel, J., and Horhold, C. (1963): Selective hydration of steroid hormones by Clostridium under anaerobic conditions. *Z. Naturforsch.*, 18b:284–286.

19. Schubert, K., Bohme, K-H., and Horhold, C. (1961): The formation of aromatization and hydration products from progesterone by Mycobacterium smegmatis. *Z. Naturforsch.*, 16b: 595–597.

20. Schubert, K., Bohme, K-H., and Horhold, C. (1964): Formation of low molecular weight degradation products from progesterone by microorganisms. *Steroids*, 4:581–586.

21. Wade, A. P., Slater, J. D. H., Kellie, A. E., and Holliday, M. E. (1959): Urinary excretion of 17-ketosteroids following rectal infusion of cortisol. *J. Clin. Endocrinol.*, 19:444–453.

22. Schubert, K., Schlegel, J., and Horhold, C. (1963): Stereospezifische Hydrierung von ^{1,4}-Androstadiendrion-(3.17)zu^1-5β-Androstendion-(3.17) und 5β-Androstanol-(3α)-on-(17) mit Clostridium paraputrificum unter anaeroben Bedingungen. *Hoppe Seylers Z. Physiol. Chem.*, 332: 310–313.

23. Schubert, K., Schlegel, J., and Horhold, C. (1965): Stereospecific hydrogenation of delta-4-, delta-1,4-, delta-4,6- and delta-1,4,3,6-ketosteroids by Clostridium paraputrificum. *Steroids (Suppl.)*, 1:175–184.

24. Laatikainen, T., and Vihko, R. (1969): Identification of 18-hydroxyandrosterone in human bile. *Steroids*, 13:615–621.

25. Gustafsson, J-A., and Sjovall, J. (1968): Steroids in germfree and conventional rats. 6. Identification of 15α- and 21-hydroxylated C_{21} steroids in faeces from germfree rats. *Eur. J. Biochem.*, 6:236–247.

26. Cooley, G., Davies, M. T., Ellis, B., and Petrow, W. (1966): Partial synthesis of 17α-acetoxy-6-acetoxymethylpregna-4,6-diene-3,20-dione and its 2α-acetoxy derivative, two acetylated metabolites of megestrol acetate. *Tetrahedron*, 22:365–367.

27. Cooper, J. M., Jones, H. E. H., and Kellie, A. E. (1965): The metabolism of megestrol acetate (17α-acetoxy-6-methylpregna-4,6-diene-3,20-dione) in the rabbit. *Steroids*, 6:255–275.

28. Cooke, B. A., and Vallance, D. K. (1968): Metabolism of megestrol acetate by rat adrenal glands in vitro. *Biochem. J.*, 109:121–125.

29. Chainey, D., McCoubrey, A., and Evans, J. M. (1970): The excretion of megestrol acetate by beagle bitches. *Vet. Rec.*, 86:287–288.

30. Martin, F., Bhargava, A., and Adlercreutz, H. (1975): Endogenous conjugated androgen metabolites in bile from male beagles: A mass-fragmentographic study. *Acta Endocrinol. (Kbh.) [Suppl.]*, 199:232.

31. Martin, F., Bhargava, A. S., and Adlercreutz, H. (1977): Androgen metabolism in the beagle. Endogenous $C_{19}O_2$ metabolites in bile and faeces and the effect of ampicillin administration. *J. Steroid Biochem. (in press)*.

Pharmacology of Steroid Contraceptive Drugs
edited by S. Garattini and H. W. Berendes.
Raven Press, New York © 1977.

Metabolism, Metabolic Clearance Rate, Blood Metabolites, and Blood Half-Life of Norethindrone and Mestranol

V. B. Mahesh, T. M. Mills, T. J. Lin, J. O. Ellegood, and W. E. Braselton

Departments of Endocrinology and Obstetrics and Gynecology, Medical College of Georgia, Augusta, Georgia 30902

Oral contraceptives constitute some of the most commonly used drugs in the United States and around the world. Recent reports point out that oral contraceptive use may be a risk factor in several thromboembolic diseases including myocardial infarction (16) and cerebral and pulmonary embolism (2,10,25). Oral contraceptives may be diabetogenic (9), alter liver function (1), and raise serum levels of triglycerides, potentially leading to vascular disease (6,23,28). The elevation in serum triglycerides and phospholipids and the fall in the α_2-antithrombin III levels is attributed to synthetic estrogens as these do not occur after administration of natural estrogens in postmenopausal women (13).

In spite of the extensive use of oral contraceptives and their reported untoward effects, only limited information was available about their blood half-life, their metabolic clearance rate (MCR), and the clearance of their metabolites from the bloodstream. Therefore studies to this effect were carried out by Mills et al., using norethindrone (17β-hydroxy-17α-ethynyl-4-estrene-3-one) (18) and mestranol [3 methoxy-17α-ethynyl-1,3,5(10)-estratrien-17β-ol] (19).

MCR AND BLOOD HALF-LIFE OF NORETHINDRONE AND MESTRANOL

The study was carried out in paid volunteers 20–37 years of age with normal menstrual histories. The volunteers had not taken any oral contraceptive medication for at least 1 year prior to joining the study. Informed consent was obtained from each volunteer. The volunteers received orally either 2.5 mg norethindrone (norethindrone study) or 80 µg mestranol (mestranol study) at 8 P.M. before the start of the study. At 6 A.M. the following morning the drug was repeated. At 9 A.M. the subject received an intravenous injection of 5.5 µCi ^{3}H-9,11-norethindrone (norethindrone study) or ^{3}H-9,11-mestranol (mestranol study). Blood samples (20 ml) were collected in heparinized tubes through a venous catheter immediately before (0 time) and 3, 6, 10, 20, 40, and 90 min and 3, 6, 12, and 24 hr after injection of the ^{3}H-drug. ^{3}H-Norethindrone and ^{3}H-mestranol were estimated in blood plasma, after adding carrier steroid, by thin-layer chromatography and measuring absorbancy in a spectrophotometer as well as counting for ^{3}H in a liquid scintillation counter. Such treatment resulted in good radiochemical purity. The methods are described in detail by Mills et al. (18,19).

After the initial study the volunteers took either 2.5 mg norethindrone per day from days 5 to 24 of each cycle (norethindrone study) or Ortho-Novum SQ (80 μg mestranol per day on days 5–18, then 80 μg mestranol plus 2 mg norethindrone per day for 5 days) (mestranol study). After six or seven such courses of treatment, the blood half-life and MCR of norethindrone and mestranol were re-evaluated as described above.

The data obtained from the blood levels of norethindrone and mestranol after the single intravenous injection of the ^{3}H-steroid was plotted using a semilogarithmic plot of the percent of injected dose per liter (ordinate) versus time after injection (abscissa), and then fitting the best line through these plots. This was accomplished statistically by the method of least squares with a program written for the Hewlett-Packard 9100B calculator (18). In constructing these plots it was assumed that the injected ^{3}H was distributed over two compartments. The intercepts and the slopes of the two lines were determined and the half-life and metabolic clearance rate calculated according to the method of Tait (26). The typical disappearance curves of norethindrone and mestranol in blood are shown in Fig. 1.

Table 1 shows the calculated half-life values for the two components of each curve represented by the lines α and β. Alpha (α) represents the slope of the first component of the disappearance curve (3–90 min), and β is the slope of the second part of the curve (3–24 hr). The MCR of norethindrone in 10 patients after acute

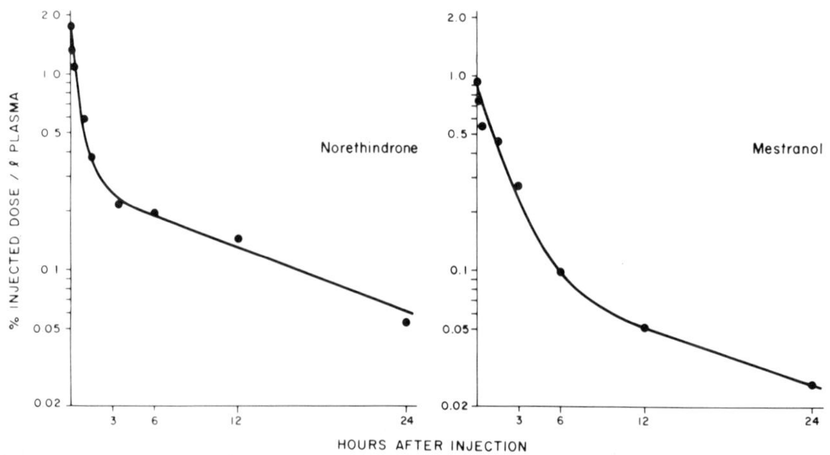

FIG. 1. Disappearance curves of native norethindrone and mestranol from blood following single intravenous injection of tritium-labeled drug.

TABLE 1. *Plasma half-life and MCR of ^{3}H-norethindrone before and after 6-month courses of norethindrone 2.5 mg/day*

Subject	Before			After		
	$T_{\frac{1}{2}\alpha}$ (min)	$T_{\frac{1}{2}\beta}$ (min)	MCR (liters/day)	$T_{\frac{1}{2}\alpha}$ (min)	$T_{\frac{1}{2}\beta}$ (min)	MCR (liters/day)
C.B.	31	708	442	39	467	505
L.B.	24	632	657	25	142	1,570
M.C.	21	465	622	23	603	483
M.B.C.	32	274	284	23	990	196
N.F.	16	545	608	16	371	1,020
S.H.	27	671	481	19	336	797
N.H.	36	366	360	55	279	461
M.M.C.	25	631	405	30	226	799
M.R.	19	181	910	28	326	1,000
V.S.	46	324	536	44	417	494
Mean ± SEM	27.7 ± 2.8	480 ± 59	531 ± 57	30.2 ± 3.9	416 ± 76	733 ± 125[a]

[a] Significantly greater than "before" value ($p < 0.01$) by paired variable t-test.

administration of the drug and after 6–7 months of drug treatment are also presented in Table 1. The mean MCR of norethindrone was 531 ± 56.8 liters/day after acute administration and increased to 732 ± 125 liters/day after 6–7 months of treatment. Using the paired t-test (one-tailed), this increase in MCR after 6–7 months of treatment with norethindrone proved to be statistically significant ($p < 0.05$). These findings extend the previous report of Mills et al. (18), who presented data earlier on a smaller number of volunteers. The increase in the MCR of norethindrone is perhaps not surprising in view of its similarity to the structure of testosterone. An increase in the MCR of testosterone in women in virilized states and after testosterone administration has been reported by several investigators (14,20–22,27).

Table 2 presents the MCR of mestranol in 10 women before and after 6- to 7-month courses of mestranol. Half-life values of α and β calculated from the mestranol disappearance curve are also shown in Table 2. The MCR of 1,265 ± 139 liters/day for mestranol after acute treatment was not different from that found after 6–7 months of treatment (1,267 ± 158 liters per day), in contrast to results with norethindrone. However, the absence of an increase in the MCR of mestranol after prolonged treatment is in agreement with the results of Lee and Chen (14), who found that feeding mestranol to rats did not alter the demethylation activity of rat liver microsomes. The results of the MCR of mestranol in this study extend the previously reported values of Mills et al. (19) in a smaller number of patients and are in agreement with the MCR of mestranol reported by Bird and Clark (4). Furthermore, it is of interest that the MCR of mestranol is similar to that of estradiol-17β in normal women (15), and the MCR of norethindrone (acute administration) is similar to the MCR of testosterone in nonhirsute and nonvirilized women (3).

TABLE 2. *Plasma half-life and MCR of ^{3}H-mestranol before and after 6-month courses of mestranol[a]*

Subject	Before			After		
	$T_{1/2\alpha}$ (min)	$T_{1/2\beta}$ (min)	MCR (liters/day)	$T_{1/2\alpha}$ (min)	$T_{1/2\beta}$ (min)	MCR (liters/day)
J.B.	24	851	1,140	20	357	1,010
K.E.	10	426	1,730	20	321	1,630
J.G.	34	414	828	27	634	751
P.H.	14	930	1,840	16	706	1,090
M.H.	17	434	1,740	23	266	2,050
T.H.	11	1,160	1,050	16	455	1,040
K.H.	38	432	1,260	32	398	1,210
S.S.	13	2,420	849	16	1,080	745
M.S.	12	1,230	617	11	368	1,020
C.W.	2	97	1,600	18	125	2,130
Mean ± SEM	17.5 ± 3.6	839 ± 211	1,265 ± 139	19.9 ± 1.9	471 ± 86	1,268 ± 158

[a] Dosage: 0.08 mg/day as Ortho-Novum SQ.

LONG HALF-LIFE METABOLITES OF NORETHINDRONE AND MESTRANOL IN BLOOD

Although native norethindrone and mestranol cleared rapidly from the bloodstream (Fig. 1), the total ^{3}H counts in plasma remained elevated for a considerable period of time. The total counts in plasma were determined (18) using an emulsifier for aqueous samples (Insta Gel, Packard Instrument Co.); the results are shown in Fig. 2. In all probability, the persistence of radioactivity in blood was due to conjugated metabolites of the steroid, because this radioactivity was in the form of water-soluble and not ether-soluble compounds. In order to deter-

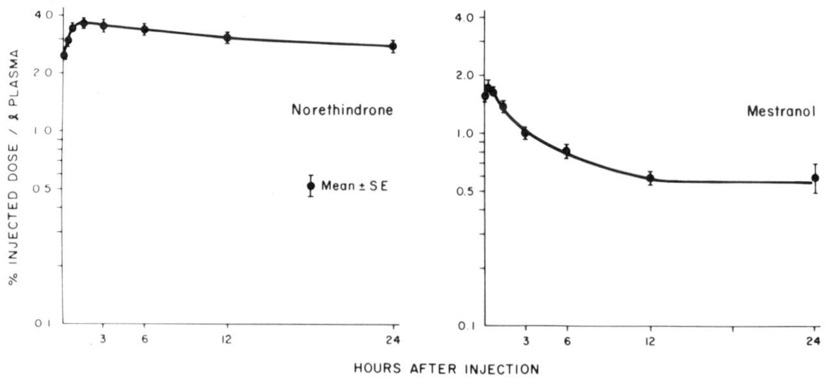

FIG. 2. Persistence of radioactivity in blood following single injection of tritiated norethindrone or mestranol in 10 volunteers.

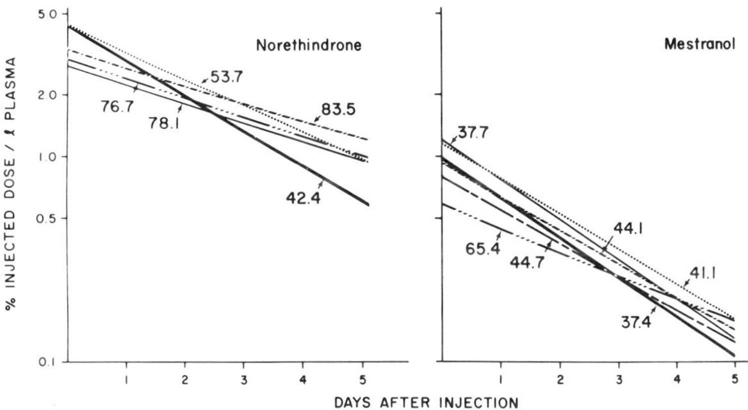

FIG. 3. Half-life of total radioactivity following single injection of tritiated norethindrone or mestranol.

mine the half-life of the metabolites in blood, ^{3}H-norethindrone (10.1 μCi) or ^{3}H-mestranol (9.6 μCi) were given as a single intravenous injection in volunteers, and blood samples were collected at several intervals ranging from 3 min to 5 days after the injection (17). The results in Fig. 3 show that the half-life of norethindrone metabolites in blood varied from 42.4 to 83.5 hr, with a mean of 66.9 hr. The half-life of mestranol metabolites varied from 37.4 to 65.4 hr, with a mean of 45.1 hr. Although it is not valid to use the expression "metabolic clearance rate of metabolites" because some of the basic assumptions of MCR determinations are not met, nevertheless one could calculate the crude clearance of metabolites from blood from the disappearance curve in Fig. 3. Such a calculation yields a mean value of 7.4 liters/day for norethindrone metabolites and 41.3 liters/day for mestranol metabolites. The MCR of a compound closely related to norethindrone [norethynodrel (17β-hydroxy-17α-ethynyl-5(10)-estrene-3-one)], calculated on the basis of disappearance of total radioactivity from blood, was reported earlier to be approximately 30 liters/day (12).

ORAL ADMINISTRATION OF NORETHINDRONE AND MESTRANOL

In view of the fact that contraceptive steroid medication is taken orally rather than by injection, the appearance of radioactivity in blood, half-life of metabolites in blood, and excretion of radioactivity in urine was studied in volunteers given a gelatin capsule containing 10.23 μCi ^{3}H-norethindrone or 10.21 μCi ^{3}H-mestranol (17). Measurable levels of the drug were present in blood within 15 min of ingestion, and the disappearance of the native drug and the metabolites from blood appeared to be similar to that found after injection. The overall average urinary excretion over a period of 5 days of radioactivity following injection of

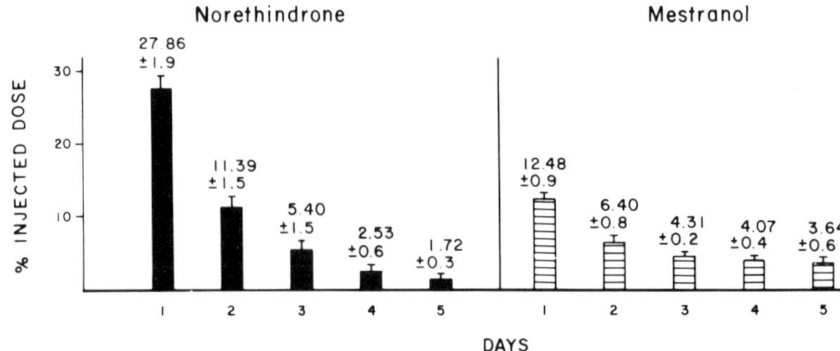

FIG. 4. Urinary excretion of radioactivity following single injection of ^{3}H-norethindrone and ^{3}H-mestranol.

[3]H-norethindrone was 48.91% of the administered dose and 31.2% of the dose of ^{3}H-mestranol (Fig. 4). After oral administration the percentage excreted and the patterns of excretion were similar.

Since oral contraceptives are taken in daily doses and the above-mentioned results indicated the presence of metabolites with a long half-life, it was of considerable interest to study the accumulation of metabolites of these drugs over a period of time. Therefore gelatin capsules containing 5.38 μCi ^{3}H norethindrone were administered daily at 12 noon for 6 days to several volunteers; blood samples were obtained immediately before and 3 hr after each capsule (17). The blood collection was continued for 4 days after the last capsule was taken. Urine was collected over the entire 10-day period. Figure 5 shows the "staircase" accumulation phenomenon of norethindrone metabolites; this pattern was not unexpected owing to the long half-life of norethindrone metabolities. Even on the sixth day of administration there was no indication of a plateau in blood levels of ^{3}H-metabolites. Once the oral drug was discontinued, the metabolite levels declined in the blood, with a half-life of approximately 70 hr. The urinary excretion of ^{3}H followed a different pattern (Fig. 6). After an initial rise in ^{3}H output on the second day of collection, urinary excretion of ^{3}H was essentially unchanged

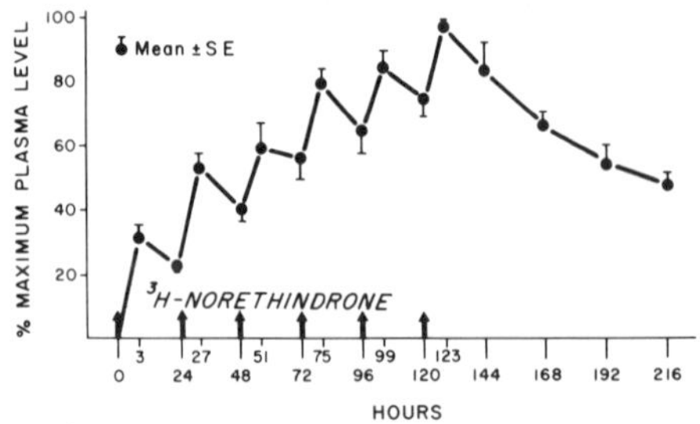

FIG. 5. Buildup of plasma radioactivity during six oral ingestions of tritiated norethindrone at 24-hr intervals and subsequent decline on 4 days without treatment.

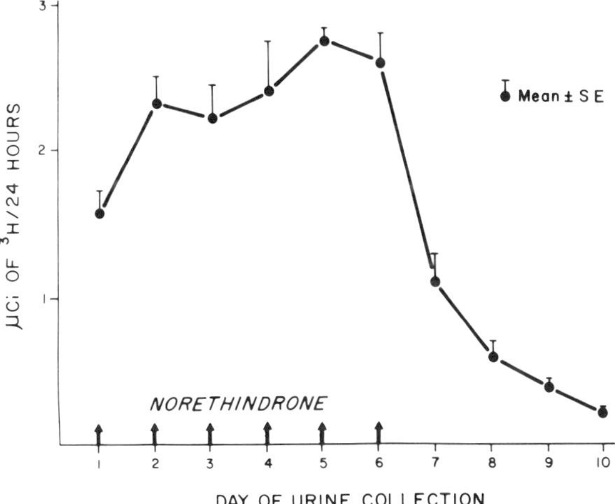

FIG. 6. Urinary excretion of radioactivity during six oral ingestions of tritiated norethindrone at 24-hr intervals (days 1–6) and subsequent decline on 4 days without treatment.

during the remaining 4 days of ^{3}H-norethindrone administration, followed by a rapid decline. Over a 10-day period 48% of the ingested radioactivity was excreted, a value comparable to that found after injection of the drug.

The expected "staircase" effect of accumulation of metabolites in blood after daily oral ingestion of ^{3}H-mestranol was also observed *(unpublished observation).*

CHARACTERIZATION AND MEASUREMENT OF NORETHINDRONE METABOLITES IN URINE AND BLOOD

In the above-mentioned studies the presence of radioactivity in the blood indicated the possibility of norethindrone and mestranol metabolites with long half-lives. It was necessary to confirm their presence unequivocally, establish their identity, and devise methods so their levels could be estimated in women taking oral contraceptive medication (5).

In order to study the urinary metabolites of norethindrone, a normal female volunteer was administered norethindrone 25 mg/day for 4 days; her urine was collected over boric acid and refrigerated. The urine was extracted with methylene chloride to obtain the free steroid fraction. It was then brought to pH 6.5 with 1 M phosphate buffer, and bacterial β-glucuronidase (360 units/ml urine) was added. After the mixture was incubated at 37°C for 24 hr, a second and a third addition of β-glucuronidase was done at 24-hr intervals. After a final incubation of 48 hr, the liberated free steroids from the hydrolysis of glucuronides were extracted with ether/ethyl acetate mixture (2 : 1) to yield the "glucuronide" fraction. The aqueous phase was acidified to pH 1 with 4 N sulfuric acid and, after saturation with sodium chloride, was extracted with ethyl acetate. After incubation at 37°C for 16 hr, the ethyl acetate extracted was neutralized, evaporated to dryness, taken up in water, and extracted with ether to yield the "sulfate" fraction. The use of bacterial β-glucuronidase rather than liver β-glucuronidase gave higher yields of hydrolysis; the details are described elsewhere. The sulfate and glucuronide fractions were further separated into neutral and phenolic fractions using the toluene/1 N NaOH partition procedure (7). The crude "free," "sulfate," and "glucuronide" fractions were further purified by silicic acid chromatography and Amberlite XAD-2 chromatography. After preparing trimethylsilyl ethers of various fractions, the compounds were chromatographed on a Finnigan 1015D gas chromatograph-mass spectrometer (GC-MS) interfaced with a System Industries System 150 data processing and control system.

Compounds were identified by their mass spectra and their gas chromatography retention times (expressed as methylene unit values) obtained on two stationary phases of different polarity, 1% XE-60 and 1% SP-2250. Four ring A-reduced metabolites, a ring A-reduced metabolite with an additional hydroxyl group, norethindrone itself, and ethynylestradiol were identified in this fashion (Fig. 7;

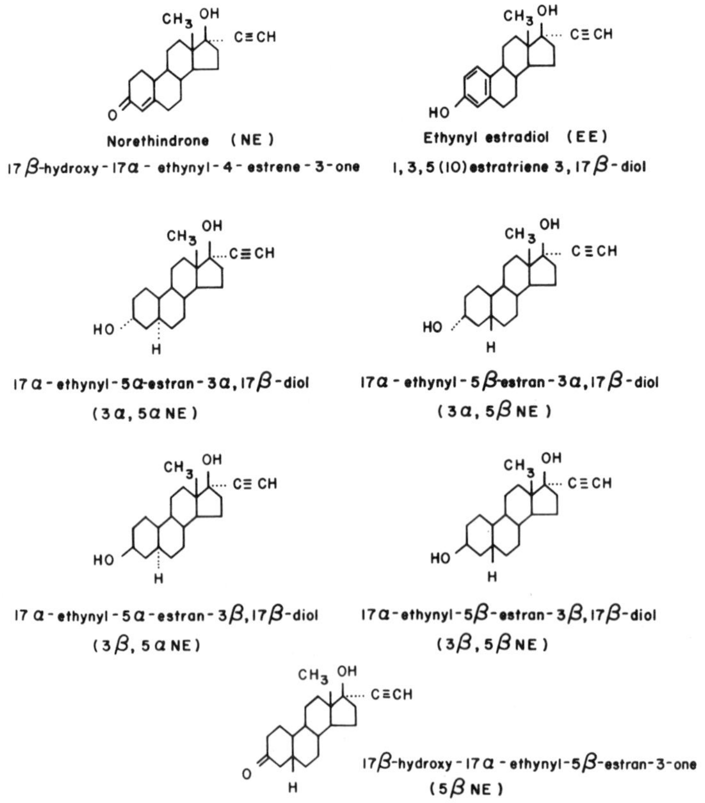

FIG. 7. Blood and urinary metabolites of norethindrone identified in urine and plasma by GC-MS.

TABLE 3. *Blood and urinary metabolites of norethindrone*

Fraction	NE	5β-NE	3α,5α-NE	3α,5β-NE	3β,5α-NE	3β,5β-NE	EE
URINARY METABOLITES (μG IN 2.5% OF URINE) AFTER 100 MG NORETHINDRONE							
Free	—	—	Trace	0.24	—	—	—
Sulfate	0.76	—	0.20	4.93	Trace	0.37	Trace
Glucuronide	1.52	—	0.56	4.09	Trace	0.24	Trace
BLOOD METABOLITES (NG/ML PLASMA) 3 HR AFTER A 25-MG ORAL DOSE							
Free	104	9	4	8	—	4	—
Sulfate	23	—	46	110	—	0.2	—
Glucuronide	69	—	5	27	—	—	—

Table 3). The presence of ethynylestradiol in the sulfate fraction was established by mass fragmentography. An example of the gas chromatographic separation of a urinary sulfate fraction is shown in Fig. 8. Tetrahydro metabolites were located by computer-reconstructed chromatograms of m/e 431 (M-15). The C_{28} and C_{32} *n*-alkanes (m/e 71) were included for calculation of methylene unit values. The mass spectrum of 3α,5βNE-bis-TMS isolated as above is compared with the reference standard in Fig. 9. To study the blood-borne metabolites of norethindrone (NE), one female volunteer was administered an oral dose of 25 mg NE, and a blood sample was obtained 3 hr later. A second female volunteer was treated with the normal regimen of Ortho-Novum (2 mg NE, 0.1 mg mestranol) daily, and blood samples were drawn 12–16 hr later. Methanol (25 ml)

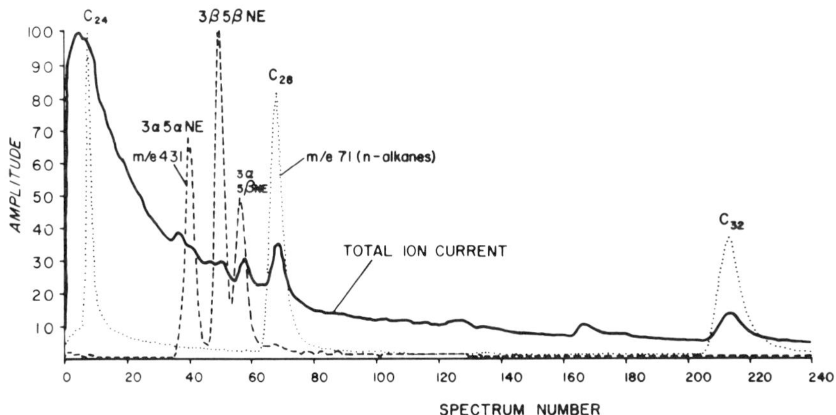

FIG. 8. Total ion current chromatogram (———) of TMS derivatives of a urinary sulfate fraction from a volunteer treated with norethindrone. The sample was chromatographed on a 1.5 meter × 2 mm column of 1% XE-60 with temperature programmed from 170° to 230° at 1°/min. The reconstructed mass chromatogram of ion m/e 431 (-------) indicates the ring A-reduced metabolites of NE; the mass chromatogram of m/e 71 (.......) indicates the *n*-alkane reference compounds used to calculate methylene unit values.

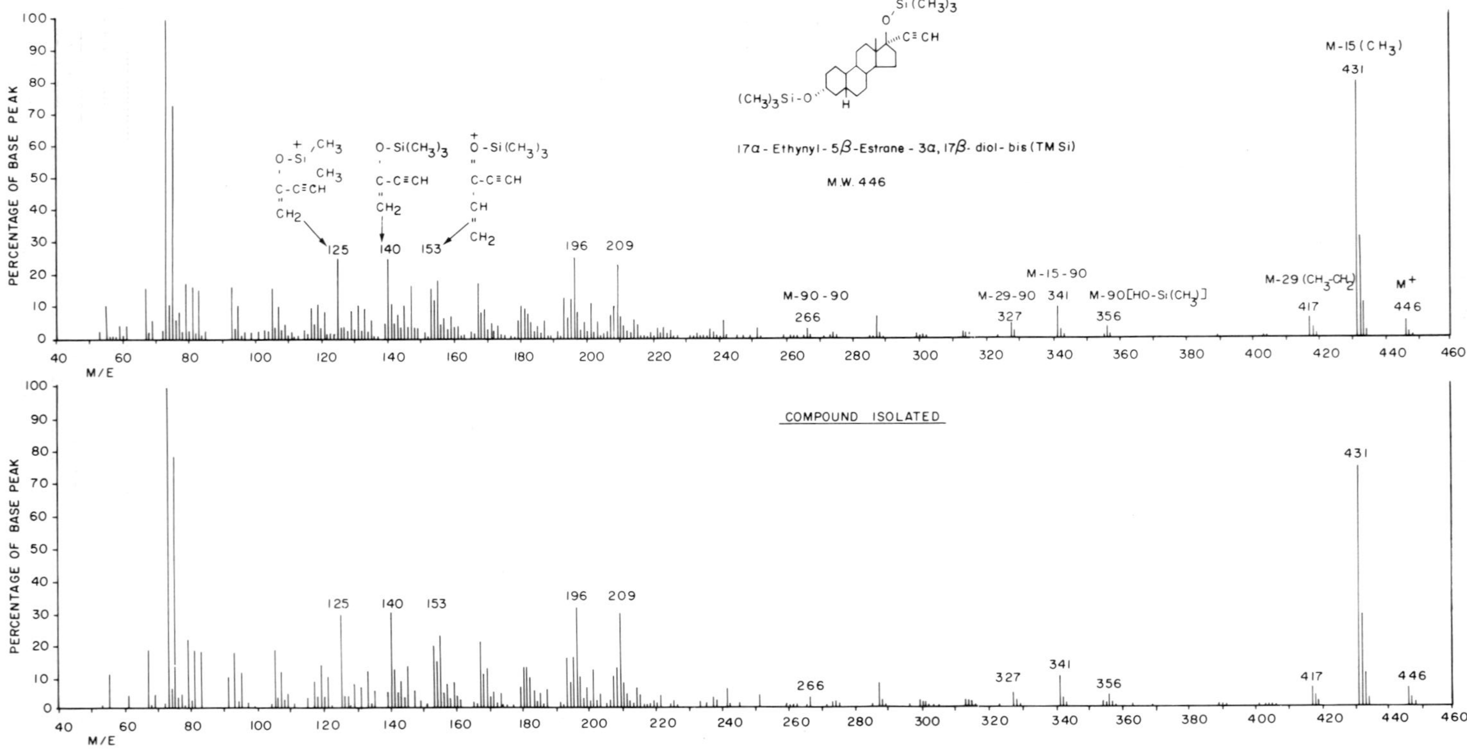

FIG. 9. Mass spectrum (70 eV) of 17α-ethynyl-5β-estrane-3α,17β-diol-bis-TMS *(top)* and the compound with retention time equal to 17α-ethynyl-5β-estrane-3α,17β-diol-bis-TMS isolated from the urinary sulfate fraction of a patient treated with norethindrone *(bottom)*.

was added to 10-ml aliquots of plasma, and the precipitated proteins were removed by centrifugation. The aqueous methanol fraction was evaporated to dryness, taken up in 5 ml water, and the free, sulfate, and glucuronide fractions prepared as described above for urine.

Mass fragmentography was used to identify and quantitate the plasma metabolites of NE following treatment with either 25 or 2 mg NE per day. Positive identification by mass fragmentography required the presence of the selected ion peak at the correct relative retention time determined on two stationary phases of different polarity: 1% XE-60 and either 1% SP-2250 or 1% SP-2100. Tetrahydro metabolites were chromatographed as TMS derivatives, with 5α-androstane-17α-vinyl-3β,17β-diol-bis-TMS as the reference compound; and 3-keto compounds were chromatographed as methoxime (MO) derivatives, with 17α-ethynylestr-5(10)-en-17β-ol-3-one MO as the reference compound. Quantitation was achieved by relative peak height measurement and interpolation from a standard curve prepared the same day.

Following treatment with 25 mg NE, 3α,5α-NE, 3α,5β-NE, and NE were found in the free, sulfate, and glucuronide fractions of plasma; 3β,5β-NE in the free and sulfate fractions; and 5β-NE in the free fraction (Table 3). The presence of 3α,5β-NE as the major metabolite of NE and 3α,5α-NE as the minor metabolite in urine was established by Stillwell et al. (24) using GC-MS methods. Using radioactive tracer techniques, 3β,5α-NE and 3β,5β-NE were also demonstrable

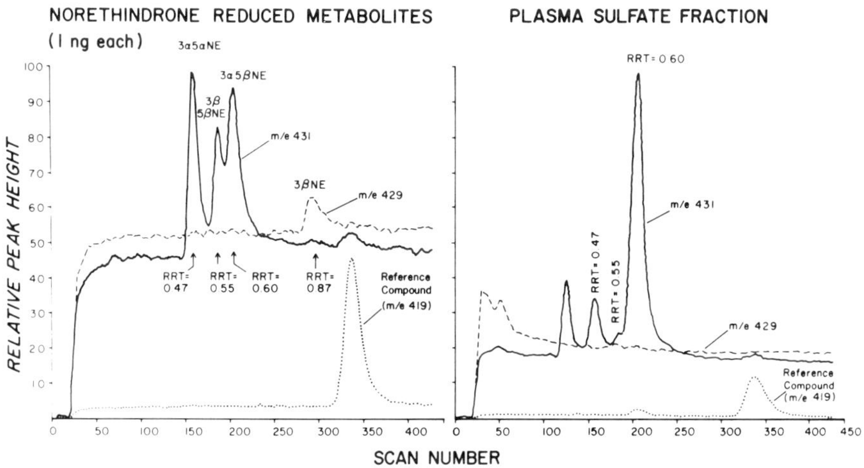

FIG. 10. Mass fragmentogram of TMS derivatives of ring A-reduced metabolites of norethindrone (m/e431),3β-NE (m/e 429), the reference compound 17α-vinyl-5α-androstane-3β,17β-diol (m/e 419), and the compounds isolated from the plasma sulfate fraction of a volunteer administered 2 mg NE daily (Ortho-Novum 2 mg). The compounds were chromatographed on a 1.5 meter × 2 mm column of 1% XE-60 at 185°, with He carrier gas flow 30 ml/min. Ions were monitored at 500-msec intervals on the space quadrupole mass spectrometer, with electron energy at 70 eV.

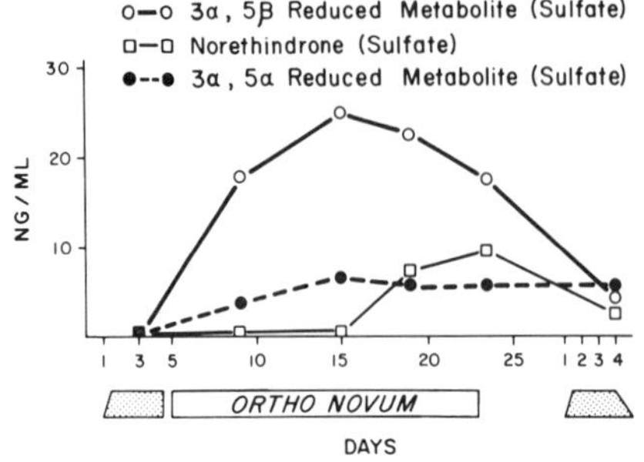

FIG. 11. Blood metabolites of norethindrone in the sulfate fraction before, during, and after a course of Ortho-Novum 2 mg.

as trace metabolites (8,11) in earlier studies. The presence of 5β-NE in blood was demonstrated for the first time by the current study.

During daily administration of 2 mg NE, ring A-reduced metabolites were found mainly in the sulfate fraction, along with some NE, whereas unchanged NE and some 5β-NE were the major compounds in the free fraction. Only traces of NE metabolites were detected in the glucuronide fraction during treatment with normal doses of NE. A representative mass fragmentogram of the plasma A ring-reduced metabolites of the volunteer treated with 2 mg NE is shown in Fig. 10 and is compared with a mass fragmentogram of 1 ng each of the reference compounds. A buildup of metabolites in the sulfate fraction during daily treatment with a normal dose of NE occurred (Fig. 11). This indicates that the sulfate esters of NE and ring A-reduced NE were at least partially responsible for the stepwise increase in plasma radioactivity seen during daily treatment with ^{3}H-NE.

SUMMARY

The MCR of norethindrone and mestranol was studied in 10 female volunteers 20–37 years of age with normal menstrual histories. The volunteers had not taken any oral contraceptive medication for at least 1 year prior to the study. Using the single intravenous injection technique, the MCR of norethindrone was found to be 531 ± 56.8 liters/day and that of mestranol 1,265 ± 139 liters/day. After 6–7 months of oral contraceptive medication, the MCR of mestranol showed no change, whereas the MCR of norethindrone increased significantly (732 ± 125 liters/day; $p < 0.05$). The native drugs disappeared rapidly from the circulation, but their metabolites appeared to persist in the bloodstream.

The radioactivity half-life in various volunteers after administration of a single injection of ^{3}H-norethindrone varied from 42.4 to 83.5 hr, with a mean of 66.9 hr. The half-life of mestranol metabolites varied from 37.4 to 65.4 hr, with a mean of 45.1 hr. Initial experiments with oral administration of ^{3}H-norethindrone and ^{3}H-mestranol indicated that the half-life of blood metabolites were similar to those obtained by injection. The oral administration of ^{3}H-norethindrone for 6 days at 24-hr intervals, in the same manner as oral contraceptives are taken, revealed a "staircase" effect in the buildup of blood radioactivity with no indication of a plateau. On discontinuation of further treatment, the norethindrone metabolites slowly cleared from the bloodstream, with a half-life of approximately 70 hr.

The identity of these metabolites as well as the development of methods by which circulating metabolites of norethindrone could be measured in the blood of users of oral contraceptives, was of considerable interest. Therefore the trimethyl silyl ethers from the free and hydrolyzed sulfate and glucuronide fractions of urine of a volunteer treated with norethindrone were examined using GC-MS with XE-60 and SP-2250 columns and selected ion recording. The presence of all four ring A-reduced metabolites of norethindrone ($3\alpha,5\alpha$; $3\alpha,5\beta$; $3\beta,5\alpha$; $3\beta,5\beta$), norethindrone itself, ethynylestradiol, and a hydroxylated ring A-reduced metabolite was detected. In the blood an additional intermediate (17β-hydroxy-17α-ethynyl-5β-estran-3-one) was also present. The GC-MS method proved sensitive enough to measure circulating metabolites of norethindrone in volunteers taking Ortho-Novum 2 mg, and a buildup of $3\alpha,5\beta$ and $3\alpha,5\alpha$ reduced metabolite of norethindrone was found.

ACKNOWLEDGMENT

This investigation was supported by NIH Contract NO1-HD-2297.

REFERENCES

1. Anonymous (1974): *Br. Med. J.,* 4:430–431.
2. Astedt, B. (1975): *Am. Heart J.,* 90:1–3.
3. Bardin, C. W., and Lipsett, M. B. (1967): *J. Clin. Invest.,* 46:891–902.
4. Bird, C. E., and Clark, C. F. (1973): *J. Clin. Endocrinol. Metab.,* 36:296.
5. Braselton, W. E., Lin, T. J., Mills, T. M., Ellegood, J. O., and Mahesh, V. B. (1977): *J. Steroid Biochem.,* 8: *(in press).*
6. Clezy, T. M., Foy, B. N., Hodge, R. L., and Lumbers, E. R. (1972): *Br. Heart J.,* 34:1238–1243.
7. Engel, L. L., Slaunwhite, W. R., Jr., Carter, P., and Nathanson, I. T. (1950): *J. Biol. Chem.,* 185:255–263.
8. Gerhards, E., Hecker, W., Hitze, H., Nieuweboer, B., and Bellmann, O. (1971): *Acta Endocrinol. (Kbh.),* 68:219.
9. Goldman, J. A. (1975): *Diabetologia,* 11:45–48.
10. Inman, W. H., and Vessey, M. P. (1968): *Br. Med. J.,* 2:193–199.
11. Kamyale, S., Fotherby, K., and Klopper, A. I. (1962): *J. Endocrinol.,* 71:639.
12. Laumas, K. R., Murugesan, K., and Hingorani, V. (1971): *Acta Endocrinol. (Kbh.),* 66:385.
13. Lebech, P. E., and Borggaard, B. (1970): In: *The Menopausal Syndrome,* edited by R. B. Greenblatt, V. B. Mahesh, and P. G. McDonough, pp. 68–74. Medcom Press, New York.
14. Lee, S., and Chen, C. (1971): *Steroids,* 18:565–575.
15. Longcope, C., Layne, D. S., and Tait, J. F. (1968): *J. Clin. Invest.,* 47:93.
16. Mann, J. I., Vessey, M. P., Thorogood, M., and Doll, R. (1975): *Br. Med. J.,* 2:241–245.
17. Mills, T. M., Lin, T. J., Braselton, W. E., Ellegood, J. O., and Mahesh, V. B. (1976): *Am. J. Obstet. Gynecol.,* 126:987–993.
18. Mills, T. M., Lin, T. J., Hernandez-Ayup, S., Greenblatt, R. B., Ellegood, J. O., and Mahesh, V. B. (1974): *Am. J. Obstet. Gynecol.,* 120:764–772.
19. Mills, T. M., Lin, T. J., Hernandez-Ayup, S., Greenblatt, R. B., Ellegood, J. O., and Mahesh, V. B. (1974): *Am. J. Obstet. Gynecol.,* 120:773–778.

20. Rosenfield, R. L. (1971): *J. Clin. Endocrinol. Metab.,* 32:717–728.
21. Southern, A. L., Gordon, G. G., and Tochimoto, S. (1968): *J. Clin. Endocrinol. Metab.,* 28:1105–1112.
22. Southern, A. L., Gordon, G. G., Tochimoto, S., Olivo, J., Sherman, D. H., and Pinzon, G. (1969): *J. Clin. Endocrinol. Metab.,* 29:1356–1363.
23. Spellacy, W. N., Buhi, W. C., Birk, S. A., and Cabal, R. (1973): *Fertil. Steril.,* 24:178–184.
24. Stillwell, W. G., Horning, E. C., Horning, M. G., Stillwell, R. N., and Zlatkis, A. (1972): *J. Steroid Biochem.,* 3:699–706.
25. Stolley, P. D., Tonascia, J. A., Tockman, M. S., Sartwell, P. E., Rutledge, A. H., and Jacobs, M. P. (1975): *Am. J. Epidemiol.,* 102:197–208.
26. Tait, J. F. (1963): *J. Clin. Endocrinol. Metab.,* 23:1285.
27. Vermeulen, A., Verdonck, L., Van der Straeten, M., and Orie, N. (1969): *J. Clin. Endocrinol. Metab.,* 29:1470–1480.
28. Weir, R. J. (1971): *Lancet,* 1:467–470.

Pharmacology of Steroid Contraceptive Drugs
edited by S. Garattini and H. W. Berendes.
Raven Press, New York © 1977.

In Vivo Metabolism of Progestins. II. Metabolic Clearance Rate of Medroxyprogesterone Acetate in Four Species

Chhanda Gupta, Neal A. Musto, Leslie P. Bullock, David Nahrwold, Juraj Osterman, and C. Wayne Bardin

Departments of Medicine, Physiology, Comparative Medicine, and Surgery, The Milton S. Hershey Medical Center, The Pennsylvania State University, Hershey, Pennsylvania 17033

A variety of animals are often used as surrogates for man in toxicity studies to determine long-term metabolic effects of contraceptive steroids. There are, however, relatively few experiments indicating which species are truly appropriate for such studies. In view of these considerations, our laboratory initiated a program to investigate the biological activity of progestins in four species. Since activity is determined in part by the rate of steroid metabolism, we thought it pertinent to determine the metabolic clearance rate (MCR) of commonly used progestins. In the present study, ^{3}H-medroxyprogesterone acetate (^{3}H-MPA) was synthesized and its MCR and volume of distribution (V_o) determined in man, monkey, dog, and rat. In addition, methodological factors such as experimental design and data reduction which were likely to influence the calculated MCR and V_o values were investigated.

SYNTHESIS OF RADIOACTIVE STEROIDS

The methods used for the synthesis of ^{14}C- and ^{3}H-MPA are described elsewhere (7). Briefly, ^{14}C-MPA was synthesized by acetylating 6α-methyl-17α-hydroxy-pregn-4-ene-3,20-dione with 1-^{14}C-acetic anhydride.

In order to synthesize ^{3}H-MPA, 6α-methyl-17-hydroxy-pregn-1,4-diene-3,20-dione acetate was synthesized from MPA. The ^{3}H-MPA was then synthesized by selective catalytic tritiation of the Δ^1-olefinic bond of the diene. ^{3}H-MPA (50–150 μCi) dissolved in 1–5 ml 10% ethanol in saline was administered intravenously to each subject or animal studied.

PATIENTS AND ANIMALS

Sixteen women volunteered for these studies. Since we initially anticipated that MPA would have a slow clearance rate, we chose a protocol similar to that used for studying cortisol metabolism in which eight blood samples were obtained

30–300 min following steroid administration (protocol A). After it was observed that MPA had a much faster MCR rate than cortisol, three additional protocols were tried in succession as follows. Protocol B: 10 blood samples obtained between 7 and 300 min; protocol C: 11 blood samples obtained between 5 and 180 min; and protocol D: 13 blood samples obtained between 3 and 180 min. For reasons discussed below, protocol D was finally selected for routine use in women.

Six rhesus monkeys were trained to sit in metabolic chairs. Following the administration of 100 μCi ^{3}H-MPA, 11 blood samples were obtained between 3 and 240 min.

Seven female mongrel dogs weighing 13–17 kg were trained to stand on a table with support straps under chest and abdomen. Following the administration of 100 μCi ^{3}H-MPA, 15 blood samples were obtained between 3 and 240 min.

Six female rats weighing 200–220 g were studied 2 weeks following gonadectomy. After the intravenous administration of 150 μCi ^{3}H-MPA, 8 blood samples were obtained under transient ether anesthesia between 5 and 720 min.

EXTRACTION AND PURIFICATION OF STEROIDS

The procedure for extraction and purification of ^{3}H-MPA from biological fluids is described elsewhere (7). Briefly, plasma or blood samples containing ^{3}H-MPA were extracted with 7 volumes of petroleum ether after addition of ^{14}C-MPA. Extracts were spotted on thin-layer plates and developed in methylene chloride/ether (80 : 20). The MPA was eluted, dried, and reacted with pyridine and acetic anhydride, and then rechromatographed in the same system. The samples were eluted into counting vials, and radioactivity was measured in a liquid scintillation spectrometer.

CALCULATION OF MCR AND V_0

Mathematical procedures for calculation of parameters representing whole-body hormone distribution and metabolism from tracer data are described elsewhere (2). In the present study a digital computer-implemented nonlinear regression analysis was employed. The computer program determined a "least square best fit" multiexponential function (1–4 terms, i.e., up to 4 pairs of real valued coefficients and exponents) by successive approximation using the Marquardt algorithm.

$$r(t) = \sum_i A_i e^{-b_i t}$$

The data were entered as fraction of dose/volume and weighted to reflect estimated constant relative error. The estimated MCR and V_0 were subsequently determined from the best multiexponential function by the standard formulas:

$$MCR = \frac{1}{\sum_i A_i / b_i}$$

$$V_0 = \frac{1}{\sum\limits_{i} A_i}$$

The algorithm and computer code have been validated by analytical test problems and have proved consistently superior to the commonly employed "peel-off" techniques (1). Four criteria were used to choose the number of exponential terms in a particular experiment: (a) random distribution of residual sign; (b) residual amplitude within estimated methodological error; (c) significant reduction in sum of squared residuals (with respect to optimum fit with one less term); (d) time of first sample, time of last sample, and estimated methodological error appropriate for computed optimum parameter values (7).

The computed MCR and V_0 values were expressed as "liters of plasma per day per kilogram body weight" and "liters of plasma," respectively.

EFFECT OF EXPERIMENTAL DESIGN ON MCR AND V_0

Several experimental protocols were evaluated for estimating MCR and V_0 in women. Initially protocol A (eight samples obtained between 30 and 300 min) was selected since MPA was thought to have a slow clearance rate. When a rapid rate of metabolism was observed, three other protocols were tested (protocols B, C, and D). Not only did these protocols shorten the time of study, they also increased the number of blood samples obtained during the first 20 min. The MCR and V_0 values determined in each of these protocols are summarized in Table 1. The V_0 and MCR were overestimated when only a few plasma samples were obtained. In addition, the results emphasize the importance of the early time points in estimating the V_0, a fact discussed previously by Bogumil (1). By contrast, the estimated MCRs were not as dependent on the early time points.

EFFECT OF NUMBER OF EXPONENTIAL TERMS ON MCR AND V_0

In a preliminary study on seven dogs, the disappearance of radioactivity as MPA was described by a function which was the sum of two exponentials in three

TABLE 1. *Effect of sample number and time on the MCR and V_0 of MPA in women*

Protocol	No. of blood samples per study	Time of sample (min)	No. of studies	MCR (liters/day/kg)	V_0 (liters)
A	8	30–300[a]	3	25–36[b]	9–746[b]
B	10	7–300	3	21–54	76–273
C	11	5–180	3	29–35	62–83
D	13	3–180	7	16–29	3–30

[a] Time after administration of ^{3}H-steroid. All samples were obtained between the times shown.
[b] Range.

TABLE 2. *Effect of the number of exponential terms on the MCR and V_o of MPA in women*

	Two exponentials		Three exponentials	
Study	MCR (liters/day/kg)	V_o (liters)	MCR (liters/day/kg)	V_o (liters)
1	22	18	20	10
2	28	20	25	9
3	15	30	16	30

dogs and the sum of three exponentials in four dogs (7). The V_o was 27 ± 13 (SD). The large variance of this estimate was due to the fact that the V_o tended to be higher in those dogs whose disappearance curves were described by two exponential terms. These studies confirmed previous observations that the V_o may be reduced significantly by increasing the number of exponential terms used for its calculation (1). In a given experiment, however, the number of terms which can be used are in part determined by biological variability. If the experimentally determined plasma steroid concentrations differ from the computer-calculated disappearance curve by as little as 2%, the number of identifiable exponentials which describe the curve may be reduced.

Variations in the estimated V_o which relate to the number of exponential terms have also been observed in women. The results from three experiments are shown in Table 2. In these studies the disappearance of radioactive MPA could be described by a function which was the sum of two or three exponentials. In studies 1 and 2 (Table 2), when two exponentials were used, the V_o values were significantly higher; whereas in study 3 (Table 2), the V_o was the same regardless of the number of exponential terms used. Interestingly, the MCRs were similar regardless of the number of terms. We conclude from these studies and those cited above that V_o is the parameter most sensitive to changes in experimental design and error. By contrast, the MCR is less affected by these errors. Therefore in comparative studies of steroid kinetics, the experimental design should be optimized to determine the MCR since this parameter may be more accurately estimated if the number of samples is limited by the size of the animal.

COMPARATIVE METABOLISM OF MPA

The MCR and V_o values of MPA in man, monkey, dog, and rat are summarized in Table 3. The MCR of this steroid in man (21 ± 2 liters/kg/day; mean $\pm$ SEM) and monkey (26 ± 3 liters/kg/day) were similar to the progesterone MCRs of 30 and 19 liters/kg/day reported for man and monkey, respectively (3–5,8). By contrast, the MCR of MPA in the dog (45 ± 2 liters/kg/day) and rat (29 ± 3 liters/kg/day) were one-half to one-third those for progesterone (6,7). The results of this study suggest that a distinctive feature of the comparative metabolism of MPA is its clearance relative to that of progesterone. It is of additional interest

TABLE 3. *MCR and V_o of MPA in different species*

Species	No. studied	MCR (liters/day/kg)	V_o (liters)
Man	7	21 ± 2[a]	20 ± 3[a]
Monkey	6	26 ± 3[a]	9 ± 1[a]
Dog	7	45 ± 2[b]	27 ± 5[b]
Rat	6	29 ± 3[a]	0.37 ± 0.05[a]

[a] Mean $\pm$ SEM of values calculated from disappearance curves which were the sums of two exponentials.

[b] Mean $\pm$ SEM of values calculated from disappearance curves which were the sums of two or three exponentials.

that the MCR of MPA of man, monkey, and rat are remarkably similar when corrected for body size, and that only the clearance rate in dogs appears to be higher.

SUMMARY

A technique for determining the comparative metabolism of progestins has been evaluated. The large variance of the estimated volume of distribution relates in part to the number of samples obtained during the early part of the disappearance curve, and in part to the number of exponentials used in the calculation. These considerations emphasize the difficulty inherent in measuring the volume of distribution of compounds that are rapidly metabolized. As a consequence, an accurate between-species comparison of this metabolic parameter may be difficult to obtain by the technique employed in the present study.

The metabolic clearance rate is a kinetic parameter that is less subject to the errors which effect the volume of distribution. In addition, only a minor overestimation of this metabolic parameter occurs when the number of blood samples is limited by the size of the animal.

The metabolic clearance rates and volumes of distribution of medroxyprogesterone acetate were estimated in man, monkey, dog, and rat. The between-species variations in the clearance rate of this steroid appears to be less than that of progesterone.

ACKNOWLEDGMENTS

This study was supported by NIH Contract No. NO1-HD-2–2730.

REFERENCES

1. Bogumil, R. J. (1975): In: *Tracer Methods in Hormone Research,* edited by E. Gurpide, p. 140. Springer-Verlag, New York.
2. Gurpide, E., editor (1975): *Tracer Methods in Hormone Research.* Springer-Verlag, New York.

3. Lin, T. J., Billiar, R. B., and Little, B. (1972): *J. Clin. Endocrinol. Metab.,* 35:879–886.
4. Lin, T. J., Lin, S. C., Erlenmeyer, F., Kline, I. T., Underwood, R., Billiar, R. B., and Little, B. (1972): *J. Clin. Endocrinol.,* 34:287–297.
5. Little, B., Tait, J. F., Tait, S. A. S., and Erlenmeyer, F. (1966): *J. Clin. Invest.,* 45:901–912.
6. Pepe, G. J., and Rothchild, I. (1973): *Endocrinology,* 93:1200–1205.
7. Runic, S., Miljkovic, M., Bogumil, R. J., Nahrwold, D., and Bardin, C. W. (1976): *Endocrinology* 99:108–113.
8. Sholl, S. A., and Wolf, R. C. (1974): *Endocrinology,* 95:1287–1292.

Pharmacology of Steroid Contraceptive Drugs
edited by S. Garattini and H. W. Berendes.
Raven Press, New York © 1977.

Studies with *d*-Norgestrel-^{3}H in Lactating Women

**W. Mützel and S. El Mahgoub*

Research Laboratories of Schering AG, Berlin/Bergkamen, FGR; and the Department of Gynecology, Ain Shams University, Cairo, United Arabic Republic

Control of conception that is as effective as possible is particularly desirable for mothers during the first year postpartum. Oral contraceptives have properties which recommend their use in principle during this period of a woman's life. However, the use of steroidal contraceptive preparations may result in side effects in the lactating woman and the breast-fed infant, whose development may thus be impaired.

One such side effect is connected with passage of the administered steroid and its metabolites via breast milk. Since the naturally occurring steroid hormones in breast milk can induce or aggravate hyperbilirubinemia and jaundice of the newborn (3), concurrent administration of synthetic steroid hormones cannot be excluded from producing these side effects also. For an assessment of the situation it is necessary to know what quantities may ultimately be transferred to the infant in addition to the natural steroid hormones.

The pathogenesis of jaundice of the newborn is caused by the relative inadequacy of the as-yet immature liver of the infant to conjugate sufficiently endogenous or exogenous substrates (4). Hence comes the hypothesis that the preparation which affords the mother effective contraception and contains the smallest quantity of steroid hormones is the one which involves the least risk for the infant. Today Microlut, a product of Schering AG, is available for monohormonal contraception. It contains 30 μg *d*-norgestrel (13β-ethyl-18,19-dinor-17α-pregn-4-en-20-yn-3-one) (Fig. 1), which is an unusually small quantity of active ingredient.

EXPERIMENTAL

The principal focus in our studies was on the passage of this progestagen and its metabolites into breast milk. For this purpose, 14,15-^{3}H-labeled *d*-norgestrel was administered in accordance with the schedule shown in Fig. 2. Each of two mothers was given 30 μg ^{3}H-labeled *d*-norgestrel on the 3rd day postpartum, and

---

* Address for correspondence: Dr. W. Mützel, Schering AG, Department of Biodynamics, P.O. Box 65 03 11, D-1000 Berlin 65, Germany.

d-Norgestrel
(13-ethyl-17-hydroxy-18,19-dinor-17α-pregn-4-en-20-yn-3-one)

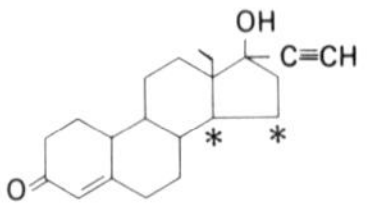

FIG. 1. Structural formula of *d*-norgestrel.

each of two mothers 30 μg ^{3}H-norgestrel on the 7th, 11th, and 15th days postpartum. On the intervening days each mother was given 30 μg nonlabeled *d*-norgestrel in the Microlut formulation.

Several times a day the mother's milk was quantitatively drawn off using a breast pump so the babies had to be fed prepared food. In addition, blood was withdrawn from the women for plasma analysis, and their urine was collected quantitatively.

The time of administration was specially chosen in order to obtain information on the effect of the milk's composition on the content of *d*-norgestrel and its metabolites. As is well known (5), the composition of colostrum with its low fat and high protein content is just as adapted to the development of the infant's enzyme systems as the transitory milk and the mature milk, in which there is a distinct increase in fat content.

	1	2	3	4	5	6	7	8	9	10	11	12	13	14	15	16	17
Subject I			●														
Subject II			●														
Subject III							●	○	○	○	●	○	○	○	●		
Subject IV							●	○	○	○	●	○	○	○	●		
Time (day post partum)	1	2	3	4	5	6	7	8	9	10	11	12	13	14	15	16	17

Type of milk	Colostrum	Transitorian milk	Ripe milk
Mean consistence:			
Fat (g/l)	29,0	35,2	45,4
Carbohydrate (g/l)	57,0	64,0	68,0
Mineral (mval/l)			
electropositive elements	68,0	55,0	41,0
electronegative elements	40,0	37,0	28,0
Protein	22,9	15,9	10,6
Rest nitrogen	910,0	479,0	324,0

● 30 μg ^{3}H-d-norgestrel
○ 30 μg d-norgestrel

FIG. 2. Scheme of application of *d*-norgestrel.

RESULTS AND DISCUSSION

Plasma *d*-norgestrel levels were measured in two young nulliparous women after administration of the same ³H-steroid preparation as was given to the lactating women (Fig. 3). The determinations were carried out with the aid of a *d*-norgestrel-specific radioimmunoassay (2). Following extremely quick absorption, 2 hr after ingestion the concentration of *d*-norgestrel and metabolites in total plasma was 2,100 ng *d*-norgestrel equivalents. Approximately 75% of this value was accounted for by unchanged *d*-norgestrel. At 6 hr after administration the ratio of *d*-norgestrel to its metabolites was 1 : 1. During the period 1–10 hr after administration, the plasma half-life for *d*-norgestrel was approximately 4–5 hr.

Figure 4 shows the plasma levels of *d*-norgestrel and nonconjugated steroids 2 hr after oral administration of *d*-norgestrel to lactating women. The plasma steroids were characterized by thin-layer chromatographic comparison with reference substances.

On the 3rd day postpartum the concentrations of roughly 6,000 ng *d*-norgestrel equivalents (corresponding to 20% of the dose in total plasma volume) were approximately three times as high as for the already mentioned nonlactating women. On the 15th day postpartum the plasma levels reached only half these values. This observation is explained by a considerable increase in the plasma protein transport capacity for steroids during the immediate postpartum period. The biological half-life of binding plasma proteins is approximately 2 weeks. In addition to *d*-norgestrel, which in each case accounted for more than half of the

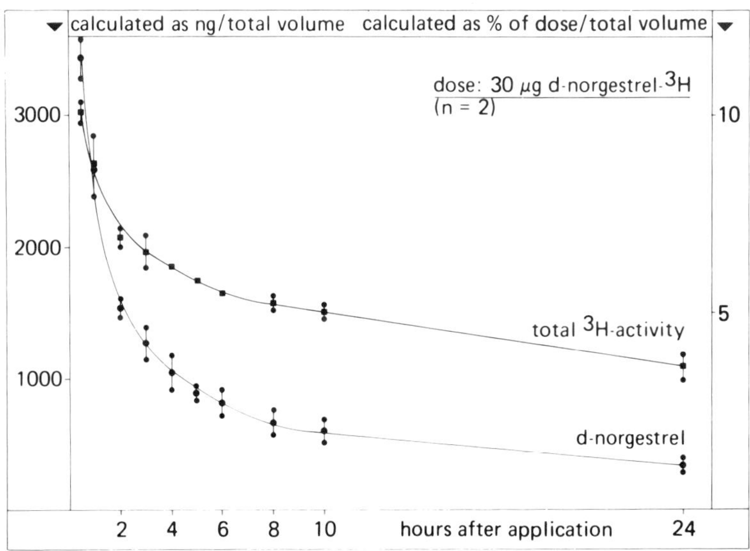

FIG. 3. Plasma levels of *d*-norgestrel and total ³H activity in normal women. (From Hümpel, ref. 2.)

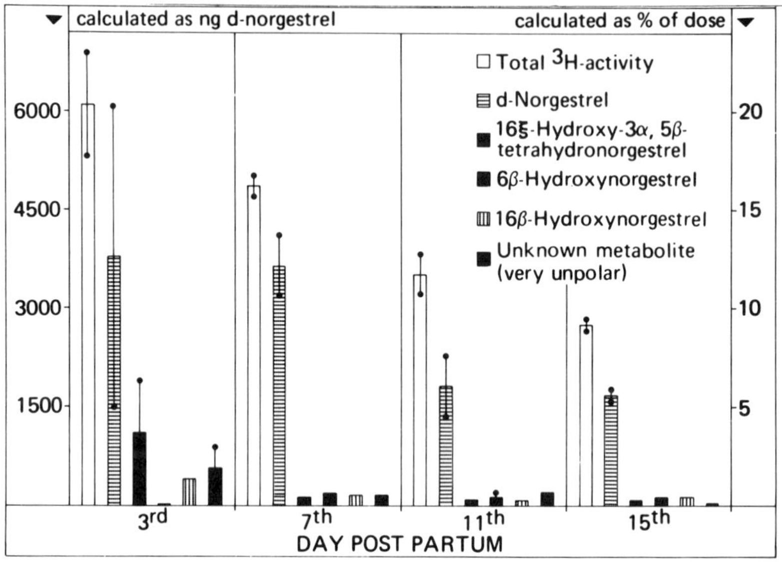

FIG. 4. Plasma levels of *d*-norgestrel-^{3}H and radioactive metabolites in lactating women. (For systematic name of steroids see text.)

total ^{3}H-steroids 2 hr after administration, 16-hydroxy-3α,5β-tetrahydronorgestrel[1]), 6β-hydroxynorgestrel, and 16β-hydroxynorgestrel, as well as a nonpolar metabolite, could be identified.

Figure 5 shows cumulative excretion of ^{3}H-steroids with total milk. The extent of excretion was extremely slight: Each day approximately 1% of the dose corresponding to 30 ng *d*-norgestrel equivalents was excreted with colostrum. In transitory milk and mature milk only 0.5% of the dose, respectively, was detected each day. For qualitative and quantitative detection of nonconjugated steroids, the milk was extracted and fractionated in accordance with the scheme shown in Fig. 6.

After adding 100-μg portions of nonlabeled *d*-norgestrel, the milk was frozen at −18°C for separation of fat and lipoproteins. The defatted milk was extracted with ether and the extract analyzed by thin-layer chromatography. The dominant fraction in the milk is that of unchanged *d*-norgestrel, which is in complete agreement with the metabolic pattern in plasma (Fig. 7). Accordingly, the quantity of progestagen transferred with breast milk to an infant in 1 day after

---

[1] In accordance with IUPAC nomenclature for steroids, the following systematic names are given to the compounds referred to in this chapter: *Norgestrel:* 13-ethyl-17-hydroxy-18,19-dinor-17α-pregn-4-en-20-yn-3-one. *16-Hydroxy-3α,5β-tetrahydronorgestrel:* 13-ethyl-18,19-dinor-5β,17α-pregn-20-yn-3α,16ξ,17-triol. *6β-Hydroxynorgestrel:* 13-ethyl-6β,17-dihydroxy-18,19-dinor-17α-pregn-4-en-20-yn-3-one. *16β-Hydroxynorgestrel:* 13-ethyl-16β,17-dihydroxy-18,19-dinor-17α-pregn-4-en-20-yn-3-one. *d-Homogonen:* 13-ethyl-*d*-homogon-4-en-3,17α-dione. *3α,5β-Tetrahydronorgestrel:* 13-ethyl-18,19-dinor-5β,17α-pregn-20-yne-3α,17-diol. *3β,5β-Tetrahydronorgestrel:* 13-ethyl-18,19-dinor-5β,17α-pregn-20-yne-3β,17-diol.

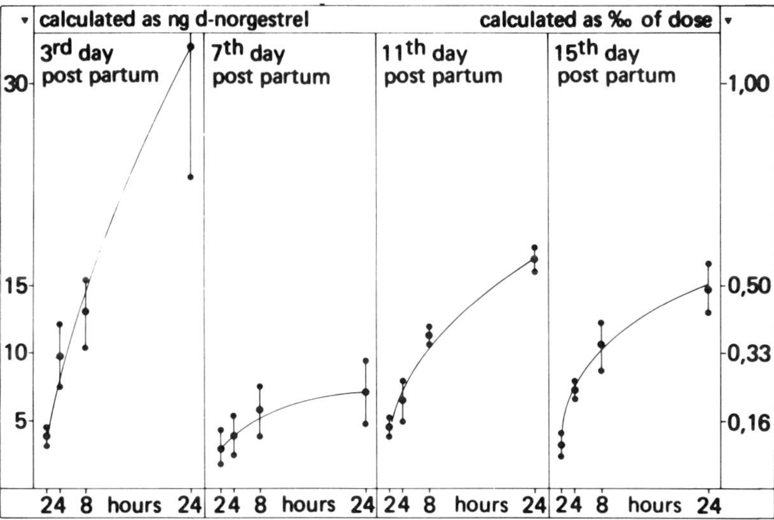

FIG. 5. Accumulative excretion of *d*-norgestrel-³H and radioactive metabolites with maternal milk.

medication with 30 μg *d*-norgestrel does not exceed 10 ng. In addition to *d*-norgestrel, very small quantities (roughly in the range of the limit of detection of 1 ng) of 16-hydroxy-3α,5β-tetrahydronorgestrel, 6β-hydroxynorgestrel, 16β-hydroxynorgestrel, and a very lipophilic metabolite were identified.

To illustrate the ratios of concentration of *d*-norgestrel and its metabolites in plasma and milk 2 hr after administration, the corresponding quotients were calculated (Fig. 8). Accordingly, the steroid concentrations present in colostrum

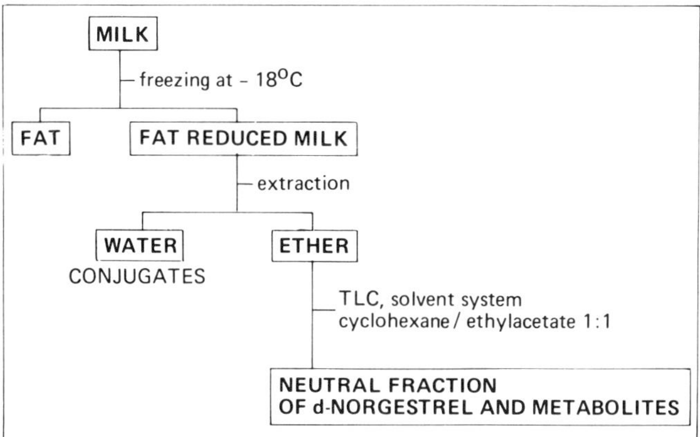

FIG. 6. Procedures employed for the extraction and fractionation of metabolites in milk after application of *d*-norgestrel-³H.

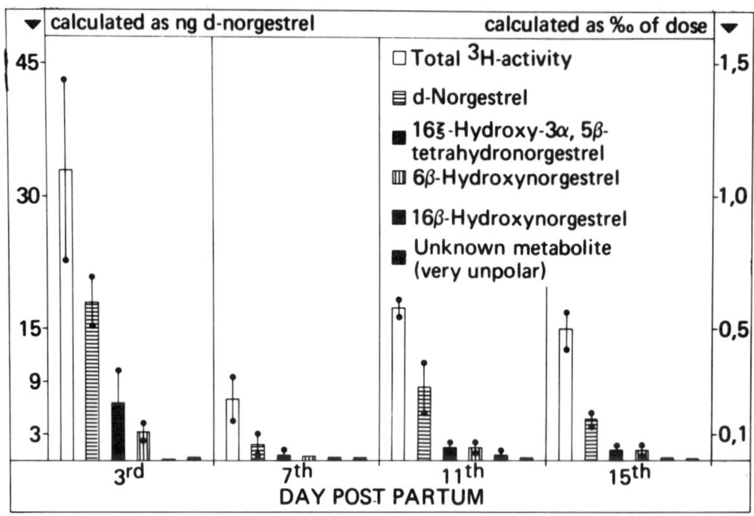

FIG. 7. Excretion of *d*-norgestrel-³H and radioactive metabolites with maternal milk within 24 hr after oral application of 30 μg *d*-norgestrel-³H.

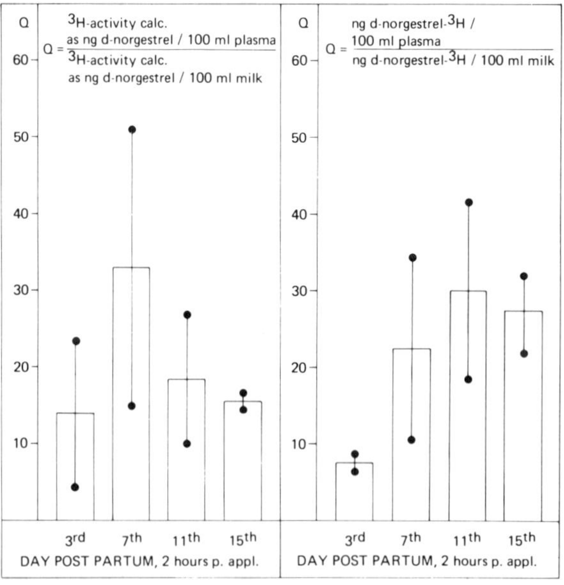

FIG. 8. Quotients of total radioactivity in plasma and milk *(left)* and *d*-norgestrel-³H in plasma and milk *(right)*, respectively, after oral application of 30 μg *d*-norgestrel-³H.

were roughly 15 times less than those in plasma at the same time. Calculated for *d*-norgestrel, the concentrations were 5–10 times less. Thus at the very high plasma concentration of *d*-norgestrel—with which there is presumably a causal association—somewhat larger quantities of steroids were excreted with colostrum than subsequently with transitory and mature milk. Two hours after administration, plasma concentrations of *d*-norgestrel were roughly 30 times as high as in mature milk obtained at the same time. The fact that more than 90% of *d*-norgestrel is bound to plasma proteins is regarded as a reason for this observation.

A synopsis of the formulas of the *d*-norgestrel metabolites we identified in lactating women and their occurrence in plasma, milk, and urine are shown in Fig. 9. It is important to note that the metabolites detected in free or conjugated form in plasma and milk were also found in urine. The plasma and urinary metabolite patterns we obtained are in accord with the results of Sisenwine et al. (6,7).

Formula	Plasma Free	Milk Free	Urine Free	Urine Gluc.	Urine Sulf.
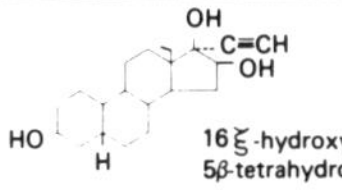 16ξ-hydroxy-3α, 5β-tetrahydronorgestrel	●	●	●	●	●
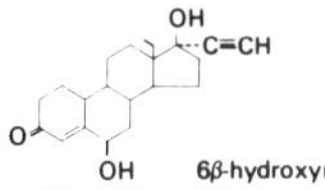 6β-hydroxynorgestrel	●	●	●	—	●
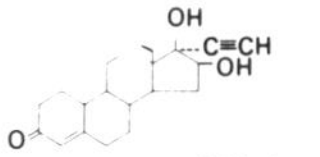 16β-hydroxynorgestrel	●	●	●	●	●
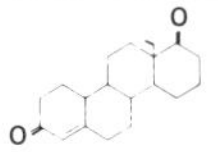 D-homo-gonen	—	—	●	—	●
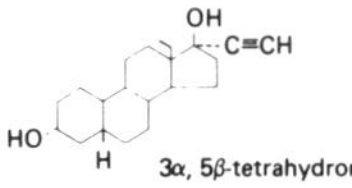 3α, 5β-tetrahydronorgestrel	—	—	●	●	●
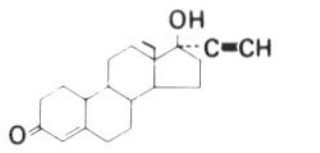 d-norgestrel	●	●	●	—	●
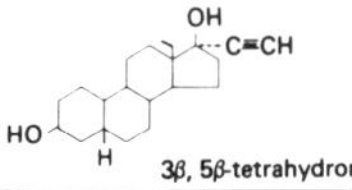 3β, 5β-tetrahydronorgestrel	—	—	●	—	●

FIG. 9. Occurrence of *d*-norgestrel-³H and radioactive metabolites in lactating women. (For systematic name of steroids see footnote 1 in text.)

CONCLUSIONS

The extent of excretion of *d*-norgestrel and metabolites with breast milk was dependent on the time postpartum when the contraceptive was taken. In this, the plasma protein transport capacity for steroids on the one hand, and on the other hand the fat content and the remaining composition of the breast milk, presumably played a part.

Unchanged *d*-norgestrel dominates quantitatively in plasma and milk compared with its metabolites, which incidentally can also be expected to appear in urine.

As a result of daily administration of 30 μg *d*-norgestrel to nursing mothers, approximately 10–20 ng *d*-norgestrel and metabolites might be absorbed daily by the infant from breast milk. These quantities of the steroids are approximately 100,000 times smaller than those which could be transferred to the infant in the form of natural steroids (e.g., pregnanediol), as described by Arias et al. (1). Therefore when an oral contraceptive such as Microlut is administered to nursing mothers, loading of the infant's glucuronyl transferase system (which is significant for the pathogenesis of jaundice of the newborn) can be regarded as negligible.

ACKNOWLEDGMENTS

We are grateful to Dr. I. Ekdawi for his prudence and help in obtaining and supplying samples. Our thanks are also due to Mrs. W. Milius for her skilled technical assistance.

REFERENCES

1. Arias, I. M., Gartner, L. M., Seifter, S., and Furman, M. (1964): Prolonged neonatal unconjugated hyperbilirubinemia associated with breast feeding and a steroid, pregnane3(alpha),20(beta)-diol, in maternal milk that inhibits glucuronide formation in vitro. *J. Clin Invest.,* 43:2037–2047.
2. Hümpel, M.: Research Laboratories of Schering AG, Berlin. Personal communication.
3. Lauritzen, Ch., and Lehmann, W-D. (1965): Die Bedeutung der Steroidhormone für Hyperbilirubinämie und Icterus neonatorum. *Geburtshilfe Frauenheilkd.,* 25:962–973.
4. Lucy, J. F., and Villee, C. A. (1962): Human fetal hepatic glucuronyl transferase activity. Proceedings of the Tenth International Congress of Pediatrics, Lisbon.
5. Macy, I. G. (1949): *Am. J. Dis. Child.,* 78:589. See also in: *Wissenschaftliche Tabellen,* edited by K. Diem and C. Lentner. Georg Thieme Verlag, Stuttgart, 1975.
6. Sisenwine, S. F., Kimmel, H. B., Liu, A. L., and Ruelius, H. W. (1973): Urinary metabolites of dl-norgestrel in women. *Acta Endocrinol. (Kbh.),* 73:91–104.
7. Sisenwine, S. F., Kimmel, H. B., Liu, A. L., and Ruelius, H. W. (1975): Excretion and stereoselective biotransformations of dl-, d- and l-norgestrel in women. *Drug Metab. Dispos.,* 3:180–188.

Pharmacology of Steroid Contraceptive Drugs
edited by S. Garattini and H. W. Berendes.
Raven Press, New York © 1977.

Plasma Hormone Profiles and Pathological Observations in Medroxyprogesterone Acetate-Treated Beagle Bitches

William Hansel, P. W. Concannon, and K. McEntee

Department of Animal Science, Cornell University, Ithaca, New York 14853

Until now, statements questioning the use of the bitch in studies evaluating the carcinogenic potency of contraceptive drugs have been unconvincing because of lack of basic information on hormonal control of reproductive processes in this species. Recent studies carried out in our laboratories (5) and others (15,16) have partially filled this gap in our knowledge. These studies emphasized that the basic hormonal mechanisms controlling estrus, ovulation, fertilization, pregnancy, and parturition in the bitch are not greatly different from those found in other species.

Hormonal and behavioral events occurring at the time of estrus and ovulation in the bitch are summarized in Fig. 1. As in other species studied, a rapid rise in plasma estrogen precedes the plasma LH peak that causes ovulation. Progesterone rises during proestrus and reaches quite high concentrations during the onset of estrus and well before ovulation. These changes in plasma progesterone reflect the early infolding and granulosa cell luteinization seen in preovulatory canine follicles (8). It has been shown in other studies that this early rise in progesterone plays an essential role in the behavioral manifestation of estrus in the bitch (4).

Figure 2 shows plasma estrogen and progesterone concentrations—corrected for the hemodilution resulting from the characteristic pregnancy anemia found in the bitch—in pregnant and nonpregnant animals during a 70-day period following ovulation. Plasma progesterone peaks at 20–25 days at concentrations of 30–35 ng/ml in both pregnant and nonpregnant bitches. Thereafter, progesterone is higher in the pregnant than in the nonpregnant bitch until a few days before parturition, at which time a rapid decline occurs. Plasma estrogen concentrations during this period are higher in pregnant than in nonpregnant bitches and, like progesterone concentrations, decline rapidly at the time of parturition. Plasma progesterone concentrations decline at quite variable rates after day 25 in nonpregnant bitches; on the average they remain above 1 ng/ml for 84 days (range 60–105) and reach a nadir at approximately day 145.

A high incidence of mammary tumors has been demonstrated in previous studies with bitches receiving progestin doses many times higher than those recommended for human contraception (1,9,14). Therefore we carried out an

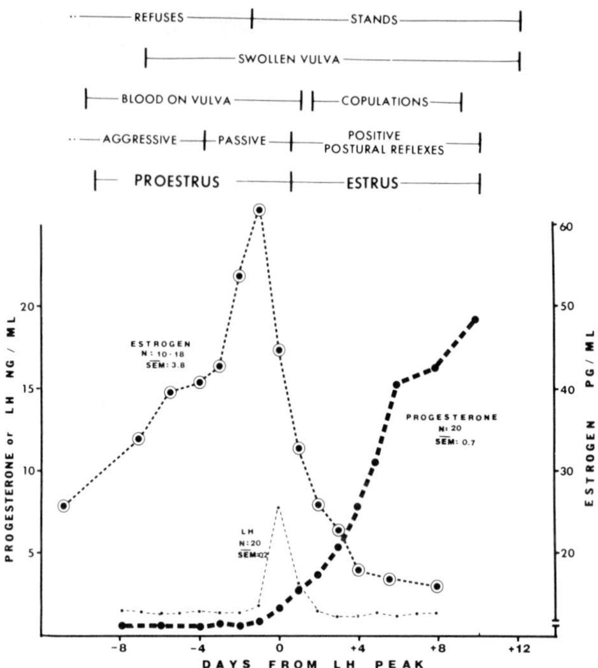

FIG. 1. Mean plasma levels of estrogen, LH, and progesterone during proestrus and estrus in beagle bitches. The vertical bars represent the mean time of onset and termination of the parameter indicated. (From Concannon et al., ref. 5.)

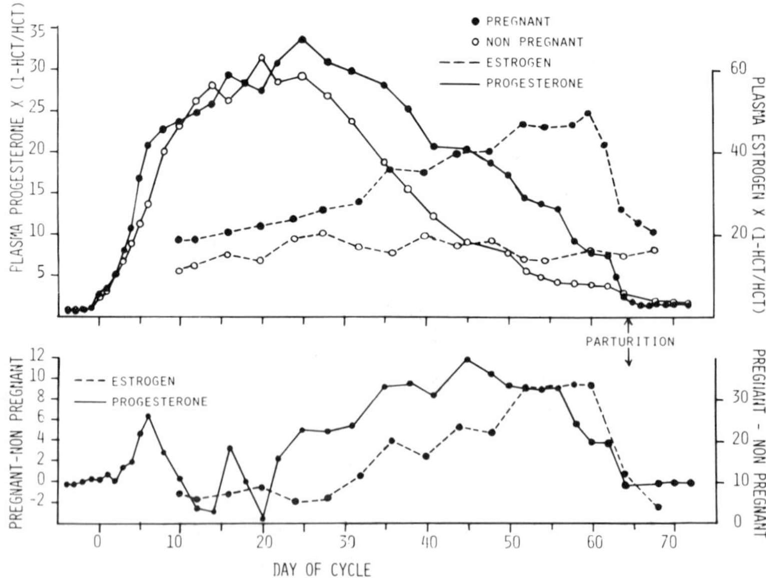

FIG. 2. Mean plasma levels of progesterone and estrogen during the luteal phases of pregnant and nonpregnant beagle bitches. Values were corrected for hemodilution resulting from pregnancy anemia **(top)**. Pregnancy-specific differences were obtained by subtraction **(bottom)**.

experiment designed to determine the effects of chronic administration of moderate doses of medroxyprogesterone acetate (MPA) on plasma hormone concentrations as related to the incidence of mammary gland tumors.

EXPERIMENTAL PROCEDURE

Treatment

As outlined in Table 1, 48 adult cycling beagle bitches were placed in four experimental groups of 12 animals each. Animals were randomized as to genetic background, stage of cycle at initiation of treatment, and body weight. In accomplishing this distribution of animals, the factor of age was compromised to a slight degree; the mean age of the control animals was slightly greater than that of the treated animals (Table 2). This age distribution, if anything, would tend to increase the incidence of mammary tumors in the control animals, since these tumors are claimed to occur spontaneously in older bitches (1,9,14).

Group A bitches were injected with 500 μl of the vehicle used to inject MPA (Depo-Provera). Group B bitches received subcutaneous implants of 3.3 $\times$ 4.6 mm Silastic tubing (Dow Corning No. 601–331) containing crystalline progesterone. The initial dose was 150 mg/kg body weight for each bitch. Six bitches in a subgroup preselected for necropsy at 20 months of study were reimplanted at 14 and again at 18 months with a dose of 60 mg/kg. MPA-treated bitches were injected intramuscularly every 90 days for 16 months at doses of 2 mg/kg (group C) or 10 mg/kg (group D). Six bitches in each of these groups were selected for necropsy at 20 months of study. These bitches received final injections of MPA at 18 months, whereas the remaining bitches received their last injection at 15 months. The 90-day MPA injection schedule is the same as that recommended for contraception in women. The doses selected (2 and 10 mg/kg) bracket the recommended human dose of 3 mg/kg and are well below the doses (30 and 75 mg/kg) recommended for toxicity studies in dogs by the US Food and Drug Administration (1).

Parameters studied during the first 18 months of hormone administration included gain in body weight, mammary gland growth, histopathology and

TABLE 1. *Experimental design*

Group treatment	No.	Study 1 subgroups: necropsy at 20 months (No.)		Study 2 subgroups: withdrawal after 15 months (No.)	
A Vehicle-injected controls	12	A-1	(6)	A-2	(6)
B Progesterone implants	12	B-1	(6)	B-2	(6)
C MPA (2 mg/kg/90 days)	12	C-1	(6)	C-2	(5)[a]
D MPA (10 mg/kg/90 days)	12	D-1	(6)	D-2	(5)[a]

[a] One bitch in the group died during treatment.

TABLE 2. *Data on beagle bitches chronically treated with progesterone or MPA*

Measurement	Group A Controls vehicle-injected	Group B Progesterone implants	Group C MPA 2 mg/kg/90 days	Group D MPA 10 mg/kg/90 days
Total bitches studied	12	12	12	12
Mean initial body weight (kg)	11.3 ± 0.7	10.7 ± 0.6	11.1 ± 0.9	10.4 ± 0.7
Mean body weight at 70 weeks (kg)	12.0 ± 0.8	12.2 ± 0.9	11.9 ± 0.8	12.9 ± 0.9
Initial age (mo) of all bitches	47 ± 7	35 ± 5	37 ± 5	32 ± 6
Initial age of bitches later developing mammary nodules	—	—	50	47 ± 8
No. of bitches cycling by				
13 months	12	0	0	0
14 months	12	1	0	0
20 months	12	0/6, 5/6[a]	0	0
Total cycles by 20 mo	36	5	0	0
Cycles with proestrous/estrous signs	33	4	—	—
No. of bitches with persistent mammary nodules by				
7 months	0	0	0	1
11 months	0	0	0	4
15 months	0	0	1	6
Total nodules palpated by 15 months	0	0	1	9
Nodules studied histologically	—	—	—	4
Nodules diagnosed as mixed mammary tumors	—	—	—	4

[a] These six bitches were not reimplanted with progesterone at 14 months.

nodule development, and circulating levels of the drug and of progesterone and luteinizing hormone (LH). External signs of proestrus and estrus, and occurrence of metestrus progesterone profiles, were used to monitor ovarian cyclicity.

Animals

Ages and weights of the beagles used are listed in Table 2. All animals were maintained indoors in individual cages, fed a standard ration at 1000 hr daily, and individually handled and observed for signs of proestrus three times a week. When proestrus was observed, bitches were checked daily for standing estrus with a male. Plasma samples were collected between 0800 and 1000 hr biweekly or more frequently from each bitch by cephalic or jugular venipuncture. Mammary glands were palpated at 3- to 4-month intervals to determine general glandular development and the presence of nodules. Subjective estimations of size and turgescence were made and animals scored on a scale of 1–5. At 0, 120, 240, and 380 days of treatment mammary tissue was surgically excised for biopsy from one of the four most caudal glands of each bitch.

Hormone Assays

Plasma MPA was radioimmunoassayed according to the procedure of Cornette et al. (6), the only modification being the use of dextran-coated charcoal to separate free from bound hormone. Plasma LH was radioimmunoassayed by the method of Boyns et al. (2), as modified by Concannon et al. (5). Plasma progesterone was radioimmunoassayed using a specific antiserum (7) to progesterone. Progesterone assays sensitive to concentrations as low as 200 pg/ml were conducted on petroleum ether extracts, prepared as previously described (5), of samples collected from control dogs during anestrus and of selected samples from treated bitches (Fig. 6, below). Values reported were not corrected for the 200–300 pg/ml estimated for ovariectomized plasma. Less-sensitive progesterone assays, measuring concentrations from 1.5 to 40 ng/ml, were conducted on 10- to 20-μl aliquots of unextracted plasma, and these values were used to determine the presence of concentrations characteristic of metestrus (Figs. 3 and 4). All hormone assays utilized had within- and between-assay coefficients of variation of less than 11%, based on triplicate or quadruplicate determinations of all samples and on two or three pools of plasma measured in each assay.

Necropsies

Six bitches from each group were preselected for necropsy in such a manner that the entire range of ages, body weights, mammary gland hypertrophy, and incidence of nodules for each treatment group were represented. During the 20th month of study each of these bitches was submitted to a complete postmortem examination immediately following administration of an anesthetic dose of Suri-

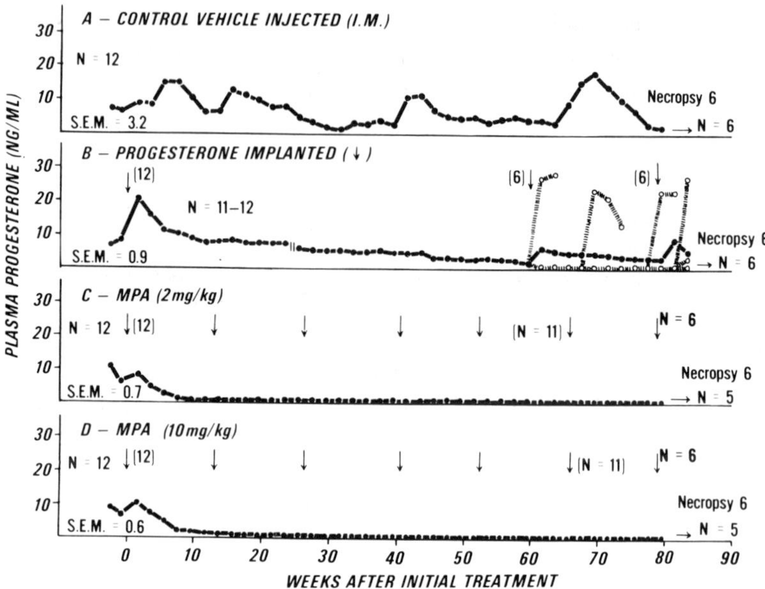

FIG. 3. Mean plasma progesterone in beagle bitches during chronic administration of progesterone and MPA.

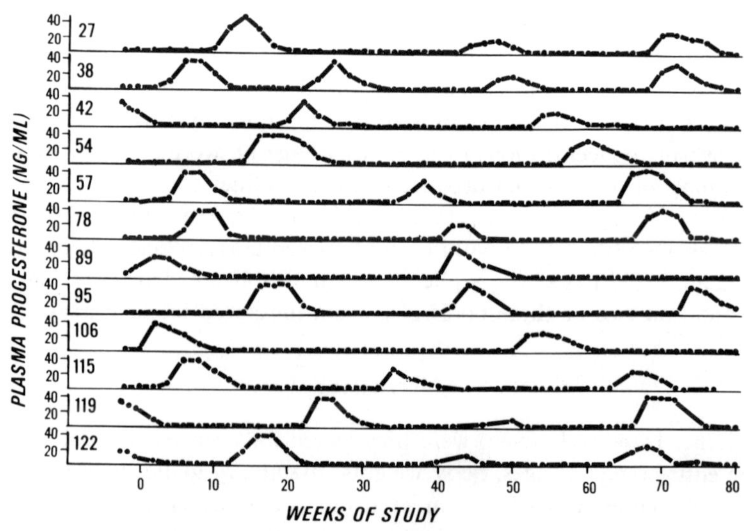

FIG. 4. Plasma progesterone for 12 untreated beagle bitches during 80 weeks of study.

tal and carotid exsanguination. One bitch in group C died as a result of overanesthesia during a scheduled collection of mammary tissue for biopsy. One bitch in group D died after 15 months of treatment (see below). The remaining control and treated bitches were not reinjected after 15 months and are currently being monitored for return of estrus.

RESULTS

Ovarian Cycles

Throughout the 20 months of study, MPA, at both doses used, effectively prevented the recurrence of proestrus and estrus (Table 2). Furthermore, the absence of progesterone levels characteristic of metestrus indicates that ovulation did not occur in any of the treated animals (Fig. 3). In contrast, during the same period of study each of the 12 control bitches showed signs of proestrus and estrus (Table 2), and each had two to four distinct metestrus progesterone profiles (Fig. 4). External morphological and behavioral signs of proestrus and estrus were exhibited for 33 of the 36 cycles diagnosed by the progesterone assays in the control bitches (Table 2). None of the bitches implanted with progesterone cycled during the initial 13 months of study. Five of the six animals in the group not reimplanted with progesterone at 14 months cycled between 14 and 20 months when their plasma progesterone concentrations fell below 1 ng/ml (Fig. 3). Four of these five bitches showed signs of estrus and were bred; three became pregnant and whelped normal litters. None of the bitches injected with MPA at 15 months had cycled by the 22nd month of the study.

Hormone Concentrations

Plasma MPA measured during the study for group C and D bitches is shown in Fig. 5. As expected, peak concentrations after each injection were dose-dependent. MPA did not disappear from the circulation prior to the second injection at 90 days in any case in either group. Small, stepwise increments in the mean residual levels prior to subsequent reinjection were noted in group D.

Four or five bitches in each group were in metestrus at the time of initial treatment. In no case was the progesterone level suppressed by MPA injections. In fact, the metestrus progesterone profiles in the bitches treated with the 10 mg/kg dose appeared to be broadened, giving the appearance of profiles seen during pregnancy, as opposed to profiles seen in nonpregnant animals (Fig. 2).

Plasma progesterone profiles determined for control bitches (Fig. 4) and for bitches cycling following previous suppression of cycles with progesterone implants were similar to those previously reported (5). More-sensitive assays of picogram concentrations of progesterone made at weekly intervals during anestrus in control bitches showed that the mean concentrations remained above 1 ng/ml for 60–105 days (mean 84 days) and reached a nadir of 420 ± 4 pg/ml

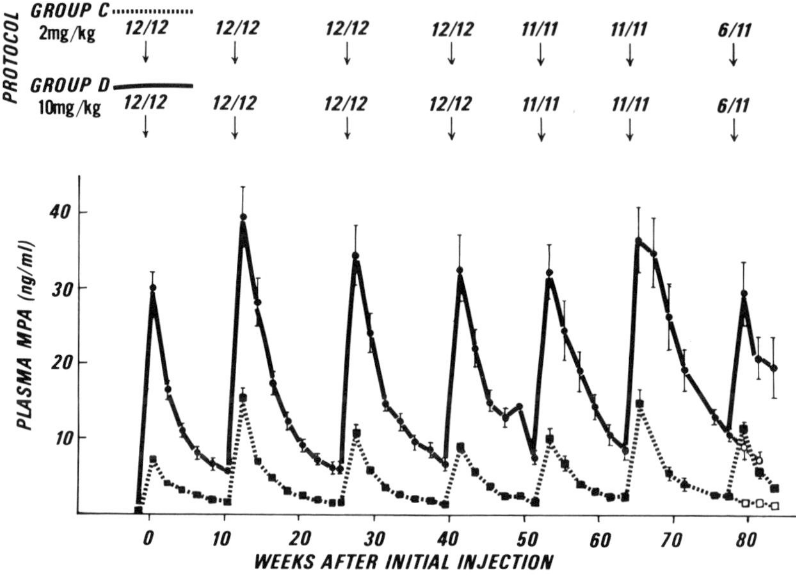

FIG. 5. Mean plasma MPA in beagle bitches injected at 90-day intervals.

around day 145. Basal (less than 600 pg/ml) levels were found for variable lengths of time in each of the 12 cycles studied. Mean basal concentrations of 410 ± 6 pg/ml were only slightly above the value of 360 ± 4 pg/ml obtained for plasma from ovariectomized bitches in the same series of assays. Viewed in terms of days prior to the next estrus, the nadir in mean levels occurred approximately 35 days prior to estrus, with a subsequent slow rise during proestrus (Fig. 6). In the same set of weekly samples from control bitches in anestrus the mean LH levels were 0.56 ± 0.06 ng/ml during the 3-week period for which the lowest mean progesterone levels were found. A small rise in LH was associated with the onset of proestrus in seven bitches, giving a mean concentration of 1.65 ± 0.4 ng/ml at the second week prior to estrus. Concentrations of progesterone and LH were also determined in three consecutive weekly samples collected after 10 or 12 months of MPA or progesterone treatment, respectively. As shown in Fig. 6, chronic MPA-treated animals had progesterone concentrations comparable to the nadir values for normal animals in anestrus. Mean LH levels in groups B, C, and D were 0.93 ± 0.13, 0.86 ± 0.10, and 1.43 ± 0.27 mg/ml, respectively. These concentrations were higher ($p < 0.02$) than the basal levels found in late anestrus in control bitches (0.56 ± 0.06 ng/ml). Additional assays for plasma estrogens are being conducted.

Mammary Gland Palpations

Digital palpations of the mammary glands of all bitches prior to treatment indicated that there were no pre-existing nodules, and that the average and range

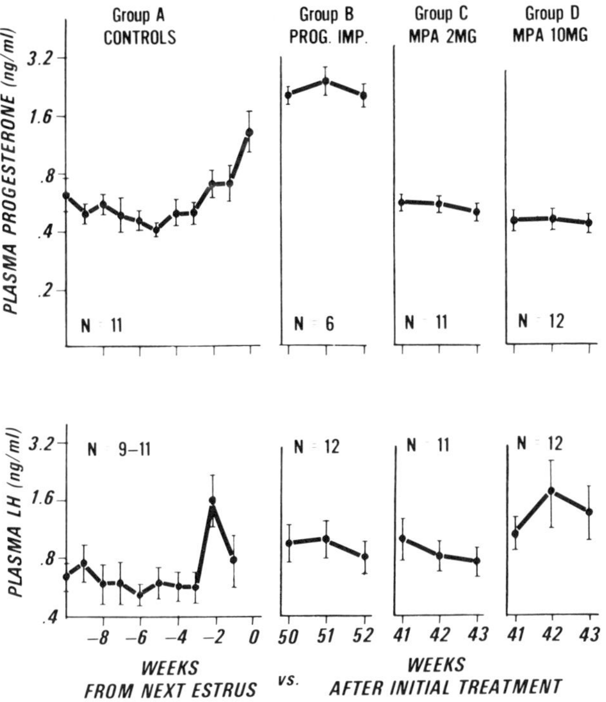

FIG. 6. Mean plasma progesterone (**top**) and LH (**bottom**) in beagle bitches during chronic administration of progesterone or MPA.

for estimated mammary gland development were similar in all groups. By the end of the first 90-day period of study, mammary development was markedly increased in several bitches that received MPA at 10 mg/kg. Thereafter at 7, 12, 16, and 18 months of treatment, the effects of MPA on mammary development were progressive and dose-dependent. Such effects are indicated in the mean palpation scores for mammary development given in Fig. 7. By 13 months of study, five of the six oldest bitches treated with the higher dose of MPA had developed one or two palpable nodules 0.5–1.0 cm in diameter. One young ($<$ 2.5 years) bitch developed a nodule. One nodule excised at 8 months, another at 12 months, and several obtained from a bitch that died after 15 months of treatment were studied histopathologically and were diagnosed as mixed mammary tumors (Table 2, Fig. 8). A persistent palpable nodule was found in only one of the bitches receiving the lower dose of MPA. None of the control or progesterone-implanted bitches developed palpable nodules similar to those found in MPA-treated bitches.

Biopsy of Mammary Tissues

Tissues removed from each bitch prior to treatment provided a range of samples representative of various stages of the cycle. Proliferative changes within this

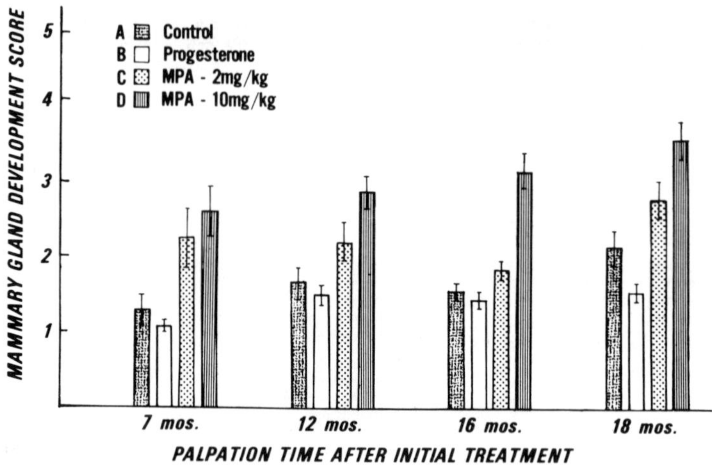

FIG. 7. Mean mammary gland development scores in beagle bitches during chronic administration of progesterone or MPA.

normal range were scored for each tissue sample collected from each bitch at 120, 240, and 380 days of treatment and are summarized in Table 3. At each biopsy time, as well as throughout the entire study, proliferative changes in alveolar, ductal, and stromal elements were greater in bitches receiving MPA than in those with progesterone implants or in control animals. The incidence of such proliferative changes was greater in MPA-treated bitches in terms of both percentage of biopsies and percentage of animals studied. The incidence of proliferative changes outside the normal range observed in control animals, but not including the excised mixed mammary tumors, are given in Table 4. A total of 11 mammopathies, including the excised mixed mammary tumors, were found in the biopsy material studied. Nine of these lesions were found in five of the six oldest bitches in the group receiving MPA at a dose of 10 mg/kg.

Body Weight and Skin Changes

Moderate weight gains were recorded for all groups of bitches over the course of treatment. After 30 weeks of treatment the increase in body weight was somewhat greater in bitches receiving the higher level of MPA; however, mean body weights at 70 weeks (Table 2) were not significantly different. Excessive skin folding, most prominent on the head and limbs, was noted in the oldest bitch (6.5 years) on the higher dose of MPA after 10 months of treatment (Fig. 8). After 14 months of treatment the second oldest bitch in this group developed the same syndrome, also at 6.5 years of age. The onset and development of this puffy, wrinkled, "basset hound appearance" was rapid in the latter bitch, and she died at 15 months of treatment. Necropsy results for these and other bitches are given below.

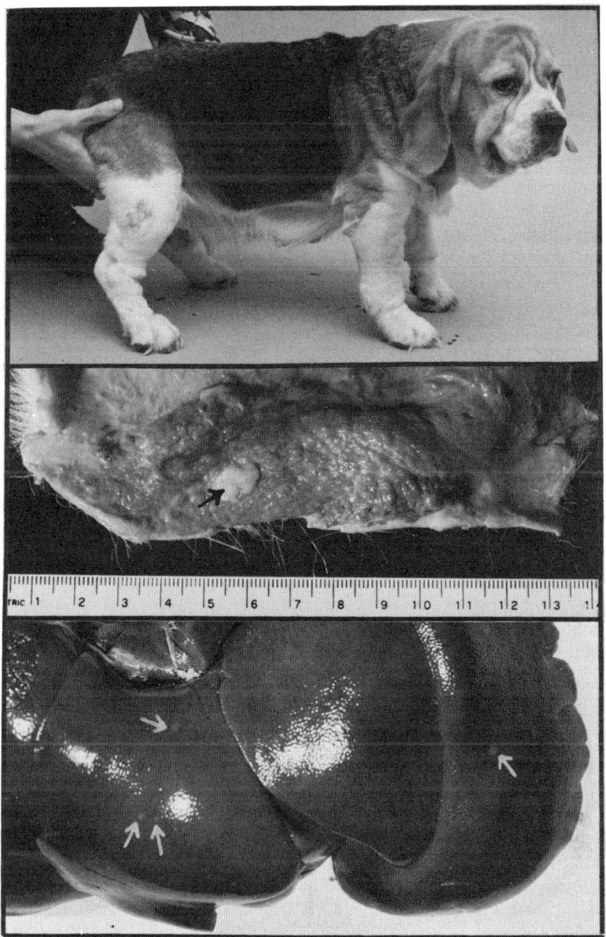

FIG. 8. Lesions observed in beagle bitches receiving injections of MPA (10 mg/kg/90 days). **Top:** Skin overgrowth in a 7-year-old bitch after 20 months of treatment. **Middle:** One of several mixed mammary tumors (*arrow*) found in a bitch that died after 15 months of treatment. **Bottom:** Liver from a bitch necropsied after 20 months of treatment. Arrows indicate hepatomas.

Necropsy Findings

Mean age, body weight, and selected organ weights for the six bitches in each group necropsied after 20 months of study are given in Table 5. The bitches chronically treated with MPA (10 mg/kg/90 days) had larger ($p < 0.05$) mammary glands and thyroids than did the controls. Gross lesions observed at necropsy of the 24 bitches and in the additional bitch from group D that died during the 15th month of treatment are reported in Table 6. Liver adenomas (Fig. 8) were larger and more extensive in MPA-treated bitches. Histologically, these

TABLE 3. *Incidence of proliferative changes in mammary tissue selected for biopsy every 120 days during treatment with progesterone or MPA for 13 months*

Measurement	Group A Control	Group B Progesterone	Group C MPA 2 mg/kg	Group D MPA 10 mg/kg
No. of bitches	12	12	12	12
Biopsies	36	36	36	36
Alveolar proliferation				
Mean score[a]	1.7	1.9	2.7	2.5
% Biopsies >2 score	5	22	69	72
% Bitches >2 score	16	50	100	100
Duct proliferation				
Mean score	1.3	1.2	2.5	2.4
% Biopsies >2 score	2	13	61	66
% Bitches >2 score	8	25	100	100
Stromal proliferation				
Mean score	1.0	1.0	2.0	1.4
% Biopsies >2 score	0	0	25	11
% Bitches >2 score	0	0	50	25

[a] Scoring: 1 = none. 2 = slight. 3 = moderate. 4 = extensive.

TABLE 4. *Incidence of mammopathies in beagle mammary tissue randomly selected for biopsy every 120 days during treatment with progesterone or MPA for 13 months*

Measurement	Group A Control	Group B Progesterone	Group C MPA 2 mg/kg	Group D MPA 10 mg/kg
No. of bitches	12	12	12	12
Biopsies (post treatment)	36	36	36	34[a]
Nodular hyperplasia	0	0	0	6
Ductal adenoma	0	0	1	2
Total mammopathies	0	0	1	8
Bitches involved	0	0	1	5

[a] Does not include mixed mammary tumors removed from two bitches in lieu of a random sample.

lesions consisted of hepatocytes with vacuolated cytoplasm. A high incidence of gallstones and gallbladder mucosal cysts was found in the MPA-treated bitches. Other evidence of liver dysfunction in the animals treated with the higher dose of MPA included green discoloration of the plasma in one bitch after 5 months of treatment and greenish discoloration of the mammary tissue removed at necropsy in two bitches. In addition, higher ($p < 0.05$) plasma cholesterol (302 ± 27 versus 224 ± 22 mg/100 ml) and creatine phosphokinase (48 ± 3 versus 36 ± 3 mg/100 ml) concentrations were found in bitches on the higher MPA dose when compared to controls at 17 months of study. Preliminary examination of skin sections suggests that the extreme skin folding was related to increased dermal collagen and did not represent hyperkeratosis. More extensive histopathological

TABLE 5. *Organ weight at necropsy after 20 months of treatment with progesterone or MPA*

Measurement	Group A Controls	Group B Progesterone	Group C MPA 2 mg/kg	Group D MPA 10 mg/kg
No. of bitches	6	6	6	6
Age (months)	61 ± 1[a]	52 ± 7	58 ± 8	49 ± 9
Body weight (kg)	11.0 ± 1.1	9.5 ± 0.5	11.8 ± 0.6	12.1 ± 1.0
Mammary glands				
Grams	41 ± 11 (5)[b]	28 ± 5 (6)	77 ± 17 (6)	144 ± 36[c] (5)
Grams/kg	3.4 ± 0.8	3.0 ± 0.6	6.5 ± 1.3	11.6 ± 2.0[c]
Livers				
Grams	288 ± 16 (6)	243 ± 25 (5)	312 ± 18 (6)	399 ± 67 (5)
Grams/kg	27 ± 2	26 ± 1	27 ± 1	32 ± 3
Adrenals				
Grams	1.3 ± 0.1 (6)	1.3 ± 0.1 (6)	1.6 ± 0.1 (6)	1.4 ± 0.2 (6)
Mg/kg	129 ± 20	138 ± 15	137 ± 9	118 ± 13
Thyroids				
Grams	0.65 ± 0.05 (6)	0.80 ± 0.07	0.92 ± 0.09	1.78 ± 0.50[c]
Mg/kg	64 ± 12	85 ± 7	79 ± 9	141 ± 33[c]

[a] All values are the mean $\pm$ standard error.
[b] Numbers in parentheses are the number of animals.
[c] Different from controls ($p < 0.05$) Student's *t*-test (group A vs. group D).

TABLE 6. *Incidence of gross lesions at necropsy of beagle bitches following 20 months of treatment with MPA*

Lesion	Group A Control N-6	Group B-1 Progesterone[a] N-6	Group C MPA 2 mg/kg N-6	MPA 10 mg/kg N-7[b]
Liver adenomas				
Dogs	0	2	2	3
Total	0	4	12	28
Size (mm)	—	1–4	1–3	1–18
Gallbladder				
With cystic mucosa	0	1	1	3[b]
With stones	0	1	5	5
Excessive skin folding	0	0	0	2[b]
Uterus—mucometra	0	0	3	6[b]

[a] Subcutaneous Silastic implants at 150 mg/kg, followed by 60 mg/kg at 14 and 18 months.
[b] Includes one bitch that died after 14 months of treatment.

examinations of these lesions, including the mammary gland lesions, are being conducted.

DISCUSSION

Endocrine Effects

Continued suppression of estrous cycles in bitches treated with a low (2 mg/kg) dose of MPA was not unexpected. Bryan (3) reported that estrus was delayed more than 4 months in bitches following single intramuscular injections of doses as low as 1.25 mg/kg. However, interestrous intervals in control animals were not reported. Results of plasma progesterone assays in the present study indicate that MPA at this low dose suppresses not only the appearance of external signs of proestrus and estrus, but ovulatory activity as well.

None of the bitches last injected with MPA 2 mg/kg at the 15th month of study have recycled during the intervening 5.5 months. However, Bryan (3) noted that half of the bitches receiving single injections of 2.5 mg/kg i.m. had returned to estrus by 5.5 months. The greater delay in chronically treated bitches suggests that the time required to recycle after cessation of treatment may be dependent on the prior duration of treatment.

The decline of progesterone during anestrus to nearly undetectable plasma concentrations approximately 35 days prior to the next estrus suggests that follicles capable of ovulation do not develop until progesterone disappears from the circulation. The bitch appears to lack an acute luteolytic mechanism, resulting in a correspondingly prolonged period of luteal regression. The artificial "luteal phases" induced by injection of MPA (2 mg/kg) may not be unphysiological, in the sense that the 1–2 ng/ml levels of MPA in the circulation 4 months after the last injection are comparable to the progesterone levels seen in normal bitches 4 months after estrus. The stepwise increases in residual plasma concentrations of MPA prior to reinjection of the 10 mg/kg dose at 90-day intervals suggests that higher doses might effect an extreme accumulation of the drug within the animal. However, it does not appear that retention of circulating levels of MPA in the bitch is any greater than in women. Women injected with approximately 3 mg/kg had detectable plasma levels for up to 7–8 months (11).

Our results in the bitch appear to reinforce the conclusions of others (11) that MPA does not depress basal gonadotropin secretion. There was no indication of suppression of luteal function in bitches treated with MPA during metestrus, as reflected by plasma progesterone levels. Furthermore, mean plasma LH concentrations measured in the bitches chronically anovulatory during progesterone and MPA treatments were significantly higher than mean levels of LH found during late anestrus in control bitches. Several of the control animals also showed episodic release of LH associated with the transition from anestrus to proestrus. It is possible that chronic progestin treatment blocks this transition. Chronic progestational activity may interfere with the ability of estrogens produced by late anestrous follicles to act on target tissues, perhaps by inhibiting the production of estrogen receptor sites.

Pathology

The proliferative lesions in both the mammary gland and liver induced by these relatively low doses of MPA are clearly a matter of concern. The liver cell adenomas and gallstones have not previously been reported in the dog. As expected, more proliferative lesions were found in dogs on the higher dose of MPA. However, the higher dose we used (10 mg/kg/90 days) is considerably lower than that recommended for toxicity studies (1). Furthermore, the incidence of proliferative lesions was greater in MPA- than progesterone-treated animals. The fact that proliferative lesions developed earliest in the older dogs indicates an interaction between age and duration of treatment in lesion development. However, it is important to point out that no lesions were found in either the livers or mammary glands of the control dogs, despite the fact that they were older than the MPA-treated dogs.

The adenomas found in the livers of the MPA-treated bitches are of particular significance since in some respects they resemble liver lesions now being reported with increasing frequency in young women on long-term oral contraceptives (12,13,18). Cytoplasmic vacuolation of the affected hepatocytes is a feature common to the dog lesions and those reported in young women (18). The very high incidence of gallstones and gallbladder cysts found in dogs on both doses of MPA is also remarkable in view of the increased incidence of gallstone formation reported in patients who have had long-term use of contraceptives (18). Elevated plasma cholesterol levels may also indicate abnormal liver function in the treated dogs. It has been suggested that the estrogenic components of the contraceptive drugs are responsible for the hepatic changes described in women and rats (17). Our finding of similar liver lesions in the dog as a result of treatment with a progestational agent (MPA) suggests that this question needs to be re-examined. Although plasma estrogen assays for our dogs have not been completed, there were no indications of hyperestrogenicity in the treated dogs. The hyperplastic changes in the endometrium were of a progestational rather than an estrogenic type. The fact that some local nodular hyperplasia was also seen in the livers of two progesterone-treated dogs further suggests that progestins alone can produce hepatic damage.

No adequate explanation can be given for the skin changes noted in two dogs on the higher dose of MPA. The gross appearance of these animals is reminiscent of the classic picture seen in dogs overdosed with growth hormone. A similar syndrome seen after treatment with chlormadinone acetate was described as "acromegaly-like" (9). However, no remarkable skeletal changes were found, nor were any gross pituitary tumors noted in our MPA-treated dogs. The major histological feature of the overgrown skin was a thick layer of collagen in the dermis. None of these observations suggests growth hormone involvement in the condition.

The MPA-induced proliferative changes in the mammary gland were dose-dependent and greater than those induced by progesterone. The abnormal proliferative changes noted in the random tissue samples obtained during the experiment were, for the most part, limited to animals on the high MPA dose (Table 3). The increasing incidence of proliferative changes with dose and time suggest that these lesions may progress to nodular hyperplasia and ductal adenomas (Table 4) under the influence of continued MPA stimulation. It is not clear if the mixed mammary tumors seen in some dogs on the higher MPA dose arise directly from ductal and stromal proliferation or if nodular hyperplasia and ductal adenomas represent intermediary stages. Jensen et al. (10) suggest that atypical lobules showing varying degrees of anaplasia between normal epithelium and carcinoma *in situ* are common preneoplastic lesions in the human mammary gland.

ACKNOWLEDGMENTS

The authors gratefully acknowledge the technical assistance provided by M. E. Powers, R. G. Cowan, and M. E. Lanieu, and the animal care provided by D. Shattuck and F. Terwilliger. We also express appreciation to Dr. K. Kirton (The Upjohn Co.) for Depo-Provera, MPA, and antisera against MPA and progesterone; to Dr. A. S. Hartree (University of Cambridge) for canine LH; to Dr. A. R. Boyns (Tenovous Institute) for antiserum against canine LH; to Dr. J. Wagner (Eli Lilly Co.) for antiserum against rabbit gamma globulin; and to Dr. J. Tasker (New York State Veterinary College) for serum chemistry analyses. This research was supported by the U.S. National Institute of Health (NICHD) Contract No. 72–2725.

REFERENCES

1. Berliner, V. P. (1974): U.S. Food and Drug Administration requirements for toxicity testing of contraceptive steroids. In: *Pharmacological Models in Contraceptive Development,* edited by M. H. Briggs and E. Diczfalusy. Bogtrykkeriet Forum, Copenhagen.
2. Boyns, A. R., Jones, G. E., Bell, E. T., Christie, D. W., and Parkes, M. F. (1972): Development of a radioimmunoassay for canine luteinizing hormone. *J. Endocrinol.,* 55:279–291.
3. Bryan, H. S. (1973): Parenteral use of medroxyprogesterone acetate as an antifertility agent in the bitch. *Am. J. Vet. Res.,* 34:659–663.
4. Concannon, P. W., and Hansel, W. (1975): Effects of estrogen and progesterone on plasma LH, sexual behavior and pregnancy in beagle bitches. *Fed. Proc.,* 34:323.
5. Concannon, P. W., Hansel, W., and Visek, W. J. (1975): The ovarian cycle of the bitch: Plasma estrogen, LH and progesterone. *Biol. Reprod.,* 13:112–121.
6. Cornette, J. C., Kirton, K. T., and Duncan, G. W. (1971): Measurement of medroxyprogesterone acetate (Provera) by radioimmunoassay. *J. Clin. Endocrinol. Metab.,* 33:459–466.
7. De Villa, G. O., Roberts, K., Wiest, W. G., Mikhail, G., and Flickinger, G. (1972): A specific radioimmunoassay of plasma progesterone. *J. Clin. Endocrinol. Metab.,* 35:458–460.
8. Evans, H. M., and Cole, H. H. (1931): An introduction to the study of the oestrous cycle of the dog. *Mem. Univ. Calif.,* 9:65–103.

9. Hill, R., and Dumas, K. (1974): The use of dogs for studies of toxicity of contraceptive hormones. In: *Pharmacological Models in Contraceptive Development,* edited by M. H. Briggs and E. Diczfalusy. Bogtrykkeriet Forum, Copenhagen.
10. Jensen, H. M., Rice, J. R., and Wellings, S. R. (1976): Pre-neoplastic lesions in the human breast. *Science,* 191:295–297.
11. Kirton, K. T., and Cornette, J. C. (1974): Return of ovulatory cyclicity following an intramuscular injection of medroxyprogesterone acetate (Provera). *Contraception,* 10:39–45.
12. Mays, E. T., Christopherson, W. M., and Barrows, G. H. (1974): Focal nodular hyperplasia of the liver: Possible relationship to oral contraceptives. *Am. J. Clin. Pathol.,* 61:735–746.
13. Mays, E. T., Christopherson, W. M., Mahr, M. M., and Williams, H. C. (1976): Hepatic changes in young women ingesting contraceptive steroids: Hepatic hemorrhage and primary hepatic tumors. *JAMA,* 235:730–732.
14. Nelson, L. W., Carlton, W. W., and Weikel, J. H. (1972): Canine neoplasms and progestogens. *JAMA,* 219:1601–1606.
15. Nett, T. M., Akbar, A. M., Phemister, R. D., Holst, P. A., Reichert, L. E., and Niswender, G. D. (1975): Levels of luteinizing hormone, estradiol and progesterone in serum during the estrous cycle and pregnancy in the beagle bitch. *Proc. Soc. Exp. Med. Biol.,* 148:134–139.
16. Smith, M. S., and McDonald, L. E. (1974): Serum levels of luteinizing hormone and progesterone during the estrous cycle, pseudopregnancy and pregnancy in the dog. *Endocrinology,* 94:404–412.
17. Smith, R. L. (1973): Biliary excretion and hepatotoxicity of contraceptive steroids. In: *Pharmacological Models in Contraceptive Development,* edited by M. H. Briggs and E. Diczfalusy. Bogtrykkeriet Forum, Copenhagen.
18. Stauffer, J. Q., Lapinski, M. W., Honald, D. J., and Myers, J. K. (1975): Focal nodular hyperplasia of the liver and intrahepatic hemorrhage in young women on oral contraceptives. *Ann. Intern. Med.,* 83:301–306.

Pharmacology of Steroid Contraceptive Drugs
edited by S. Garattini and H. W. Berendes.
Raven Press, New York © 1977.

Contraceptive Steroids and Mammary Gland Growth in Rats and Beagles

R. von Berswordt-Wallrabe, M. Mehring, K-J. Gräf, S. Beier, and W. Elger

Department of Endocrine Pharmacology, Schering AG Berlin/Bergkamen, 1000 Berlin 65, West Germany

When growth-stimulating hormones act chronically on particular target organs, tumors are inducible within their receptive sites (1). After long-term exposure to estrogens and/or gestagens, mammary tumors have occurred in rodents and dogs. The aim of this investigation was twofold: first to find out how much contraceptive steroids (CSs) were *directly* involved in mammary tumor development; and second, to what extent they could have exerted such influence *indirectly,* possibly by means of, or together with, increased prolactin secretion. The animal models used were rats treated chronically with norethisterone enanthate (NE) (17α-ethynyl-17β-heptanoyloxy-4-estren-3-on) and beagles given hydroxy-progesterone derivatives.

Our first insights and general endocrinological findings from toxicity tests on the use of depot contraceptives were reported earlier (2). Since that report, data from extensive studies on male and female rats given NE chronically have been analyzed. The aim of the rat study reported here was to shed light on the mechanisms which cause tumors in the mammary glands. The dog studies with hydroxyprogesterone derivatives are not yet completed. There are still many unresolved methodological problems, in addition to which, studies must first be done to establish basic endocrinological knowledge.

The two species reported here had in common the working hypothesis that prolactin could play a key role in the development of mammary and pituitary tumors when synthetic gestagens were tested chronically in pharmacological doses.

EXPERIMENTS WITH RATS: LONG-TERM MAMMARY TUMOR-INDUCING DOSES OF DEPOT NE

A total of 450 randomly selected rats of both sexes, weighing 200–220 g, were used as follows: 149 rats were grafted with four hypophyseal homotransplants (4HT) under the kidney capsules to induce hypersecretion of prolactin; 201 were hypophysectomized to eliminate pituitary secretions; and 100 were left intact. NE

10 mg/100 g body weight per week was injected intramuscularly into 248 animals for up to 70 weeks.

The rats, provided by Carworth-Europe, were carefully palpated twice a week. The palpable mammary nodules (PMNs) were noted on individual sheets. Moribund animals and those which survived the test period were given to the pathologist for inspection. The animals were kept and killed under standardized laboratory conditions.

The experimental design and the experimental groups are described in Tables 1 and 3 and in Fig. 1. The test compound, NE, was dissolved in sesame oil by gently raising its temperature to 68°–70°C; 10 mg NE was given in 0.1 ml. Injection sites were the upper thighs, used alternately.

After killing 10 animals for miscellaneous reasons and 47 for prolactin determinations between days 325 and 362, 393 rats remained for the total test period of 435–492 days. Sixty-eight NE-treated and 100 other rats survived, whereas 154 NE-treated and 71 untreated ones had to be excluded because of death or moribund condition. With two exceptions, none of the NE-treated hypophysectomized (HE) rats survived longer than 213 days; they were thus dead before PMNs were found in the reference groups.

The PMNs appeared in the males approximately 60 days after they were seen in the females, but ultimately the males had the highest incidence of PMNs and histologically verified tumors when 4HT was done in association with NE treatment. There were seven tumors in the females with 4HT, and none in the corresponding group of males. With NE alone, the males had three tumors plus two cases of mastitis, and the females showed one tumor. However, the combined influence of additional hypophyseal secretions derived from the 4HT plus NE generated 12 tumors plus four cases of mastitis in the males and 8 tumors in the females, which never had mastitis.

The palpatory findings (41 nodules in 23 females and 53 in 35 males) were confirmed histologically as mammary adenomas, adenocarcinomas, cystadenomas, and fibroadenomas in only 16 females and 15 males. After NE injections and under the influence of 4HT, respectively, proliferation of the lobuloalveolar system had taken place distinctively in both sexes; with both treatments, all rats had abundant secretory material in addition. In the NE-treated rats the pituitaries showed stimulation of the so-called prolactin-producing cells. Nine pituitary tumors composed of chromophobic elements were found, distributed erratically.

Pituitary homografts stimulated the mammary glands of the female rat and finally led to an increased incidence of PMNs. The concomitant NE treatment generated no further increase in PMNs. This points to the decisive role of the hypophyseal homotransplants for mammary tumor development in *female* rats.

In contrast, the 4HT *male* rats had a low rate of PMNs and no tumors. However, NE treatment abolished this sex difference and even elevated the PMN rate distinctively over the rate in the corresponding female group. The data point to a hypophyseal-ovarian steroid hormone synergism in the mammary gland which can also activate tumor development. The assumption of such a "tumorigenic complex" explains the supplementation of 4HT in females; in males, however, addition of NE increased the risk of PMN development. Since NE exerts gestagenic and estrogenic activity, it becomes clear why this compound induced PMNs so readily in rats in the presence of hypophyseal secretion(s); nonestrogenic gestagens are supposed not to induce mammary tumors under the same experimental conditions. It remains to be shown how far the 4HT and the estrogenic gestagens, respectively, produce the expected increase of serum prolactin. This will help to focus on whether prolactin, perhaps in concert with other hypophyseal hormones, plays a still-hypothetical key role in mammary tumor development in rats.

EXPERIMENTS WITH DOGS: LONG-TERM MAMMARY TUMOR-INDUCING DOSES OF HYDROXYPROGESTERONE DERIVATIVES

The mammary glands of dogs were stimulated after the animals had been given 4,6-dichlor-17-acetoxy-16α-methyl-4,6-pregnadiene-3,20-dione 5 mg/kg p.o. for 30 weeks. The beagles' pituitaries were affected also. Moreover, eosinophils, the cells thought to be the prolactin-producing elements, were markedly increased. These first hints pointing to the possibility of a positive feedback between hydroxyprogesterone derivatives and prolactin and/or growth hormone must be confirmed by prolactin determinations or experiments with prolactin-inhibiting compounds.

RESULTS

Body Weight

After treatment with NE, the body weight gain slowed. This effect was more pronounced in the males. The same trend was true for the 4HT-bearing animals, although the hypophyseal homografts—particularly in the females—exerted anabolic effects. The HE control rats remained within the range typical after this operation (Table 1). If exposed to NE the body weight losses were dramatically enhanced.

Survival Rate

None of the HE plus NE-treated rats survived the entire experimental period (Fig. 1). The HE male controls and the intact male controls, respectively, had the next better rates of survival. Otherwise, the male rats tolerated the NE treatment better than the females (Tables 2 and 3).

TABLE 1. *Body weight of rats at beginning and end of long-term NE treatment*

Experimental group[a]	Females				Males			
	Beginning		End		Beginning		End	
	No. of rats	Body wt. (g ± SEM)	No. of rats	Body wt. (g ± SEM)	No. of rats	Body wt. (g ± SEM)	No. of rats	Body wt. (g ± SEM)
Intact controls	25	206 ± 0.9	14	304 ± 5.2	25	210 ± 1.5	6	508 ± 9.5
Intact plus NE	25	206 ± 0.6	10	281 ± 10.9	25	213 ± 1.0	18	347 ± 6.2
4 HT controls	39	206 ± 0.6	28	345 ± 7.3	33	210 ± 1.2	24	524 ± 10.0
4 HT plus NE	37	206 ± 1.1	17	296 ± 7.4	40	212 ± 1.0	23	342 ± 4.7
HE controls	40	208 ± 0.7	26	192 ± 4.0	40	210 ± 1.0	2	185 ± 8.0
HE plus NE	60	208 ± 0.06	—	—	61	212 ± 1.0	—	—
Total	226		95		224		73	

[a] NE: Each animal received norethisterone enanthate 10 mg/100 g body wt/week i.m. 4HT: four hypophyseal homotransplants under the kidney capsules. HE: Hypophysectomized. PMN: Palpable mammary nodules.

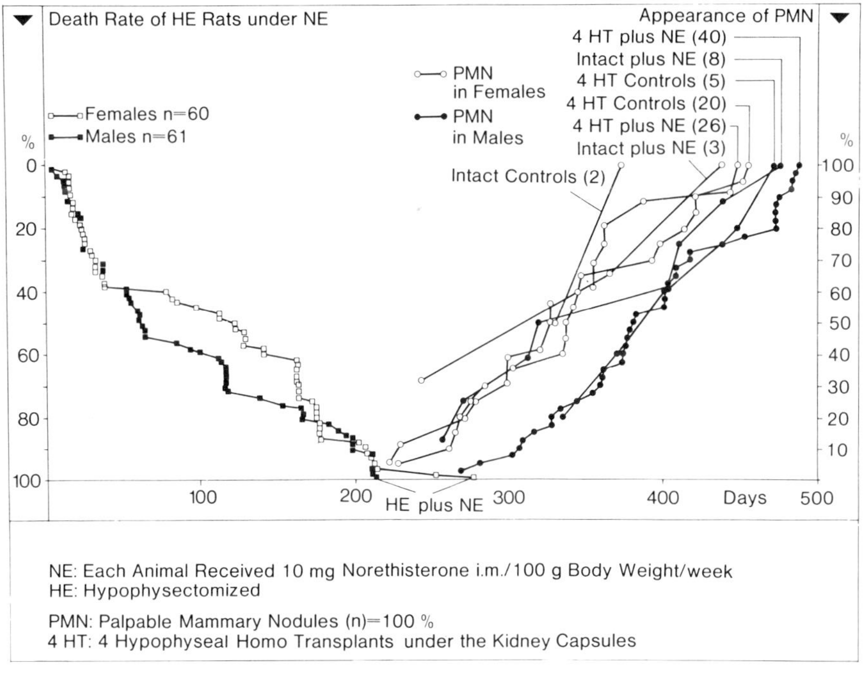

Fig. 1. Rats given long-term NE treatment.

Palpable Mammary Nodules

PMNs were found between day 222 and 487 of the experiment (Table 4). They appeared earlier in females than in males (Fig. 1). The highest rate (40 PMNs) was recorded in males with 4HT plus NE. The male 4HT controls were less affected, with only five PMNs. No such difference was seen in the corresponding female groups: There were 20 PMNs in the 4HT controls and 16 in the 4HT plus NE-treated animals (Tables 5 and 6). No statement can be made about the HE plus NE-treated rats (Fig. 1); however, none of the 73 HE controls (males and females, corrected numbers) had any PMNs (Tables 3, 5, and 6).

Mammary Tumor Identification

After killing the animals it was found that many of the manually located nodules were irritated, swollen lymph nodes, perhaps a result of the many times the rats were carefully palpated (Tables 4–6). In the females roughly 40% and in the males approximately 28% of the PMNs were tumorigenic; the male rats had six PMNs that were histologically proved cases of mastitis (Table 6). There were no correlations between the size of a PMN and the histologically determined type of mammary tumor.

TABLE 2. *Fate of surviving rats after long-term NE treatment*

		Females							Males						
		No. of rats Top: with PMN Bottom: without PMN		Transferred alive for						No. of rats Top: with PMN Bottom: without PMN		Transferred alive for			
							Histopathological inspection							Histopathological inspection	
Experimental group[a]	Total No. of rats		Dead in cage	Miscellaneous reasons	Prolactin determination	Sick	End of experiment	Total No. of rats		Dead in cage	Miscellaneous reasons	Prolactin determination	Sick	End of experiment
Intact controls	25	2	—	—	—	—	2	25	—	—	—	—	—	—
		23	1	1	5	4	12		25	4	—	5	10	6
Intact plus NE	25	3	—	1	—	—	2	25	6	—	1	—	—	5
		22	1	—	5	7	8		19	1	—	5	—	13
4 HT controls	39	10	—	3	—	—	7	33	5	—	—	—	—	5
		29	2	1	5	1	21		28	3	—	5	1	19
4 HT plus NE	37	8	—	—	—	2	6	40	24	2	—	1	3	18
		29	1	1	5	11	11		16	—	2	4	5	5
HE controls	40	—	—	—	—	—	—	40	—	—	—	—	—	—
		40	8	—	—	6	26		40	18	—	7	13	2
HE plus NE	60	—	—	—	—	—	—	61	—	—	—	—	—	—
		60	23	—	—	37	—		61	25	—	—	36	—
Totals	226	23	—	4	—	2	17	224	35	2	1	1	3	28
		203	36	3	20	66	78		189	51	2	26	65	45

[a] See footnote to Table 1 for explanation.

TABLE 3. *Rats that did not survive the test period*[a]

Experimental group[b]	Females		Males	
	Corrected No. of rats[c]	%	Corrected No. of rats[c]	%
Intact controls	19	26	20	70
Intact plus NE	18	45	19	5
4 HT controls	31	9	28	15
4 HT plus NE	31	45	33	30
HE controls	40	35	33	93
HE plus NE	60	100	61	100
Total	199		194	

[a] Dead in cage and moribund condition.
[b] See footnote to Table 1 for explanation.
[c] Total number minus animals eliminated for prolactin determinations and miscellaneous reasons.

In the male rats mammary tumors were seen after NE treatment only: 3 in intact rats and 12 in animals with 4HT. The female 4HT controls had 7 mammary tumors, practically the same number (8) as the females with 4HT plus NE treatment. Finally, one such tumor was found in an intact female NE-treated control rat (Tables 5 and 6). The morphology of the tumors revealed them to be adenomas, adenocarcinomas, fibroadenomas, and cystadenomas. The distribution of these types was erratic (Tables 5 and 6). In a few cases mammary tumors had not been located as PMNs by palpation.

Pituitary Weight

After NE treatment pituitary weight was reduced in the intact females and, in contrast, elevated in the intact males, compared with untreated intact control animals. Slight pituitary weight reductions were registered in the 4HT-bearing animals of both sexes, compared with the untreated control animals; this effect was somewhat more pronounced in the females that had received the NE treatment in addition to 4HT (Table 7).

Pituitary Tumors

Nine pituitary tumors composed of chromophobic cells were found: six in NE-treated rats, two in intact female controls, and one in a 4HT female control rat. The wet weights of these pituitary tumors were not included in Table 7.

Tumors in NE-treated rats were distributed as follows: one in an intact female rat, two in intact males, two in 4HT males, and one in a 4HT female rat. Thus in the male rats these pituitary tumors were restricted to NE-treated animals, whereas in the females they occurred in control animals as well.

TABLE 4. *PMN development in rats after long-term NE treatment*

	Females					Males				
		PMNs were found					PMNs were found			
Experimental group[a]	No. of rats	In % of rats	Per rat (No.)	Between days	Duration of experiment (days)	No. of rats	In % of rats	Per rat (No.)	Between days	Duration of experiment (days)
Intact controls	25	8	1.0	330–372	435	25	—	—	—	478
Intact plus NE	25	12	1.0	242–437	445	25	24	1.3	256–474	486
4 HT controls	39	26	2.0	228–454	450	33	15	1.0	335–471	485
4 HT plus NE	37	22	2.0	222–447	455	40	60	1.7	268–487	490
HE controls	40	—	—	—	448	40	—	—	—	492
HE plus NE	60	—	—	—	277	61	—	—	—	213
Total	226					224				

[a] See footnote to Table 1 for explanation.

TABLE 5. *Comparison of manually detected PMNs with histological findings in female rats after long-term NE treatment*

				PMN size						Analysis of the histological inspection of PMNs							
Experimental group[a]	Total No. of rats	No. of rats with PMNs	Total No. of PMNs	Head of pin	Lentil	Pea	Nodule	Total No. of rats	Total No. (1)–(3)	(1) Lost speci- men	(2)[b] No find- ings	(3) Masti- tis	No. of tumors (4)–(6)	(4) Adeno- mas	(5) Fibro- cyst- adeno- mas	(6) Adeno- carci- nomas
Intact controls	25	2	2	1	—	1	—	25	2	—	2	—	—	—	—	—
Intact plus NE	25	3	3	3	—	—	—	25	2	—	2	—	1	—	1	—
4 HT controls	39	10	20	5	9	—	6	39	13	—	13	—	7	3	3	1
4 HT plus NE	37	8	16	10	6	—	—	37	8	1	7	—	8	6	—	2
HE controls	40	—	—	—	—	—	—	40	—	—	—	—	—	—	—	—
HE plus NE[c]	60	—	—	—	—	—	—	60	—	—	—	—	—	—	—	—
Total	226	23	41	19	15	1	6	226	25	1	24	—	16	9	4	3

[a] See footnote to Table 1 for explanation.
[b] Including multiple PMNs per rat.
[c] Of the 60 NE-treated HE females, 58 died before PMNs were found in the reference groups.

TABLE 6. *Comparison of manually detected PMNs with histological findings in male rats after long-term NE treatment*

| | | No. of | | PMN size | | | | | | Analysis of the histological inspection of PMNs | | | | | | | |
| | | | | | | | | | | | (1) | (2)[b] | (3) | No. | (4) | (5) | (6) |
Experimental group[a]	Total No. of rats	rats with PMNs	Total No. of PMNs	Head of pin	Lentil	Pea	Nodule	Total No. of rats	Total No. (1)–(3)	Lost speci-men	No find-ings	Masti-tis	of tumors (4)–(6)	Adeno-mas	Cyst-fibro-adeno-mas	Adeno-carci-nomas
Intact controls	25	—	—	—	—	—	—	25	—	—	—	—	—	—	—	—
Intact plus NE	25	6	8	5	2	—	1	25	5	—	3	2	3	1	1	1
4 HT controls	33	5	5	3	1	—	1	33	5	—	5	—	—	—	—	—
4 HT plus NE	40	24	40	17	16	2	5	40	28	3	21	4	12	4	4	4
HE controls	40	—	—	—	—	—	—	40	—	—	—	—	—	—	—	—
HE plus NE[c]	61	—	—	—	—	—	—	61	—	—	—	—	—	—	—	—
Total	224	35	53	25	19	2	7	224	38	3	29	6	15	5	5	5

[a] See footnote to Table 1 for explanation.
[b] Including multiple PMNs per rat.
[c] All NE-treated HE males died before PMNs were found in reference groups.

TABLE 7. *Pituitary weight in rats after long-term NE treatment*

Experimental group[a]	Pituitary			
	Females		Males	
	No.	Wet wt. (mg ± SEM)	No.	Wet wt. (mg ± SEM)
Intact controls	14	15.5 ± 0.9	5	11.7 ± 0.5
Intact plus NE	9	10.0 ± 0.9	16	14.9 ± 0.8
4HT controls	25	13.4 ± 0.5	24	10.4 ± 0.7
4HT plus NE	15	12.5 ± 0.3	23	10.4 ± 0.5

[a] See footnote to Table 1 for explanation.

HISTOLOGY

Pituitaries

All animals (females and males) that had been given NE had clear stimulation of the so-called prolactin-producing cells, stained by carmosine L, orange G, and wool green. The cells of the pituitary nodule tumors were of the characteristic chromophobe nature. Almost all of the rats grafted with 4HT had healthy, successfully transplanted pituitaries.

Mammary Glands

In the intact female and male control rats, the mammary gland was built up to the level of small ducti lactiferi and very small alveolar complexes (single or a few) (Figs. 2a and b). Proliferation of the lobuloalveolar system occurred to almost the same extent in female and male rats given NE (Figs. 3a and b); these characteristics were also found in the experimental animals that had received only 4HT (Figs. 2c and d).

In addition to this development, the dual treatment of 4HT plus NE resulted in abundant secretory material (Figs. 3c and d). In the HE rats the mammary glands were completely involuted, even after NE treatment; they exhibited the typical picture that occurs after ablation of the pituitary gland, as shown earlier (2).

DISCUSSION

None of the HE rats given the test compound survived longer than approximately 200 days, i.e., before a mammary nodule was detected in reference groups by palpation. NE reduced the body weight, especially in all HE animals and in the intact males, indicating catabolic effects at this dose level of 10 mg/100 g/week.

It is not clear why NE, in the absence of the pituitary, reduced the body weight

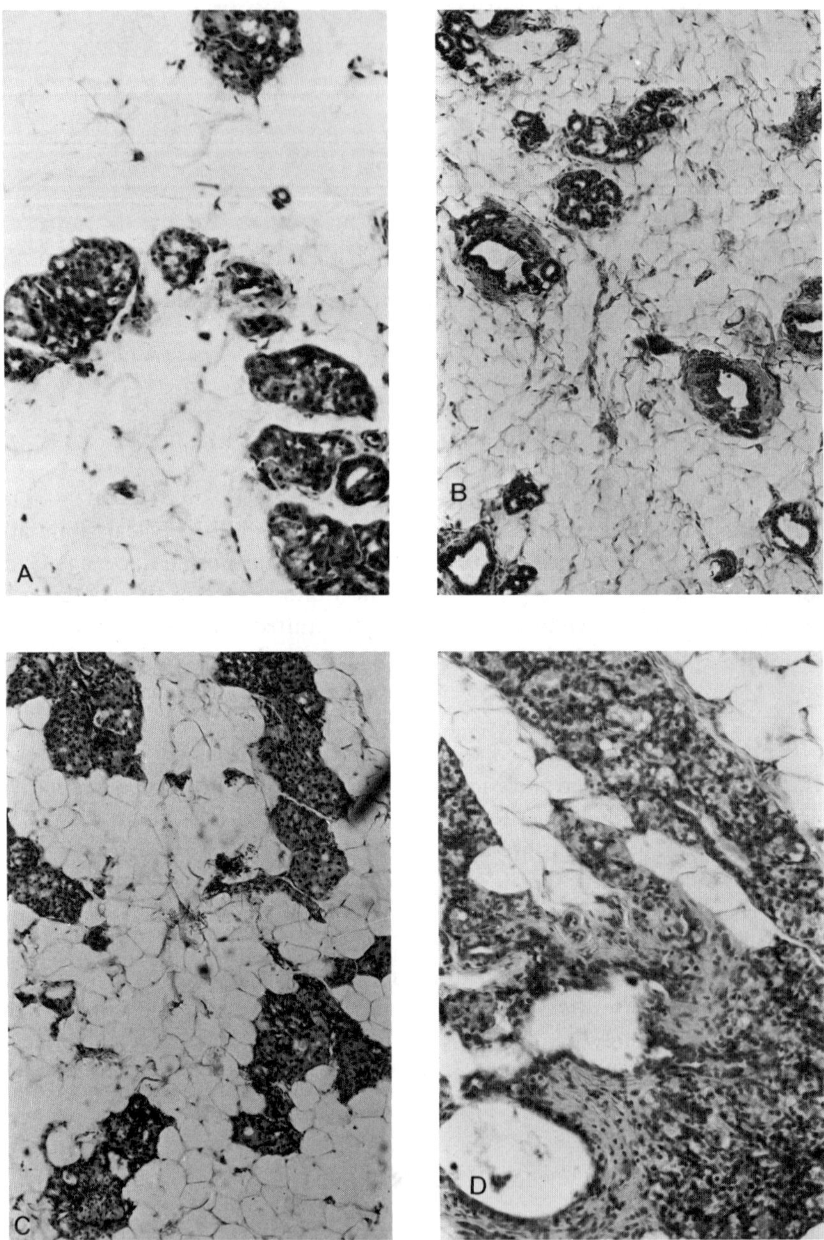

Fig. 2. Histology of the mammary gland of control rats. Duration of the experiment: intact male controls, 478 days **(A)**; intact female controls, 435 days **(B)**; male controls with four hypophyseal homotransplants, 485 days **(C)**; female controls with four hypophyseal homotransplants, 455 days **(D)**. H & E. X163.2.

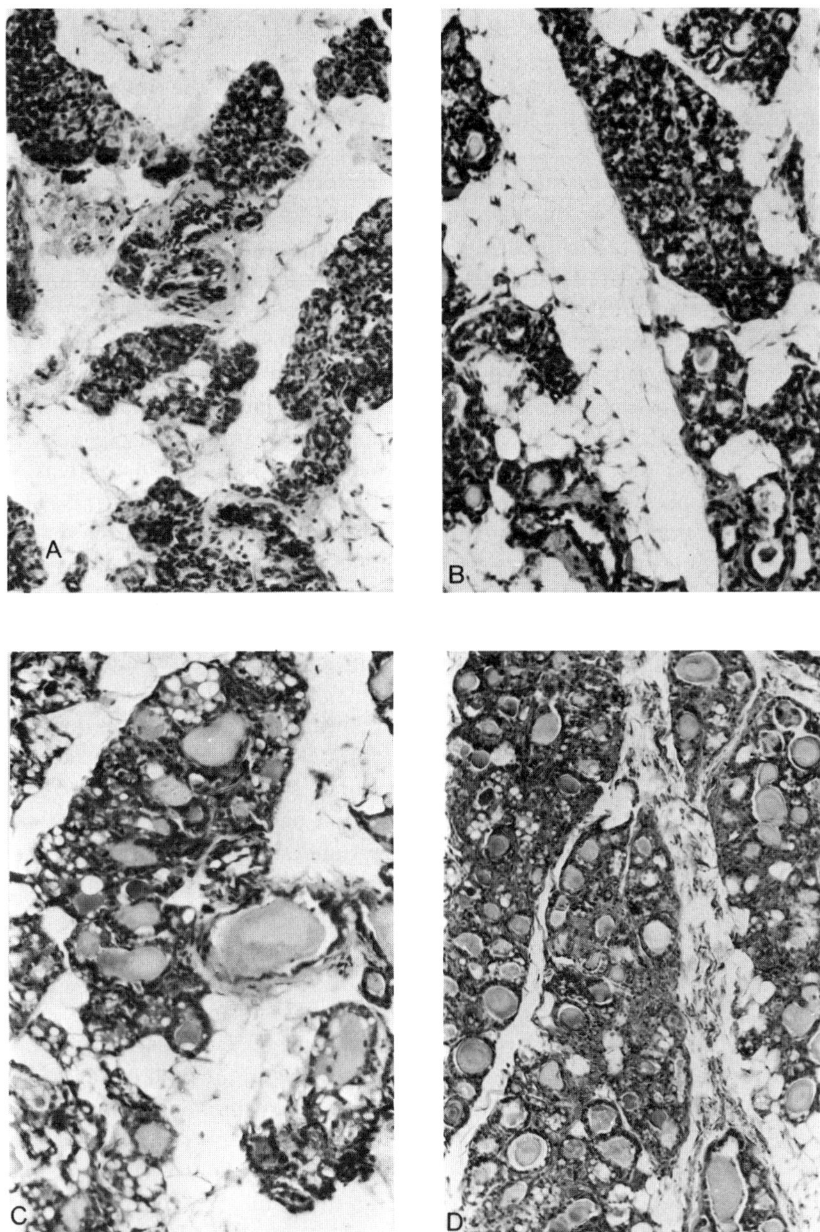

FIG. 3. Histology of the mammary gland of NE-treated rats. Weekly injection of NE: 10 mg/100 g body weight, i.m. Duration of the experiment: intact males, 486 days (**A**); intact females, 445 days (**B**); males with four hypophyseal homotransplants, 490 days (**C**); females with four hypophyseal homotransplants, 455 days (**D**). H & E. ×163.2.

so dramatically and why it led to an irrevocably moribund condition. Probably body weight enhancing and/or protecting effects were derived from the additional secretory activity of the pituitary homografts. Male rats of the same strain after hypophysectomy tolerated "anabolic" testosterone propionate 5 mg/day s.c. chronically. With this pharmacological dose, the animals were in good condition up to 40 weeks, with maintained and/or restored fertility (3). Therefore the catabolic effect of the NE might have been linked to its estrogenic power, which was described in rats (2). This effect was more pronounced in the nonhypophysectomized males, compared with the corresponding females, possibly as a consequence of simultaneously reduced testosterone secretion.

Palpation gave no chronological or qualitative information on mammary tumor development: only one-third of the PMNs were tumors. Before the PMN developed, in both sexes there was the following tendency within the mammary glands: involution in HE rats, no development in the untreated controls, and mammary growth in intact NE-treated animals. Under 4HT influence there was somewhat enhanced stimulation. Finally, still more signs of mammogenic effects, including secretion, had been noted under the dual treatment of 4HT plus NE.

However, some of our results were in conflict with earlier interpretations: The elevated prolactin levels were not found in NE-treated female rats by Gräf (4) after rats were given 4.0 mg NE per day for 41 consecutive days of treatment. In spite of this, there were intensive mammary gland growth-stimulating effects as measured by total DNA.

In confirmation of Welsch et al. (5) the 4HT-bearing *female* controls developed mammary tumors as expected with no additional treatment. Somewhat unexpected was the finding that this mammary tumor rate was not increased in the 4HT females with concomitant chronic addition of NE. In contrast, the *male* 4HT control rats did not develop mammary tumors at all, probably because of the absence of suitable amounts of ovarian steroids. The highest number of changes within the mammary glands (four cases of mastitis and 40 PMNs, 12 of which were confirmed as mammary tumors) occurred in the males given the dual treatment 4HT plus NE.

These data raise speculation about a "tumorigenic hormone complex" in the mammary glands. One could surmise that the chronic overstimulation, in concert with appropriate amounts of hypophyseal secretions and the dual gestagenic and estrogenic influence of the NE, mimicking the ovarian steroids, probably forced the normally unexposed, resting male mammary gland to react intensively. Growth, secretion, and mastitis were recorded first, and later PMNs and mammary tumors appeared. Mastitis was restricted to the male rats, perhaps because they have no cannulating milk ducts and no nipples to evacuate secretory material. In summary: No visible stimulation or overstimulation of the male mammary gland had taken place when the proposed "tumorigenic hormone complex" had not been fully administered chronically.

There was a hint of the expected enhanced hypophyseal activity after NE treatment in the intact males: elevated pituitary weight. This should be confirmed by further investigation. The histology of this structure favored enhanced prolactin stimulation as well. This is of course an interpretation of conventional staining techniques, which are believed to indicate the so-called "prolactin" cells. In contrast—and not understood as yet—the intact females reacted differently after the same NE treatment, as regards the pituitary.

Hence the ideas proposed here to explain divergent results must be considered with caution; many facts remain unresolved. This field deserves more investigation to clarify the role of synthetic steroids with multiple biological actions within their various target sites. Undesirable and/or ultimately even fatal so-called side effects—regardless of whether they are direct or, together with endogenous secretions, of an indirect, synergistic nature—must be brought into focus and understood.

REFERENCES

1. Mühlbock, O., and Boot, L. M. (1959): The mechanism of hormonal carcinogenesis. In: *Ciba Foundation Symposium on Carcinogenesis,* pp. 83–94.
2. Neumann, F., von Berswordt-Wallrabe, R., Elger, W., Gräf, K-J., Hasan, S. H., Mehring, M., Nishino, Y., and Steinbeck, H. (1973): Special problems in toxicity testing of long acting depot contraceptives. In: *Acta Endocrinologica, Separatum: Pharmacological Models in Contraceptive Development.* WHO Symposium, Geneva.
3. Von Berswordt-Wallrabe, R., and Mehring, M. (1976): Fully maintained, restored fertility of hypophysectomized (HE) male rats under long term androgen replacement therapies (Reg. No. 481). In *V International Congress of Endocrinology, Hamburg, July 1976 (in press).*
4. Gräf, K-J.: Personal communication.
5. Welsch, C. W., Jenkins, T. W., and Meites, J. (1970): Increased incidence of mammary tumors in the female rat grafted with multiple pituitaries. *Cancer Res.,* 30:1024–1029.

Pharmacology of Steroid Contraceptive Drugs
edited by S. Garattini and H. W. Berendes.
Raven Press, New York © 1977.

Oral Contraceptive Use and Breast Diseases

Howard W. Ory

Family Planning Evaluation Division, Bureau of Epidemiology, Center for Disease Control, Atlanta, Georgia 30333

From 1972 to 1976 at least eight epidemiologic analyses were published on the association between oral contraceptive use and breast disease (1–8). This report reviews the findings of these studies and highlights consistencies and inconsistencies among the results.

The upper portion of Table 1 presents a summary of the major findings of the reports (1–7) that analyzed the association between oral contraceptive use and benign breast disease. The risk of disease, by years of oral contraceptive use, was either taken directly from the published reports or calculated from the data presented. However, in the case of the Royal College of General Practitioners Study (4), I converted into numbers the results which they displayed graphically; this undoubtedly resulted in slight inaccuracies. Also, I had difficulty converting matched pair-analysis data of Kelsey et al. (5) into risk of disease by years of oral contraceptive use. Again, although the risk values may be slightly inaccurate, I believe the trend is correctly portrayed.

The most consistent finding is that oral contraceptive use for 2 years or more is associated with at least a 50% reduction of chronic cystic disease of the breast. With the exception of the Sartwell study (2), the 50% reduction is also consistent for fibroadenomatous disease.

For a number of reasons cause and effect are the most likely explanation of this finding. Were the findings due to some form of bias, that bias would have to have been operative in both case–control and cohort designs in seven different studies by seven different investigators in widely separated locations. Moreover, the association is present only with extended use of oral contraceptives. Were bias the explanation, it would have to affect long- and short-term users differentially. Furthermore, one study (4) noted that the protective effect was related to increasing dosages of progestagens. These types of differential associations with varying dosages and durations of use are more likely to be acutal pharmacological effects than effects due to bias. In short, the consistency of the association in many studies and the increasing strength of association with increasing duration and dose of use of oral contraceptives make it very likely that this is a cause-and-effect association. From published data (7), I estimate that, for every 100,000 women who use oral contraceptives for two years or more, 240 fewer women will be hospitalized for breast biopsy per year than for a similar number of women who are nonusers.

TABLE 1. *Summary of epidemiologic analyses of association between oral contraceptive use, benign breast disease, and cancer*

| Type of study[a] | Disease[b] | No. of cases | Relative risk of disease by years of OC use[c] | | | | | | Does effect persist after stopping OCs | Association between disease and | |
			0	0–1	1–2	2–3	3–4	4+		Late age at first delivery	Low parity
Benign breast disease											
Hospital-based case-control (1)	BBD	255	1.0		←1.0→		←0.3→		No	Yes	N/A
Hospital-based case-control (2)	CCD	300	1.0		←1.3→		←0.5→		N/A	Yes	No
	FAD	73	1.0		←1.0→		←1.8→		N/A	Yes	Yes
Hospital-based case-control (3)	BBD	98	1.0			←0.5→			N/A	N/A	N/A
Practice-based cohort (4)	BBD	859	1.0	0.9	0.9	0.8	0.6	0.5	N/A	N/A	N/A
Hospital-based case-control (5)	CCD	209	1.0	1.3	1.0		←0.5→		N/A	No	Yes
	FAD	123	1.0	1.2	1.0		←0.6→		N/A	No	Yes
Hospital-based case-control (6)	BBD	446	1.0		←1.4→		←0.4→	0.5	Yes/no	No	Yes
Population-based cohort (7)	CCD	499	1.0	0.9	0.7		←0.4→		Yes	No	Yes
	FAD	83	1.0		←1.2→		←0.5→				
Malignant breast disease											
Hospital-based case-control (1)	Cancer	90	1.0			No increased risk			N/A	Yes	N/A
Hospital-based case-control (3)	Cancer	23	1.0			No increased risk			N/A	N/A	N/A
Practice-based cohort (4)	Cancer	23	1.0			←1.1→			N/A	N/A	N/A
Hospital-based case-control (8)	Cancer	322	1.0			←1.0→			N/A	N/A	N/A
Hospital-based case-control (6)	Cancer	452	1.0		←1.5→		←2.5→	1.3	No	Yes	Yes
Population-based cohort (7)	Cancer	137	1.0		←0.7→		←0.7→		N/A	Yes	No

[a] Numbers in parentheses are references.
[b] BBD = all benign breast diseases.
    CCD = chronic cystic disease of the breast.
    FAD = fibroadenoma.
[c] The risk in nonusers is set to 1.0. OC = oral contraceptive.

In the three studies that looked at whether this protective effect persisted after stopping oral contraceptive use, differing conclusions were reached. Vessey et al. found the effect did not persist (1); we found it did persist (7); and Fasal and Paffenbarger (6) found mixed results depending on how they analyzed the data. I have no basis for hypothesizing an explanation for these differences.

The relationship between oral contraceptive use and risk of breast cancer is less well studied than that of oral contraceptive use and benign breast disease. In general, for up to 4 years' duration of oral contraceptive use there is no increased risk of breast cancer. However, Fasal and Paffenbarger (6) show that oral contraceptive use of 2–4 years' duration increases the risk of breast cancer 2.5 times over that of nonusers. One explanation of this is that they stratified their data many different ways and performed multiple statistical tests, thus making this result a chance finding. Another possible explanation is based on the differential oral contraceptive use by their medical and surgical control groups. The medical controls were less likely to use oral contraceptives than the surgical group (see Table 4 in their report). It appears likely that this finding would be weakened if only surgical controls were used.

Another intriguing finding of the Fasal and Paffenbarger report (6) is the 11-fold increased risk of breast cancer for women who had used oral contraceptives for 6 years or more and who had a history of "prior biopsy for benign breast disease." However, the 11-fold risk must be based on small numbers because I calculated an approximate 95% confidence interval extending from 1.1 to 112 (9). On the other hand, Hoover observed a similar increased risk of breast cancer for postmenopausal women using estrogen who developed benign disease while on long-term estrogen therapy (10). These associations must be confirmed (or refuted) before any conclusions can be drawn. The bulk of the evidence to date suggests that oral contraceptive use of up to 4 years' duration is not associated with any increased risk of breast cancer.

The studies (1,6–8) which examine the association between breast cancer and "age of first delivery" found results supporting the inverse association described by MacMahon et al. (11). With respect to the association between breast cancer and low parity, the two studies (6,7) that looked at this association yielded conflicting results. The studies (1–7) examining the association between benign breast disease and pregnancy-related events suggest there is some association, the nature of which remains to be clarified.

I believe the decreased risk of benign breast disease for oral contraceptive users is well demonstrated and is an association of cause and effect. This should result in fewer hospitalizations for oral contraceptive users. A small amount of evidence suggests that women with persistent chronic fibrocystic breast disease have a substantially increased risk of developing breast cancer (12,13). However, not all types of fibrocystic disease are associated with increased risk of breast cancer (12). It is possible that the types of fibrocystic diseases not prevented by oral contraceptives could be the types that become malignant.

This suggests an area for further study: identification of those types of benign breast disease whose incidence is reduced in oral contraceptive users. This would begin to answer the question of whether oral contraceptives are preventing the types of fibrocystic disease that have malignant potential. Only a long-term follow-up of the natural history of benign breast disease in oral contraceptive users could firmly resolve the issue.

There is substantial evidence that short-term use of oral contraceptives (up to 4 years) does not promote the development of an already existing malignancy. However, one published report suggests the opposite (6). There are no epidemiologic data on the long-term effects of oral contraceptive use on the breast. On the basis of the fibrocystic disease data, it appears that a minimum of 2 years of oral contraceptive use is necessary to induce an effect on the breast. If this effect is induction of carcinoma, at least 10 (and probably 20) years must lapse before a final conclusion can be reached. Considering that oral contraceptives came into common usage in the United States during the late 1960s, it will probably be the mid-1980s before we begin to know their long-term effects on the breast.

Future studies of the association between use of oral contraceptives and breast cancer should take into account the now well-documented association of "late age at first birth" and increased risk of breast cancer. All contraceptives, if used early in life, can delay the age of first birth. In this sense, there may be a cost of increased breast cancer incidence as women in the United States continue to delay having their first child. The differential effect on breast cancer risk of delaying first birth with oral contraceptive use compared with other methods of contraception remains to be determined. Oral contraceptives could hormonally substitute for pregnancy and confer the benefits of early pregnancy on women who use them at a young age. Alternatively, they could have a more harmful effect than that of delaying "age at first birth" with a nonhormonal contraceptive. It seems appropriate to consider this issue as we undertake new studies on the oral contraceptive–breast cancer relationship.

SUMMARY

Published reports touching on the association of oral contraceptive use and benign and malignant breast diseases are reviewed. Oral contraceptive use appears to decrease the risk of benign breast disease by approximately 50% for women who meet both of the following conditions: (a) They are free of benign breast diseases (or a history of same) when they initiate oral contraceptive use; and (b) they continue oral contraceptive use for 2 years or more. In addition, the limited evidence available suggests that there is no association between oral contraceptive use and breast cancer. Future studies should: (a) identify those specific histologic types of benign breast disease that are reduced by oral contraceptive use; and (b) examine the interaction between delay of "age at first birth," contraception, and breast cancer.

REFERENCES

1. Vessey, M. P., Doll, R., and Sutton, P. M. (1972): Oral contraceptives and breast neoplasia: A retrospective study. *Br. Med. J.,* 3:719–724.
2. Sartwell, P. E., Arthes, F. G., and Tonscia, J. A. (1973): Epidemiology of benign breast lesions: Lack of association with oral contraceptive use. *N. Engl. J. Med.,* 288:551–554.
3. Boston Collaborative Drug Surveillance Program (Greenblatt, D. J., Ory, H. W., and Levy, M.) (1973): Oral contraceptives and venous thromboembolic disease, surgically confirmed gallbladder disease, and breast tumors. *Lancet,* 2:1399–1404.
4. Royal College of General Practitioners (1974): *Oral Contraceptives and Health.* Pitman, New York.
5. Kelsey, J. L., Lindfors, K. K., and White, C. (1974): A case control study of the epidemiology of benign breast diseases with reference to oral contraceptive use. *Int. J. Epidemiol.,* 3:333–340.
6. Fasal, E., and Paffenbarger, R. S. (1975): Oral contraceptives as related to cancer and benign lesions of the breast. *J. Natl. Cancer Inst.,* 55:767–773.
7. Ory, H. W., Cole, P., MacMahon, B., and Hoover, R. (1976): Oral contraceptives and reduced risk of benign breast diseases. *N. Engl. J. Med.,* 294:419–422.
8. Vessey, M. P., Doll, R., and Jones, K. (1975): Oral contraceptives and breast cancer. *Lancet,* 2:941–944.
9. Miettinen, O. S. (1974): Simple interval estimation of risk ratio (abstract). *Am. J. Epidemiol.,* 100: 515–516.
10. Hoover, R., Gray, L. A., Cole, P., et al. (1976): Menopausal estrogens and breast cancer. *N. Engl. J. Med.,* 295:401–405.
11. MacMahon, B., Cole, P., and Brown, J. (1973): Etiology of human breast cancer: A review. *J. Natl. Cancer Inst.,* 50:21–42.
12. Monson, R. R., Yen, S., and MacMahon, B. (1976): Chronic mastitis and carcinoma of the breast. *Lancet,* 2:224–226.
13. Donnelly, P. K., Baker, K. W., Carney, J. A., and O'Fallon, W. M. (1975): Benign breast lesions and subsequent breast carcinoma in Rochester, Minnesota. *Mayo Clin. Proc.,* 50:650–656.

Pharmacology of Steroid Contraceptive Drugs
edited by S. Garattini and H. W. Berendes.
Raven Press, New York © 1977.

Pathologic Changes in Mammary Glands and Uteri from Beagle Bitches Receiving Low Levels of Medroxyprogesterone Acetate: An Overview of Research in Progress

Edward H. Fowler, Thurma Vaughan, Frances Gotcsik, Patricia Reichhart, and Carolyn Reed

University of Rochester Cancer Center, Division of Laboratory Animal Medicine, and Department of Pathology, University of Rochester School of Medicine and Dentistry, Rochester, New York 14642

Canine mammary glands and uteri, recognized as target organs for steroid hormones, develop pathologic changes in bitches exposed to high levels of synthetic progestins (3,12,18,22,23,30), progesterone (7), or synthetic estrogens (18,30) administered either to prevent ovulation *per se* (3) or as part of a drug-testing program (7,12,18,22,23,30). The latter finding has evoked much interest in canine mammary glands and uterine pathophysiology during recent years and is the stimulus for this research. Our primary objective is to elucidate the nature and pathogenesis of the changes produced in these two target organs by low doses of one of the synthetic progestins, medroxyprogesterone acetate (MPA), administered at levels below, near, and above an ovulation-suppressing dose.

MATERIALS AND METHODS

One hundred and four beagle bitches 6–14 months old having shown evidence of at least one estrous cycle were purchased from a commercial breeder, housed in stainless steel cages in a controlled environment with a 12-hr light-dark cycle, and fed a commercial lab chow *ad libidum,* supplemented occasionally with canned meat if weight loss or periodic anorexia was noted. Vaginal smears were obtained weekly on all bitches; a dry sterile cotton swab was used to obtain the specimen, which was then rotated onto a cleaned glass slide, immediately fixed in equal parts of ether and 95% ethanol, and stained with the Papanicolaou procedure. The stages of estrus were determined using established criteria (14). Mammary glands and uteri were obtained from 26 control bitches during anestrus, proestrus, estrus, metestrus, pregnancy, pseudopregnancy, and lactation.

Three groups of 26 bitches were injected intramuscularly with MPA every 13 weeks at dosages of 0.3, 1.5, and 3.0 mg/kg, which, respectively, are below the dose necessary to suppress ovulation, near the ovulation-suppressing dose, and above the ovulation-suppressing dose. Only five of the 1.5 mg/kg dosage group have cycled thus far, whereas all of the low-dose bitches have cycled approximately as many times as the controls. Mammary glands were obtained at 3, 6, 9, 12, 15, 19, 24, 32, and 40 months postinjection, and uteri were obtained at 4, 8, 12, 16, 22, 30, and 38 months postinjection.

Mammary glands were usually removed from one of the posterior two pairs, but occasionally a gland from the middle (anterior abdominal) pair was used. Either one-half or an entire uterine horn was removed. Biopsies were performed following preanesthesia with atropine, initial anesthesia with Surital, and maintenance with halothane.

Tissues were immediately placed in cold Hank's balanced salt solution for transportation to another laboratory for processing. Samples fixed in Carnoy's fixative were subsequently paraffin-embedded, sectioned, and stained with hematoxylin and eosin, periodic acid-Schiff (21) controlled with amylase digestion of glycogen (20), and methyl green-pyronin (27) for demonstration of RNA and DNA. Other histologic and histochemical techniques were performed when required. Additional samples were fixed in cold formol-calcium and stored in cold gum sucrose for subsequent cryostat sectioning at 8 μm, incubation for acid phosphatase activity (1), and staining with hematoxylin and eosin. Other samples were frozen and stored in liquid nitrogen and subsequently cryostat-sectioned at 10 μm for demonstration of free lipid (8), alkaline phosphatase (5), glucose-6-phosphate dehydrogenase activity (9), α-glycerophosphate dehydrogenase activity (29), lactate dehydrogenase activity (9), NAD and NADP cytochrome C reductase activities (9), and staining with hematoxylin and eosin. Minced tissue fragments were fixed in 4% glutaraldehyde, postfixed in osmium tetroxide, embedded in Epon (19), sectioned, and stained with uranyl acetate and lead citrate (24) for ultrastructural evaluation.

Some of the morphologic, histochemical, and ultrastructural evaluations were coded on computer forms and included in a computer file on each animal so comparisons can be made between parameters and with different stages of estrus. Clinical information, including weight and vaginal cytologic evaluation, was also coded and included in the files on each animal. Genetic information and previous clinical data relating to the genital system for both sire and dam were obtained for each bitch and were used to open each file; these may prove useful for comparisons between bitches.

RESULTS

Mammary Glands from Control Bitches

Mammary gland *morphology* changed considerably during the estrous cycle, reflected by a change in lobular size and the appearance of epithelium, myoepithelium, and lobular connective tissue within individual lobules. We computed these data as percent gland in each piece of tissue and general activity using a

TABLE 1. *Percent gland and general activity in control mammary glands*

Stage of estrus	No. of bitches	No. of tissues[a]	% Gland (mean)	Activity[b] (mean)
Anestrus	10	34	30.0	1.5
Proestrus	4	14	26.2	1.4
Estrus	5	31	19.1	1.7
Early metestrus	3	9	15.0	2.0
Late metestrus	3	16	43.3	2.8
Pregnant	3	10	48.0	3.1
Pseudopregnant	2	2	60.0	4.0
Early lactation	2	6	85.0	4.5
Midlactation	3	8	88.1	4.8
Late lactation	2	8	86.4	5.0

[a] More than one piece of mammary gland was examined from each biopsy.
[b] Activity was rated on a 5-point scale where 1 = involuted and 5 = very active (e.g., lactating).

5-point scale: from involuted (score 1) to very active, e.g., lactating (score 5) (Table 1).

The glands became progressively more involuted during *anestrus* until each lobule appeared as a small cluster of collapsed alveoli and ductules embedded in dense connective tissue containing numerous pigment-laden macrophages and scattered mononuclear inflammatory cells. Interlobular ducts appeared either collapsed or dilated and filled with acidophilic material. The gland consisted primarily of interlobular connective tissue and fat, with occasional foci of lymphocytes and plasma cells adjacent to the ducts.

During *proestrus* and *estrus* there were few apparent histologic changes in the gland. The methyl green-pyronin procedure illustrated that the amount of cytoplasmic RNA increased in the alveolar epithelial cells during these periods. Occasionally a gland began to proliferate during estrus. Glycogen generally increased in the alveolar and ductular epithelial cells prior to the proliferative phase.

Metestrus was the most active period of growth and regression. Mitotic figures were numerous in ducts, ductules, and alveoli during the first 4 weeks of metestrus as the alveolar number increased in each lobule. During this phase the lobular connective tissue appeared loose and immature. By the 5th week of metestrus alveoli were nearly all formed, and lumina containing homogeneous acidophilic material were usually seen (Fig. 1A). Ducts were collapsed during early metestrus and began to dilate as acidophilic material formed in the alveolar epithelium. The latter contained much stainable RNA, little glycogen, and no lipid during early metestrus. Ductules were indistinguishable from alveoli at this stage. During late metestrus alveolar epithelium began to accumulate lipid in large amounts, whereas ductular epithelium could be distinguished by its lack of stainable lipid. Lipid accumulation accompanied involutionary changes, and central alveoli of a lobule appeared to involute first. At the end of metestrus peripheral alveoli in lobules were the only ones which possessed stainable lipid, and central alveoli

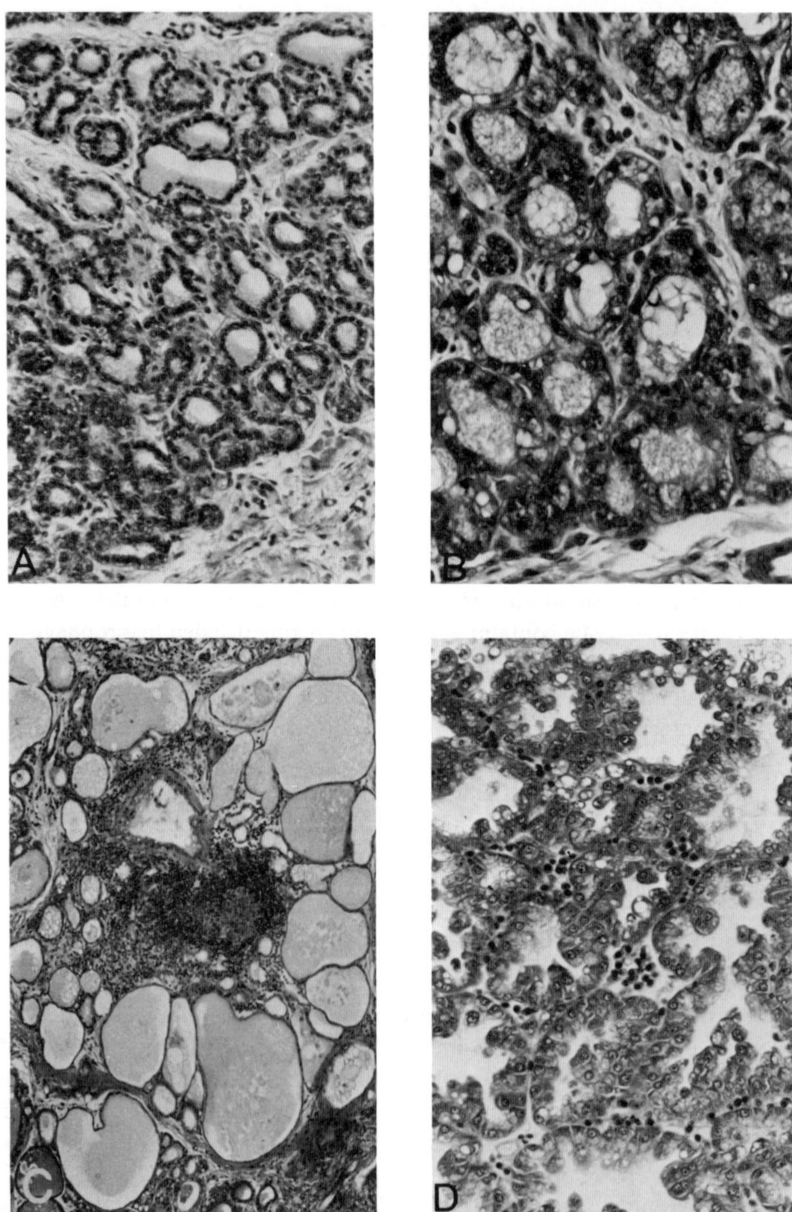

FIG. 1. A: Well-developed mammary gland lobule from a control bitch in metestrus. The alveoli, lined by cuboidal epithelial cells, contain some acidophilic secretion. H & E. ×210. B: Secretory alveoli lined by very active epithelium in a control lactating mammary gland. H & E. ×340. C: Lymph nodule in the center of a mammary gland lobule composed of extensively dilated alveoli from a bitch treated 32 months with MPA 3.0 mg/kg. H & E. ×85. D: Active epithelial cells lining alveoli from a hypersecretory lobule found in a mammary gland removed from a bitch treated 19 months with MPA 3.0 mg/kg. H & E. ×210.

appeared collapsed. Glycogen increased during involution. At the height of activity the lobular connective tissue contained virtually no pigment-laden macrophages and only little inflammation, both of which increased during involution.

During *pregnancy* the gland continued to proliferate beyond the 4th week of metestrus. Each lobule possessed many patent alveoli that contained a small amount of acidophilic material. *Lactating* glands contained large lobules composed of large secretory alveoli containing basophilic material and lipid (Fig. 1B). Involuting lactational glands had abundant hyalinized lobule connective tissues containing much basement membrane material, collagen, mononuclear inflammatory cells, and pigment-laden macrophages.

Control glands occasionally had a few lobules that appeared quite different from other lobules in the gland. These lobules contained: dilated alveoli and ductules filled with acidophilic material which sometimes had undergone inspissation and mineralization; hypersecretory lobules composed of large alveoli and ductules lined by tall, active-appearing epithelium that contained lipid droplets, the lumina of which contained lipid and basophilic material similar to that seen in lactation; increased infiltration of mononuclear inflammatory cells into the connective tissue sometimes nearly replacing the epithelium; and bridging of epithelium across some ducts.

Ultrastructural changes in mammary glands during the estrous cycle were significant. Involuted *anestrous* glands contained epithelial cells with much nuclear heterochromatin and virtually no active organelles in the cytoplasm (Fig. 2A). *Proestrous* and *estrous* gland nuclei appeared more euchromatic with prominent nucleoli, and the cytoplasm contained many free ribosomes, polysomes, and increased numbers of active mitochondria.

Early metestrous and *midpregnant* glands had more developed rough endoplasmic reticulum (rER), sometimes containing lightly osmiophilic secretory product and a well-developed but nonfunctional Golgi apparatus. As the rER developed, the nuclei appeared less active. During *late metestrus,* as cells began to involute, cytoplasmic lipid and glycogen increased, free ribosomes and rER decreased, mitochondria became swollen or condensed, nuclear envelope and other membranes sometimes dilated, and lysosomes and pigment granules increased. Macrophages and lymphocytes were often present between epithelial cells or were free in the lumina. Plasma cells were present in lobular connective tissue.

Lactating gland rER greatly increased and formed parallel arrays. The Golgi apparatus was large and sometimes contained dense osmiophilic material resembling casein micelles (Fig. 2B). During late lactation cytoplasmic lipid droplets increased significantly. No glycogen was found in the lactating gland.

Histochemically demonstrable *acid phosphatase* (AcP) activity was never very strong in mammary glands. Alveolar and ductular epithelia possessed only moderate AcP activity even during the most active involution. After involution was completed or during active stages of the cycle, no lysosomes could be demonstrated in these epithelia. Myoepithelial cells were consistently more reactive than epithelia in all stages of estrus as well as in all dosage groups. Macrophages were

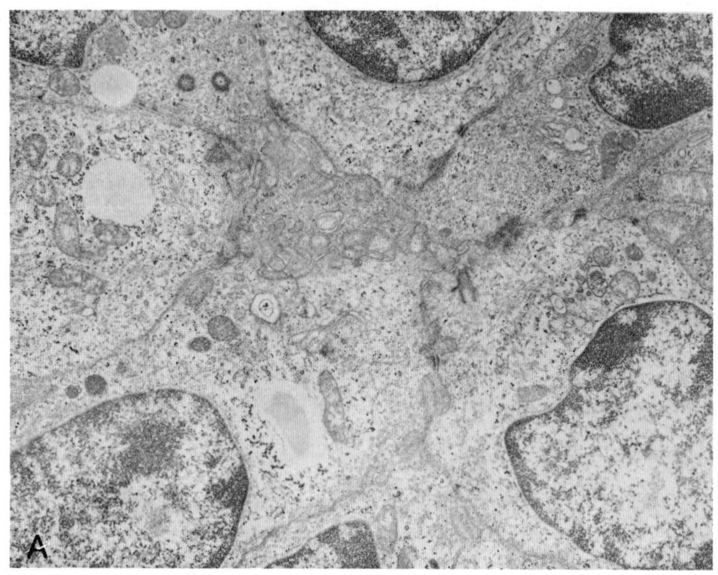

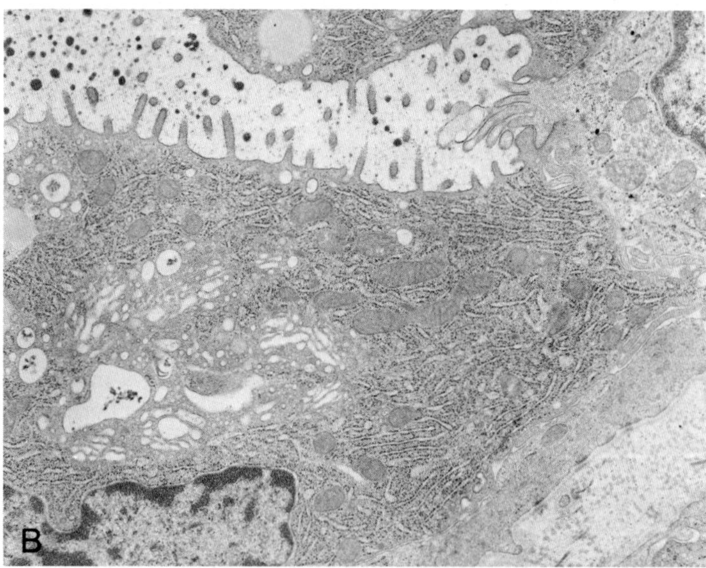

FIG. 2. A: Inactive epithelial cells lining a collapsed alveolus in an anestrous control mammary gland. ×8,925. **B:** Very active alveolar epithelial cells secreting casein into the lumen of an alveolus from a lactating control mammary gland. ×8,925.

demonstrable between duct or alveolar epithelial cells during proliferative stages and were found in the lumina of alveoli and ducts during involution. AcP activity in these cells was strong (3+) to intense (4+). During proliferation the immature connective tissues in the lobules showed weak (1+) AcP activity. Otherwise the connective tissues were unreactive.

Alkaline phosphatase (AlP) activity was demonstrable in myoepithelial cells surrounding alveoli, ductules, and ducts. Myoepithelial cells were multilayered around the ducts, single-layered and continuous around small alveoli, or discontinuous around dilated alveoli. AlP activity was generally moderate (2+) to strong (3+) around alveoli and ductules and increased to intense (4+) during active stages of proliferation and development. In involuted alveoli the only cells demonstrable in many lobules were small clumps of AlP-positive myoepithelial cells. Capillaries in lobular connective tissue of proliferating and active glands were also AlP-positive.

Histochemically demonstrable *dehydrogenases* varied with the stage of estrus. In involuted glands glucose-6-phosphate dehydrogenase (G6PD) activity in all epithelia was weak (1+) to moderate (2+). Alveoli were less reactive than ductules or ducts. During estrus, early metestrus, pregnancy, and lactation, G6PD activity in these cells became strong (3+) to intense (4+) and was also present in adjacent connective tissues. α-Glycerophosphate (α-GPD) activity occurred in alveoli (1+) and ducts (2+) of involuted glands, but as the gland became active the alveolar activity diminished and was nonexistent except in occasional cells in lobular connective tissue or myoepithelia. Duct activity remained the same or became more intense, especially in myoepithelial cells. Lactate dehydrogenase (LDH) activity was generally strong in most epithelia and lobular connective tissues but increased during active stages of development and involution.

Mammary Glands from MPA-Treated Bitches

MPA delayed involution and stimulated activity depending on the dosage level and length of administration (Table 2). Lobular size was increased, and abnormalities in lobular development occurred. The 0.3 mg/kg group continued to cycle, and fluctuation in lobular size and activity is evident (Table 2). It should also be noted that MPA was administered every 3 months, and biopsies removed at 12, 15, and 24 months coincided with the end of the 3-month interval, whereas those removed at 19, 32, and 40 months were removed 1, 2, and 1 month, respectively, after MPA administration. The shorter intervals after drug administration were characterized by increased mitotic activity in alveolar and ductular epithelia, but alveoli were smaller and contained less secretory product than was seen 3 months after drug administration. The largest lobules and most glandular activity were found in glands removed from the two higher-dosage groups 2 months after MPA injection (32 months). In all groups there was evidence of cyclic activity due to drug administration, but only in the 0.3 mg/kg group was there evidence of much cyclic variation due to different estrous cycles. Occasion-

TABLE 2. *Percent gland and general activity in mammary glands of MPA-treated bitches*

Months post injection	MPA 0.3 mg/kg				MPA 1.5 mg/kg				MPA 3.0 mg/kg			
	No. of bitches	No. of tissues[a]	% Gland (mean)	Activity[b] (mean)	No. of bitches	No. of tissues[a]	% Gland (mean)	Activity[b] (mean)	No. of bitches	No. of tissues[a]	% Gland (mean)	Activity[b] (mean)
12	6	8	36.6	2.5	8	9	37.6	2.6	8	10	56.0	3.0
15	10	21	52.6	2.0	10	20	46.2	2.6	8	15	51.7	2.8
19	9	20	31.5	2.2	8	17	36.5	2.6	7	13	54.6	2.7
24	10	72	46.7	2.3	10	63	48.2	2.6	10	75	64.1	3.3
32	10	73	50.9	2.7	9	78	71.4	3.7	9	65	73.3	3.4
40	2	14	61.0	3.0	2	13	55.0	3.0	3	19	63.4	3.0
Total	47	208	47.9	2.5	47	200	55.9	3.0	45	199	65.2	3.2

[a] More than one piece of mammary gland was examined on most bitches.
[b] Activity was rated on a 5-point scale where 1 = involuted and 5 = very active (e.g., lactating).

ally one of the 1.5 mg/kg bitches cycled, and morphologic changes in the mammary gland reflected this cyclic activity. Most of the 1.5 mg/kg and all of the 3.0 mg/kg bitches were in anestrus from the outset.

Morphologic changes in mammary glands of MPA-treated bitches were quantitatively and qualitatively different from controls. Quantitative differences included: variation in lobular size, inflammation in lobular connective tissue, dilatation of alveoli and ductules with homogeneous acidophilic secretory material (Fig. 1C), hypersecretory lobules containing secretory dilated alveoli (Fig. 1D), inspissation and mineralization of luminal contents, duct hyperplasia, bridging of epithelium across lumina of ducts and ductules that were beginning to dilate with acidophilic material, and focal accumulation of lymphocytes and plasma cells adjacent to ducts. The above changes were dose- and time-related in that they appeared earlier and more frequently in the higher-dosage groups. Small to moderate involuted lobules in the 1.5 and 3.0 mg/kg groups were negligible at 40 months postinjection, whereas such lobules could still be found in the 0.3 mg/kg group.

Lesions in mammary glands of MPA-treated bitches that were qualitatively different from controls included lobular epitheliosis, adenomas (Figs. 3A and B), mixed mammary tumors (Fig. 3C), and an intraductal papilloma (Fig. 3D) found in glands from the two highest-dosage groups but not in the 0.3 mg/kg group (Table 3). Neoplasms were few but striking when encountered. Epitheliosis occurred much more frequently, especially in the highest-dosage group, but is not included in Table 3.

Ultrastructural changes of glands from MPA-treated bitches reflected increased stimulation. Nuclei were less involuted in many glands, and the cytoplasm contained more free ribosomes and rER than was found in anestrous controls. Glycogen and lipid were often present in the cells. The 0.3 mg/kg bitches had glands that reflected cyclic variation of estrus, except that involution was delayed in anestrous glands and the proliferative stage was lengthened in metestrous glands. Casein micelles were seen in one anestrous gland at 3 months postinjection, a feature not seen in controls except during lactation. Large digestive vacuoles were present in many gland epithelia. During estrus in one bitch 9 months postinjection there was evidence of rER development and a cilium was seen. More macrophages and lymphocytes were present than were found in controls. Occasionally whorls of endoplasmic reticulum (ER) were found in the alveolar epithelial cells, and many myelin figures were seen within and even between cells.

Anestrous glands of the *1.5 mg/kg* and *3.0 mg/kg* groups appeared much more active than corresponding controls, with many free ribosomes, rER-containing secretion (Fig. 4A), and a larger, more active Golgi apparatus. Glycogen and lipid were usually present in many cells, sometimes in excessive amounts. Myoepithelial cells in a mixed tumor were producing not only excessive basement membrane material (Fig. 4B) but also fibrils resembling collagen and organized material in the intercellular space resembling cartilage. Cells containing whorls of ER,

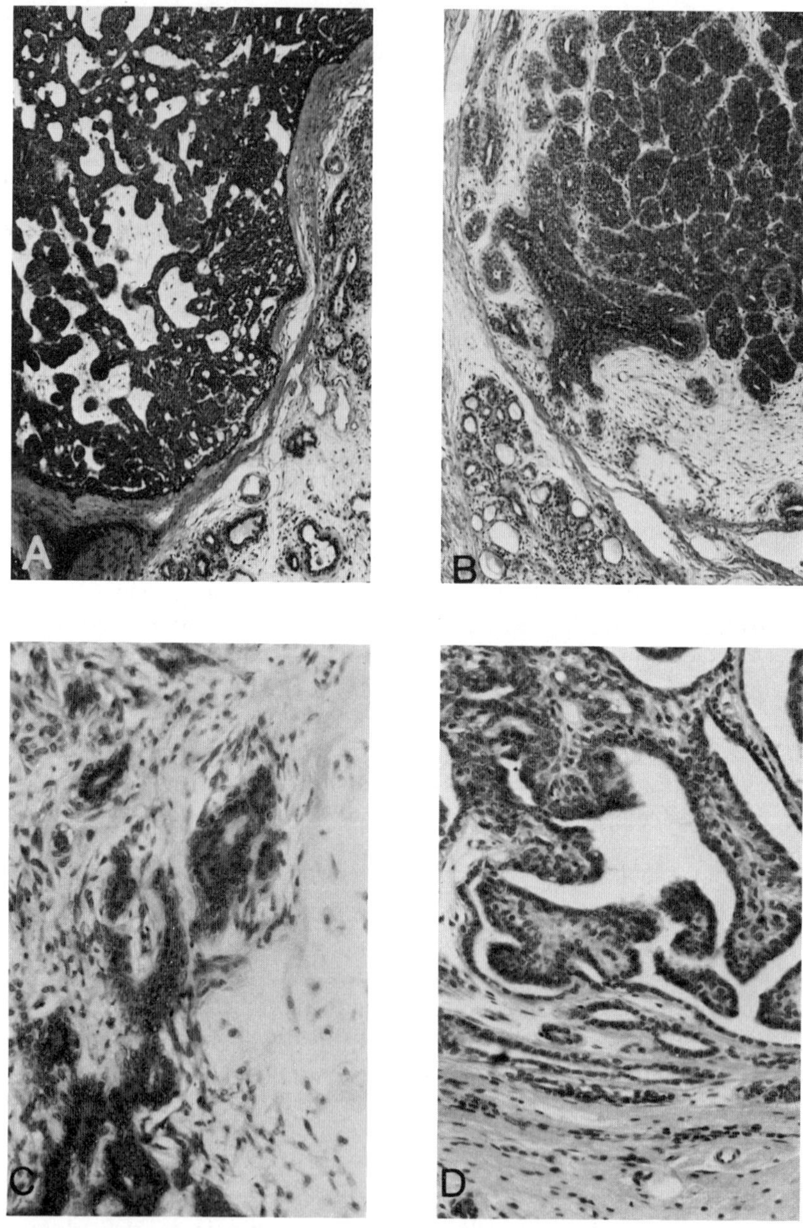

FIG. 3. A: Fibroadenoma found in the mammary gland of a bitch treated 40 months with MPA 3.0 mg/kg. H & E. X85. **B:** Adenoma present in the mammary gland of a bitch treated 40 months with MPA 3.0 mg/kg. H & E. X85. **C:** Mixed tumor present in the mammary gland of a bitch treated 32 months with MPA 1.5 mg/kg. H & E. X210. **D:** Intraductal papilloma present in the mammary gland of a bitch treated 24 months with MPA 3.0 mg/kg. H & E. X210.

TABLE 3. *Neoplastic and hyperplastic lesions in mammary glands of MPA-treated bitches*

Months postinjection	Lesion[a]		
	MPA 0.3 mg/kg	MPA 1.5 mg/kg	MPA 3.0 mg/kg
9			3 HsL
12			1 HsL
15		2 HsL	2 HsL
19		1 HsL	1 HsL
24	1 HsL	1 HsL	1 IdP, 1 HsL, 1 MT
32	1 HsL	2 MT, 1 HsL	1 DA, 4 HsL
40		1 HsL	1 FA, 1 LA

[a] HsL, hypersecretory lobules. IdP, Intraductal papilloma. MT, mixed tumor. DA, duct adenoma. FA, fibroadenoma. LA, lobular adenoma.

cilia, and large digestive vacuoles similar to those seen in the 0.3 mg group were found in the higher-dosage groups.

Acid phosphatase activity in mammary glands of MPA-treated bitches was generally greater in involuting alveoli of the 0.3 mg/kg groups, but was minimal (1+) to occasionally moderate (2+) in alveolar and duct epithelia of the higher-dosage groups. This activity was similar to late-metestrous controls, which is how the cells appeared ultrastructurally. Occasional macrophages were encountered in alveolar and duct lumina as described in control glands. Secretory epithelium in alveoli of some lobules and in hypersecretory lobules was negative for AcP activity. There was more variation in AcP activity than in the controls, which reflected the variability in lobular development. Epithelial cells in the mixed tumor were strongly reactive for AcP activity (Fig. 5A).

Alkaline phosphatase activity increased in myoepithelial cells in MPA-treated bitches compared with anestrous controls, which reflected increased activity in alveoli and ducts. Involuted alveoli present in some lobules were similar to those found in control anestrous glands, but many lobules contained secretory alveoli surrounded by 4+ myoepithelial cells. Hyperplastic ducts often had AlP-positive cells in their lumina resulting from myoepithelial cells undergoing hyperplasia along with epithelial cells and being carried into lumina with papillary infoldings. Myoepithelial cells of the mixed mammary tumor had greatly reduced AlP activity compared to normal myoepithelial cells, and some areas were negative (Fig. 5B).

Dehydrogenase activity was generally increased in mammary glands from MPA-treated bitches. Secretory alveoli had intense G6PD activity (Fig. 5C), and virtually no α-GPD activity, whereas involuted alveoli in the same lobules reacted quite differently, resulting in a patchy distribution in most glands, especially those from the higher-dosage groups. There was even greater G6PD activity in some glands than was seen in control glands at any time other than during lactation (Fig. 5C). Duct hyperplasia was characterized by intense α-GPD

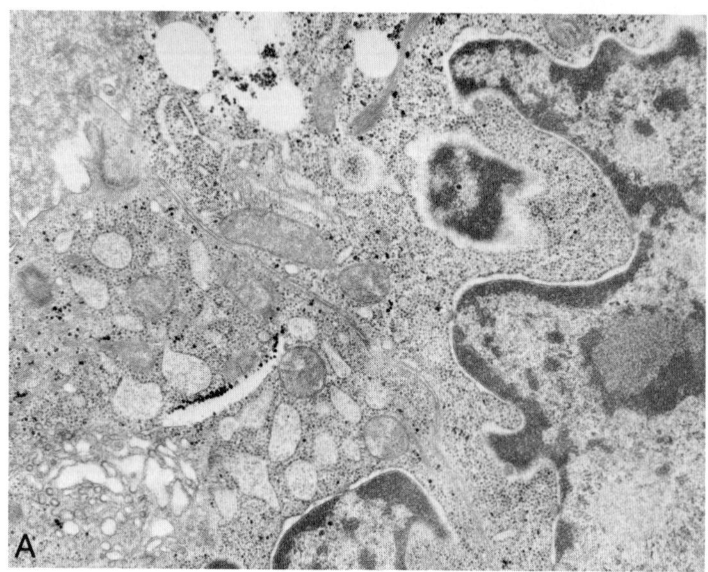

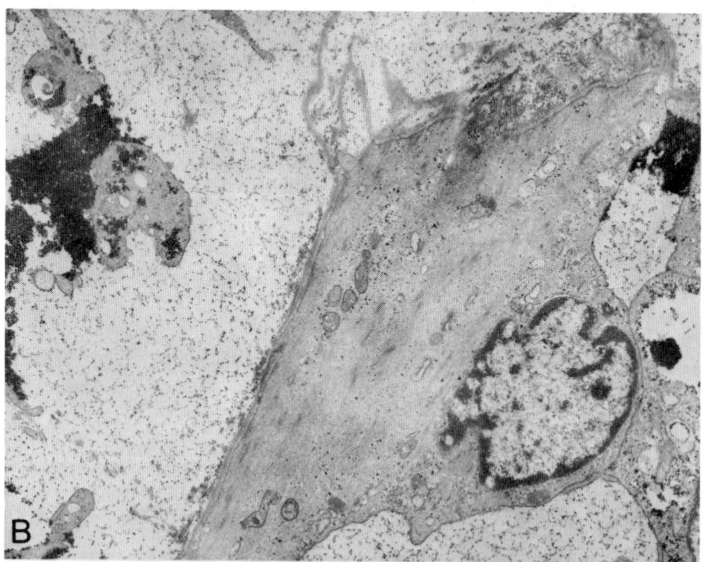

FIG. 4. A: Active rER containing lightly stained material in alveolar epithelial cell from a mammary gland removed from a bitch 15 months after treatment with MPA 3.0 mg/kg. X16,362. **B:** Neoplastic myoepithelial cells surrounded by basement membrane material from a mixed tumor present in the mammary gland of a bitch treated 32 months with MPA 1.5 mg/kg. X8,925.

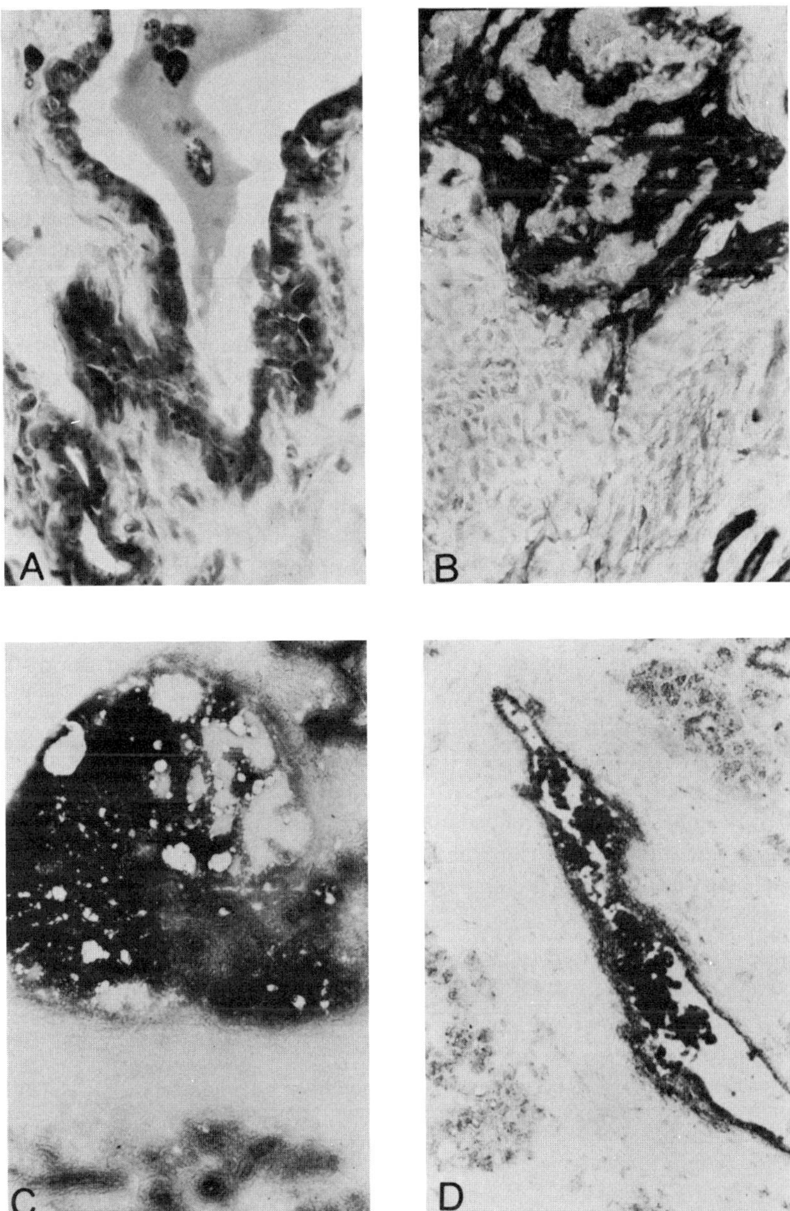

FIG. 5. A: Strong AcP activity in the duct epithelium of a mixed mammary tumor (as in Figs. 2C and 4B). AcP. X340. **B:** AIP activity in some myoepithelium and not in other cells of a mixed mammary tumor (as in Figs. 2C, 4A, and 5A). AIP. X210. **C:** Intense G6PD activity in a hypersecretory lobule in the mammary gland from a bitch treated 9 months with MPA 3.0 mg/kg. G6PD. X85. **D:** Intense α-GPD activity in hyperplastic duct epithelium in a mammary gland removed from the same bitch as in C. α-GPD. X85.

activity (Fig. 5D). LDH, NADP, and NAD cytochrome C reductase were increased in hypersecretory lobules and neoplasm, and more reactive than in involuted control glands.

Uteri from Control Bitches

Endometrial glandular development and endometrial activity were evaluated at different stages of the estrous cycle, during pregnancy, and postpartum in control uteri (Table 4). Proestrus, estrus, and early metestrus were the most active periods during a normal cycle, but pregnant and early postpartum uteri were even more active than those in other stages. Pseudopregnancy was not sufficiently evaluated in control bitches to make any firm statements, but it appeared that endometrial activity and gland development were at least as great as in the more active stages of the cycle and greater than were found during late metestrus or anestrus.

The *morphologic* appearance of anestrous uteri was characterized by markedly involuted endometrium containing a few small collapsed glands embedded in dense stroma and lined by flattened to low cuboidal epithelium. Small gland lumina often contained densely acidophilic material. The uterine cavity, which often was totally collapsed, was lined by cuboidal to low columnar epithelium containing large lipid droplets during early anestrus and no lipid during late anestrus. The myometrial layers were quite involuted and appeared very cellular owing to the reduction of cytoplasmic volume.

Proestrus was characterized by a tremendous increase in both number and size of glands as well as thicker endometrium due to stromal increase. During this proliferative phase, which extended into *estrus,* many mitotic figures were present in glands and the myometrium underwent initial hypertrophic changes. The uterine cavity still remained collapsed and occasionally was adherent from side

TABLE 4. *Endometrial glandular development and activity during estrus, pregnancy, and postpartum in control bitches*

Stage of estrus	No. of bitches	No. of tissues	Gland development[a] (mean)	Activity[b] (mean)
Anestrus	4	9	1.3	1.6
Proestrus	2	4	3.5	3.0
Estrus	2	8	3.9	3.0
Early metestrus	1	1	6.0	4.0
Late metestrus	1	2	2.0	3.0
Pregnancy	3	10	8.7	5.0
Pseudopregnancy	1	1	4.0	3.0
Early postpartum	1	2	6.0	4.5
3 Weeks postpartum	2	4	4.3	3.5

[a] Glandular development: score of 1 (small and few) to 6 (large and many) and 9 (pregnant).
[b] Activity: score of 1 (inactive) to 5 (very active—pregnant).

to side. Cells lining the cavity also increased in number and size. The proliferative stage reached its maximum during *early metestrus* (Fig. 6A), at which time the surface epithelium and lining of the upper glands began to appear secretory. Secretory epithelium was characterized by nuclear migration toward cell apices, usually residing approximately midway between base and apex, and the abundant homogeneous acidophilic cytoplasm changing to a more vacuolated lacy appearance. Involution began fairly quickly if implantation did not occur and by 7 weeks had progressed considerably (Fig. 6B). Deep glands involuted more quickly than surface and upper glands, which retained much lipid in their cytoplasm. Involuting deep glands were dilated and often contained considerable granular acidophilic material in their lumina. The lining epithelium was quite flattened, however.

Pregnancy was characterized by great changes in endometrial morphology. The surface of the endometrium became very villous, and these villi, lined by tall columnar epithelium, projected into the uterine cavity and supported the fetal portion of the placenta at placental-attachment sites. Underlying the villi was a region of very active endometrial stroma, which was virtually gland-free. Deep glands were numerous, dilated, and lined by cuboidal epithelium. The myometrium appeared extremely hypertrophic.

Early *postpartum* uteri resembled pregnant uteri at placental-attachment sites, except that there was hyalinization of stroma accompanied by extensive inflammatory cell infiltrate and lipid accumulation in epithelial cells lining the villi. Deep glands remained dilated and were filled with debris. Late postpartum, hyalinized material was present in the uterine cavity and pigment-laden macrophages were often very numerous in the endometrial stroma. *Pseudopregnant* uteri retained dilated endometrial glands, and lipid-filled cells lining the upper glands and surface were characteristic of involuting pregnant uteri.

More *ultrastructural* changes occurred in gland epithelium than in epithelium lining the uterine cavity. Involuted *anestrous* glands were lined by epithelium with inactive nuclei and few cytoplasmic organelles except lysosomes. In contrast, proestrous and estrous glands had active nuclei and abundant rER containing fibrillar-appearing secretion product (Fig. 7A), which sometimes was seen being extruded into the lumina. Organelles in the cytoplasm of proestrous and estrous gland epithelia were numerous and active.

Metestrous involution was characterized by increased lysosomal activity, with involuting cells containing large digestive vacuoles and many myelin figures. Surface and upper gland epithelia had large lipid droplets in otherwise inactive cytoplasm. Lipid was generally not found in cells that appeared to be synthesizing and secreting material. Gland and surface epithelia in *pregnant* uteri possessed much rER and active organelles but did not appear to be secreting any products. Gland epithelia from *pseudopregnant* uteri, on the other hand, were characterized by long microvilli extending into the lumina, tortuous rER, and many cytoplasmic organelles including vacuoles, vesicles, and filaments (Fig. 7B).

The most striking *histochemical* features of control uteri were changes in

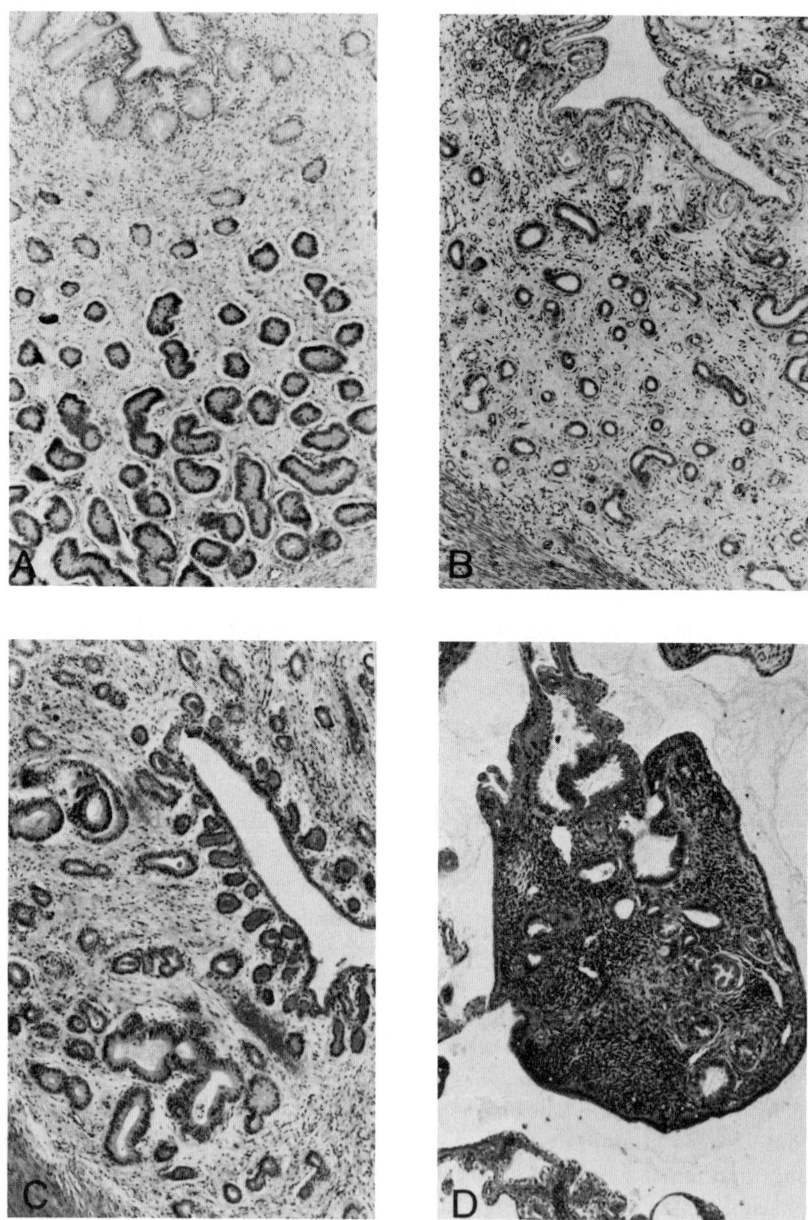

FIG. 6. A: Proliferative and early secretory endometrium in the uterus from a control bitch in early metestrus. H & E. X85. **B:** Lipid-filled surface epithelium and involuted deep glands in the uterine endometrium from a control bitch during metestrus. H & E. X85. **C:** Focal gland hyperplasia in uterine endometrium from a bitch treated 30 months with MPA 3.0 mg/kg. H & E. X85. **D:** Cystic endometrial hyperplasia and endometrial stromal hyperplasia in the uterus of a bitch treated 38 months with MPA 3.0 mg/kg. H & E. X85.

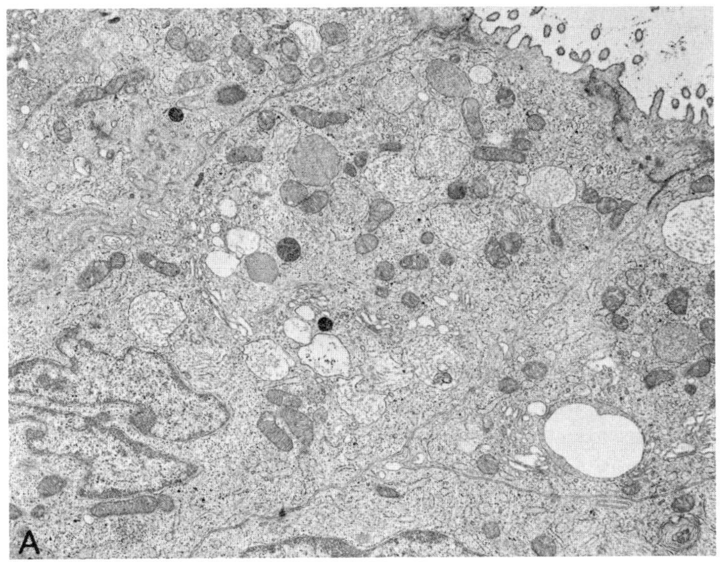

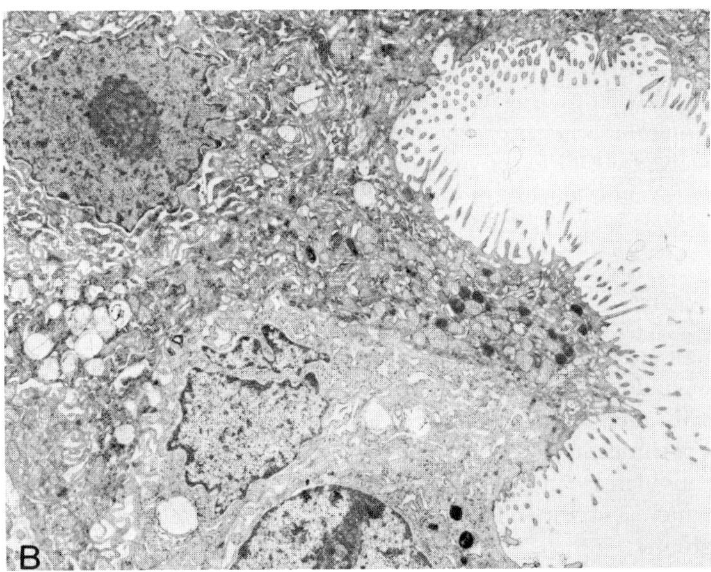

FIG. 7. **A:** Active deep gland epithelium with secretory material present in cisternae of ER from the uterus of a control bitch in estrus. X8,925. **B:** Abundant rER and long surface microvilli in upper gland epithelium from the uterus of a pseudopregnant control bitch. X6,247.

phosphatase histochemistry consistent with different stages. *Alkaline phosphatase* increased greatly in gland and stroma cells during early metestrus (Fig. 9A) and occurred throughout the cytoplasm of early secretory epithelial cells in upper glands and surface. While gland and surface cells were proliferating, however, absolutely no AlP activity was present. Capillaries in myometrium and endometrium were usually intensely (4+) AlP-positive, and in involuted uteri they were found encircling the glands and lying immediately beneath the surface epithelium. Upper levels of endometrial stroma varied in AlP activity depending on the stage of estrus, reaching maximum concentrations during early metestrus and pregnancy, and being least demonstrable during late anestrus, proestrus, and estrus. The apical surface of gland and surface epithelia were often intensely reactive for AlP activity, and in glands the entire luminal area appeared filled with intense AlP activity. This was more prominent during metestrus and anestrus than during proestrus or estrus.

Acid phosphatase activity was intense (4+) in actively involuting glands during early metestrus and in glands of pseudopregnant uteri (Fig. 9C). Actively proliferating gland and surface epithelia and quiescent anestrous endometrium were only moderately AcP-positive. In deep glands of pregnant and postpartum uteri, AcP activity was very intense, involving uterine contents as well as epithelial cells. Myometrial cells never contained much AcP activity, but more was present during involution than during other stages.

Dehydrogenases also varied with the stage of estrus. G6PD was most intense in actively proliferating gland and surface epithelia, whereas α-GPD was less active during these stages except in deep gland epithelia. The upper stroma was more reactive for G6PD activity during active stages of the cycle. LDH activity was more reactive during metestrus and anestrus than during proestrus and estrus.

Uteri of MPA-Treated Bitches

The most striking features in all groups of MPA-treated bitches were delayed involution and resemblance of some uteri to pregnant and pseudopregnant control animals. Glandular development and activity in different groups at various intervals postinjection are presented in Table 5. Not only did gland development and activity increase in general related to time postinjection, but the amount of variation increased, especially with respect to gland development in the higher-dosage groups.

The *morphology* of the uteri in the *0.3 mg/kg* group was characterized by delayed involution during anestrus, with some glands still undergoing mitosis while others were still very secretory in appearance. Villous projections into the uterine cavity characteristic of pregnant uteri were found. Deep glands were sometimes quite involuted, whereas upper glands and surface epithelia appeared more active. Myometrial involution was also delayed during anestrus. Proliferative endometrium during proestrus and estrus underwent secretory transforma-

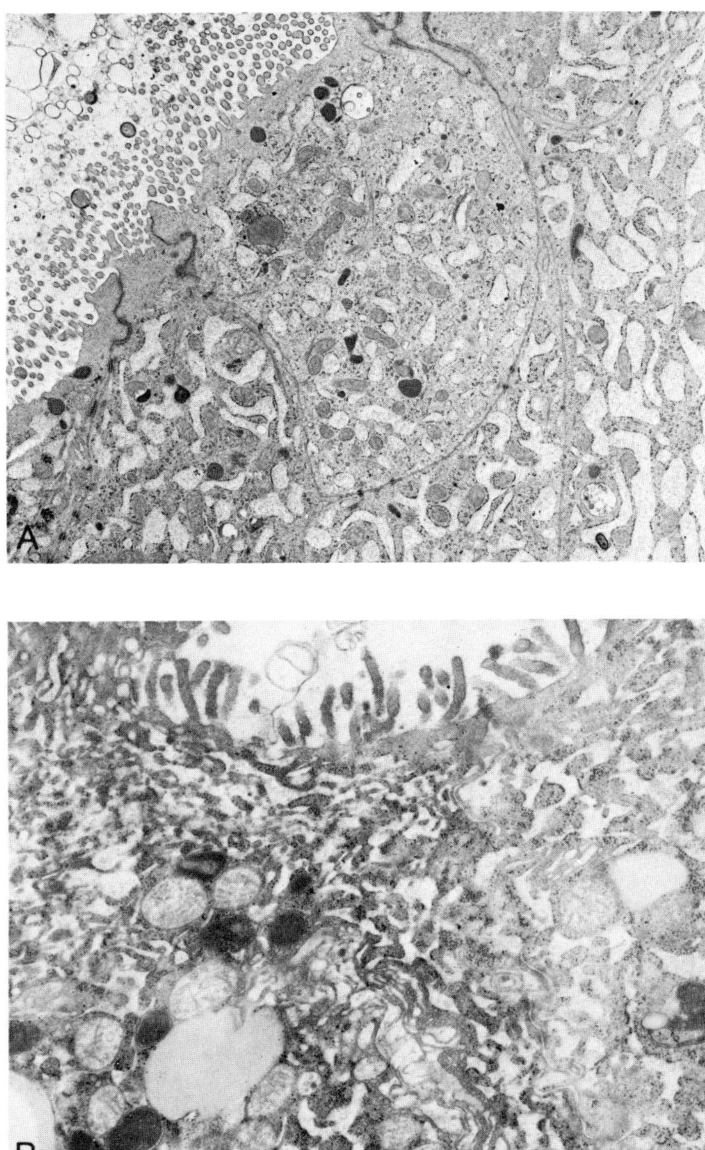

FIG. 8. A: Active endoplasmic reticulum containing some secretory product in deep gland epithelium of the uterus from a bitch treated 22 months with MPA 3.0 mg/kg. X8,925. **B:** Very active cytoplasm containing abundant rER and long microvilli on the surface of upper gland epithelium from the uterus of a bitch treated 12 months with MPA 3.0 mg/kg. X14,280.

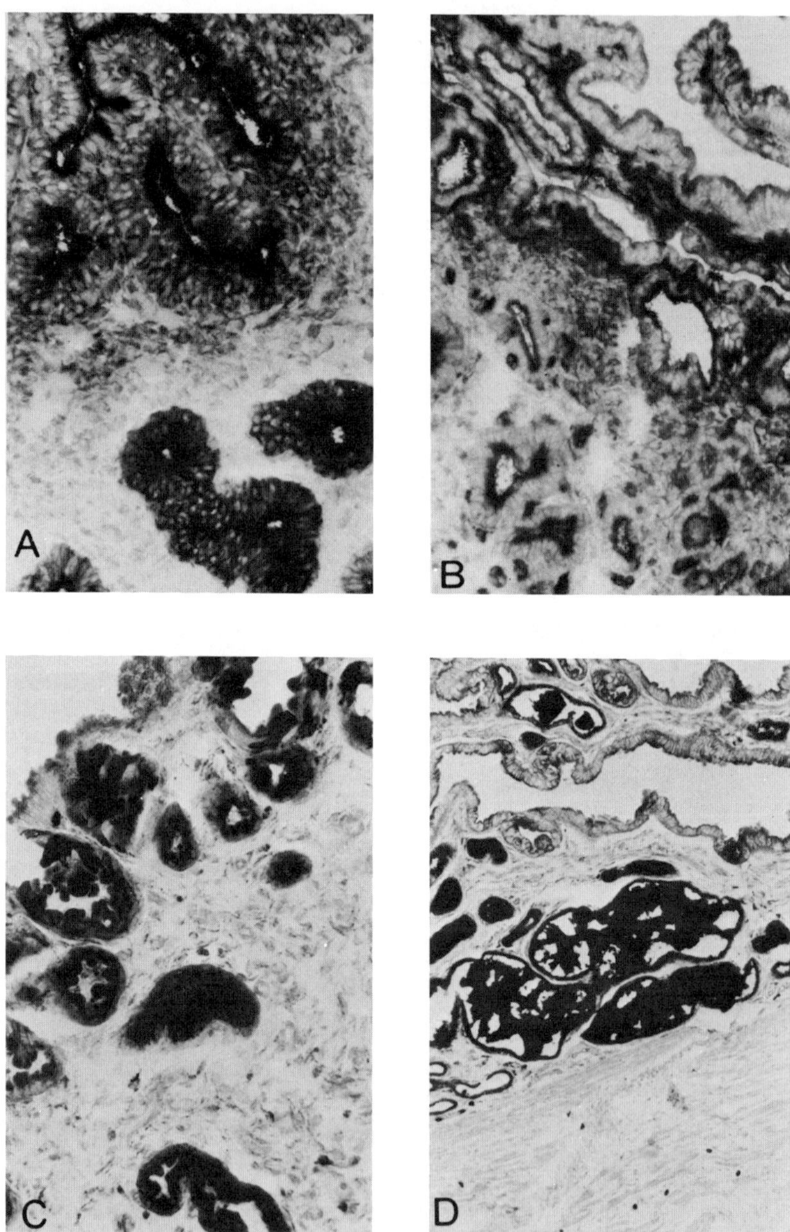

FIG. 9. A: Intense AlP activity in upper endometrial glands and stroma in the uterus from a control bitch in metestrus less than 1 week. AlP. X210. **B:** Intense AlP activity in endometrial stroma and glands of the uterus with cystic endometrial hyperplasia removed from a bitch treated 22 months with MPA 3.0 mg/kg. AlP. X210. **C:** Intense AcP activity in deep endometrial glands of the uterus from a control bitch in pseudopregnancy. AcP. X210. **D:** Intense AcP activity in deep glands of the uterus from a bitch treated 12 months with MPA 0.3 mg/kg. AcP. X85.

TABLE 5. Endometrial glandular development and activity in MPA-treated bitches at different intervals postinjection

Months post injection	MPA 0.3 mg/kg				MPA 1.5 mg/kg				MPA 3.0 mg/kg			
	No. of bitches	No. of tissues	Gland devel.[a] (mean)	Activity[b] (mean)	No. of bitches	No. of tissues	Gland devel.[a] (mean)	Activity[b] (mean)	No. of bitches	No. of tissues	Gland devel.[a] (mean)	Activity[b] (mean)
12	4	6	2.5	2.0	2	3	1.3	1.7	2	4	1.5	1.5
16	6	13	2.5	2.2	6	12	2.3	2.5	4	10	2.8	2.3
22	6	14	2.1	2.5	6	12	1.6	1.8	6	22	4.8	3.4
30	6	25	3.2	3.0	6	24	3.5	2.6	5	21	3.3	3.5
38	4	13	3.2	2.5	4	13	3.1	2.5	4	21	3.2	4.0

[a] Glandular development: score of 1 (small and few) to 6 (large and many) and 9 (pregnant).
[b] Activity: score of 1 (inactive) to 5 (very active—pregnant).

tion earlier in the cycle than would be expected in controls. Adenomyosis (gland structures present in myometrium) was encountered regularly in all MPA-treated bitches (Table 6), and epithelium lining the myometrial cysts reacted similarly to that lining the endometrial glands.

Endometrial hyperplasia, sometimes becoming cystic with extensive mucous production, was encountered in the two higher-dosage groups (Table 6). Early lesions of hyperplasia were recognized as unusual individual or focal proliferative changes in endometrial glands while the remainder of the endometrium was involuted (Fig. 6C), or there was focal secretory transformation of upper glands or surface epithelium. Unilateral or focal dilatation of glands with mucous production was seen in both higher-dosage groups especially during earlier time periods, but progressive development of lesions which ultimately involved the entire thickness of endometrium was found in both groups (Fig. 6D). Occasionally the endometrial stroma was extremely cellular (Fig. 6D), which was interpreted as hyperplasia of connective tissues rather than infiltration of inflammatory cells. Mucous production was more pronounced in the 3.0 mg/kg group, and in one uterus 275 ml of mucus was removed. There have never been any bacteria cultured from the mucus, and only occasionally have there been a sufficient number of inflammatory cells in the product to make it appear as pyometra. When cystic hyperplasia and mucometra occurred in the endometrium, it also involved all areas of adenomyosis. In one bitch there were cysts of endometriosis outside the uterine wall which also were filled with mucus.

Ultrastructural evidence of increased production and secretion of material was found in glands of MPA-treated bitches (Fig. 8A), but the material in the rER appeared different from that seen in proliferative endometrium of proestrus and estrus (Fig. 7A). The rER was extensively developed in gland epithelia from bitches with endometrial hyperplasia (Fig. 8B) and resembled that seen during pseudopregnancy (Fig. 7B). In addition to long microvilli and increased rER of hyperplastic gland cells, there appeared to be many more cytoplasmic filaments and organelles in these cells, and the number of desmosomal attachment sites

TABLE 6. *Hyperplastic lesions in uteri of MPA-treated bitches*

Months post injection	Lesion[a]		
	MPA 0.3 mg/kg	MPA 1.5 mg/kg	MPA 3.0 mg/kg
4			1 A
8	2 A		1 CEH
12	1 A	2 CEH	2 A, 3 CEH
16	1 A	1 A, 2 CEH	1 A, 2 CEH
22		1 A, 1 CEH	3 A, 4 CEH
30		2 A, 3 CEH	3 A, 4 CEH
38	2 A	1 A, 2 CEH	2 A, 4 CEH

[a] CEH, cystic endometrial hyperplasia. A, adenomyosis.

between cells appeared increased. The nuclei had unusual, dispersed heterochromatin, which differed from involuted control glands. Surface cells had many lipid droplets in addition to more-active cytoplasm.

Alkaline phosphatase activity in epithelia and stroma of bitches with endometrial hyperplasia was markedly increased (Fig. 9B) compared with involuted control glands, and resembled that found during early metestrus (Fig. 9A) or pregnancy. Focal hyperplasia of endometrial glands present in some uteri were also intensely AlP-positive, unlike involuted glands in the rest of the endometrium.

Acid phosphatase activity was very intense in hyperplastic glands, especially cystic dilated glands, and included the contents within lumina. AcP activity was also very intense in uterine glands from the low-dosage group, which resembled pregnant uteri (Fig. 9D), and was similar to the activity seen in pseudopregnant controls (Fig. 9C). Focal hyperplastic glands present in some uteri were intensely reactive for AcP activity, unlike the proliferative glands and surface epithelium in proestrous and estrous controls. Macrophages present in the stroma of some uteri with endometrial hyperplasia were very reactive for AcP activity. AcP activity in cycling 0.3 mg/kg bitches usually resembled that of the controls except for the greater activity in involuting uteri.

Activity of all *dehydrogenases* was elevated in gland and surface epithelia in areas of cystic endometrial hyperplasia. Stroma surrounding these areas was also intensely reactive. Uninvoluted endometrial and myometrial tissues were more reactive than corresponding anestrous controls in the two higher-dosage groups, but the 0.3 mg/kg group had cyclic variation in dehydrogenase activity similar to that in the controls.

DISCUSSION

This study has shown that MPA administration to bitches at levels that suppress ovulation results in mammary gland hyperplasia and neoplasia as well as cystic endometrial hyperplasia and mucometra. Hyperplastic and neoplastic lesions of canine mammary glands have been found with several other synthetic progestational and estrogenic hormones either alone or in combination (18, 22,23,30) and have even been induced using high levels of progesterone (17). The significance of our findings is that a dosage of MPA, one of the more potent progestins (2), determined to be very near the minimal ovulation-suppressing dose is capable of producing the same lesions that much higher dosages of progestins have produced—with the exception that no malignant neoplasms have yet been found, as reported in some dog studies (30). Even with a level below the ovulation-suppressing dose there is increased hyperplasia of mammary glands, but no neoplasms have been found. Hyperplastic and inflammatory nodules are commonly found in mammary glands of old beagles that have not had hormone treatment (6), and MPA may act as a stimulus to earlier development of these "spontaneous" lesions.

Contraceptives reportedly do not influence either qualitative or quantitative aspects of benign breast disease in women (15,16), and it has been suggested that neoplasms developing in beagle bitches receiving contraceptives are probably of little significance in predicting potential tumorigenesis in women anyway, because the tumors produced are different (22). In this study, however, we found some tumors similar to those found in women (16).

A stronger argument against the bitch being a suitable model for predicting response to these progestins in women is that the bitch has a markedly different reproductive cycle and a peculiar sensitivity to certain progestins (12). This can be illustrated best with respect to the uterine response. MPA has been successfully used in women as a contraceptive (13) and as a therapeutic agent for adenomatous hyperplasia and endometrial adenocarcinoma (26), where it generally causes involution of the endometrium (26). In the bitch, however, although MPA effectively eliminates estrus (4), it stimulates the uterus (25) and may result in cystic endometrial hyperplasia with mucometra (3), which limits its usefulness.

In this study cystic endometrial hyperplasia, not unlike that seen "spontaneously" in bitches (11), consistently resulted after even minimal ovulation-suppressing doses of MPA. The amount of endometrial hyperplasia and mucous production are definitely dose- and time-related with few exceptions. The largest uteri with the most mucous production were seen in the high-dose group. The ultrastructural appearance of the endometrial gland epithelium is not very dissimilar from findings in women treated with other progestins (17), but the overall response is much different. MPA administration to rats produces no untoward effect when used to suppress ovulation (10). It therefore appears that the bitch, which normally has a quiescent period (anestrus) lasting several months in its estrous cycle, cannot tolerate continued stimulation of either target organ by this potent progestin.

Our morphologic, histochemical, and ultrastructural evaluations indicate that each MPA injection induces a pseudopregnant-like response in both target organs which does not return to baseline before the next administration, and the effects are compounded until pathologic hyperplasia results. MPA effects may be mediated in part through the anterior pituitary via stimulation of increased growth hormone levels, as has been suggested for the bitch (28). Evaluation of growth hormone levels in bitches receiving synthetic progestins may shed more light on this problem.

SUMMARY

Relatively low levels of MPA stimulated pathologic hyperplasia and neoplasia in mammary glands and cystic endometrial hyperplasia and adenomyosis in uteri of beagle bitches. Tissues removed at different times after treatment with three levels of MPA—below, near, and above the minimal ovulation-suppressing dose—revealed changes which are dose- and time-related. The two dosage levels that suppressed ovulation were associated with neoplastic transformation in mammary glands and cystic endometrial hyperplasia in uteri, neither of which have been found thus far in age-matched controls.

Morphologic, ultrastructural, and histochemical studies of mammary glands and uteri from all treated bitches revealed hyperplastic changes in both target organs which resembled tissues removed from pregnant and pseudopregnant bitches. It was suggested that MPA alone, or possibly in combination with increased polypeptide hormones from the anterior pituitary (e.g., growth hormone), stimulates a pseudopregnant-like condition in these target organs which continues to compound until pathologic hyperplasia and neoplasia result.

ACKNOWLEDGMENTS

The authors wish to express appreciation for the excellent technical assistance of Mrs. Nalini Makhijani, Mrs. Joan Dubin, and Miss Michele Marquardt, and the secretarial skills of Mrs. Kathie Winner. This work was supported by contract NICHD 73-2705 from the Center for Population Research, National Institute of Child Health and Human Development, N.I.H.

REFERENCES

1. Barka, T., and Anderson, P. J. (1962): Histochemical methods for acid phosphatase using hexazonium pararosanilin as coupler. *J. Histochem. Cytochem.*, 10:741–753.
2. Boris, A., and DeMartino, L. (1971): The utilization of uterine weight as an adjunct to histology in the evaluation of progestational steroids. *Steroidologia*, 2:57–64.
3. Brodey, R. S., and Fidler, I. J. (1966): Clinical and pathological findings in bitches treated with progestational compounds. *J. Am. Vet. Med. Assoc.*, 149:1406–1415.
4. Bryan, H. S. (1973): Parenteral use of medroxyprogesterone acetate as an antifertility agent in the bitch. *Am. J. Vet. Res.*, 34:659–663.
5. Burstone, M. S. (1958): Histochemical comparison of naphthol AS-phosphates for the demonstration of phosphatases. *J. Natl. Cancer Inst.*, 20:601–615.
6. Cameron, A. M., and Faulkin, L. J., Jr. (1971): Hyperplastic and inflammatory nodules in the canine mammary gland. *J. Natl. Cancer Inst.*, 47:1277–1287.
7. Capel-Edwards, K., Hall, D. E., Fellowes, K. P., Vallance, D. K., Davies, M. J., Lamb, D., and Robertson, W. B. (1973): Long-term administration of progesterone to the female beagle dog. *Toxicol. Appl. Pharmacol.*, 24:474–488.
8. Chayen, J. (1968): Histochemistry of phospholipids and its significance in the interpretation of the structure of cells. In: *The Interpretation of Cell Structure*, edited by K. F. Ross and S. McGee-Russell, pp. 149–156. Arnold, London.
9. Chayen, J., Bitensky, L., and Butcher, R. (1973): *Practical Histochemistry*. Wiley, New York.
10. Dickmann, Z. (1973): Short-and long-term effects of a single injection of depo-medroxyprogesterone acetate (Provera) on the vaginal smear, ovulation and mating in the rat. *J. Reprod. Fertil.*, 32:447–451.
11. Dow, C. (1959): The cystic hyperplasia-pyometra complex in the bitch. *J. Comp. Pathol.*, 69: 237–250.
12. Drill, V. A. (1973): Some metabolic actions and possible toxic effects of hormonal contraceptives in animals and man. *Acta Endocrinol. (Kbh.)* [*Suppl. 185*], 75:169–202.
13. El-Mahgoub, S., Karim, M., and Ammar, R. (1972): Long-term use of depo-medroxyprogesterone acetate as a contraceptive. *Acta Obstet. Gynecol. Scand.*, 51:251–255.
14. Evans, H. M., and Cole, H. H. (1931): *An Introduction to the Oestrus Cycle in the Dog*. University of California Press, Berkeley.
15. Fechner, R. E. (1970): Fibrocystic disease in women receiving oral contraceptive hormones. *Cancer*, 25:1332–1339.

16. Fechner, R. E. (1970): Fibroadenomas in patients receiving oral contraceptives: A clinical and pathologic study. *Am. J. Clin. Pathol.,* 53:857–864.

17. Flowers, C. E., Jr., Wilborn, W. H., and Enger, J. (1974): Effects of quingestanol acetate on the histology, histochemistry, and ultrastructure of the human endometrium. *Am. J. Obstet. Gynecol.,* 120:589–612.

18. Hill, R., and Dumas, K. (1973): The use of dogs for studies of toxicity of contraceptive hormones. *Acta Endocrinol. (Kbh.) [Suppl. 185]*, 75:74–84.

19. Luft, J. (1961): Improvement in epoxy resin embedding methods. *J. Biochem. Biophys. Cytol.,* 9:409–414.

20. Luna, L. G., editor (1968): *Manual of Histologic Staining Methods of the A.F.I.P.,* 3rd ed. McGraw-Hill, New York.

21. McManus, J. F. A. (1948): Histological and histochemical uses of periodic acid. *Stain Technol.,* 23:99–108.

22. Nelson, L. W., Carlton, W. W., and Weikel, J. H., Jr. (1972): Canine mammary neoplasms and progestogens. *JAMA,* 219:1601–1606.

23. Nelson, L. W., Weikel, J. H., Jr., and Reno, F. E. (1973): Mammary nodules in dogs during four years' treatment with megestrol acetate or chlormadinone acetate. *J. Natl. Cancer Inst.,* 51: 1303–1311.

24. Reynolds, E. S. (1963): The use of lead citrate at high pH as an electron-opaque stain in electron microscopy. *J. Cell Biol.,* 17:208–212.

25. Sokowlowski, J. H., and Zimbelman, R. G. (1974): Canine reproduction: Effects of multiple treatments of medroxyprogesterone acetate on reproductive organs of the bitch. *Am. J. Vet. Res.,* 35:1285–1287.

26. Steiner, G. J., Kistner, R. W., and Craig, J. M. (1965): Histological effects of progestins on hyperplasia and carcinoma in situ of the endometrium—further observations. *Metabolism,* 14: 356–386.

27. Taft, E. B. (1951): The problem of a standardized technic for the methyl green-pyronine stain. *Stain Technol.,* 26:205–212.

28. Tucker, M. J. (1971): Some effects of prolonged administration of a progestogen to dogs. In: *Proceedings: European Society for the Study of Drug Toxicology,* Vol. 12, pp. 228–238. Excerpta Medica, Amsterdam.

29. Wattenberg, L. W., and Leong, J. L. (1960): Effects of coenzyme Q 10 and menadione on succinic dehydrogenase activity as measured by tetrazolium salt reduction. *J. Histochem. Cytochem.,* 8:296–303.

30. Wazeter, F. X., Geil, R. G., Cookson, K. M., Berliner, V. R., and Lamar, J. K. (1974): Five year progress report on long term oral contraceptive studies in female dogs and monkeys. Presented before the Society of Toxicology, 13th Annual Meeting, Washington, D.C.

Pharmacology of Steroid Contraceptive Drugs
edited by S. Garattini and H. W. Berendes.
Raven Press, New York © 1977.

Preliminary Analysis of Oral Contraceptive Use and Risk of Developing Premalignant Lesions of the Uterine Cervix

*Howard W. Ory, †S. Beach Conger, ‡Zuher Naib, *Carl W. Tyler, Jr., and §Robert A. Hatcher

Family Planning Evaluation Division, Bureau of Epidemiology, Center for Disease Control, Atlanta, Georgia 30333; †South of Market Health Center, San Francisco, California; ‡Cytology Department, Grady Memorial Hospital, Atlanta, Georgia; and §Emory University Family Planning Program, Emory University School of Medicine, Atlanta, Georgia

Hormonal steroids are capable of promoting the development of cervical neoplasia in animals (1–4). That steroid-containing contraceptives have a similar effect in women has not been firmly ruled out (5–8). Three previous case–control studies found no association between continued oral contraceptive use and risk of developing cervical changes (5–7). However, one of these studies used data obtained between 1965 and 1969 (7). The author correctly noted that the use of oral contraceptives doubled between 1965 and 1969, yet he did not state when data on cases and controls were collected. If controls were chosen from the later years and cases from the early years of the study period, an association between oral contraceptives and cervical neoplasia may have been obscured. When comparing cases with controls, another study (6) revealed major differences with respect to variables known to predict risk of cervical neoplasia (9). Since this study does not control for these variables, its results are difficult to interpret.

The fourth study is stated to be a double-blind trial whose major conclusion is that there are no significant differences in the pattern of progression and regression (of cervical abnormalities) between oral and nonoral groups (8). To arrive at this conclusion the investigators group all women whose cytologic results changed from one diagnostic category to another, irrespective of whether they went from normal to atypical or from dysplasia to carcinoma *in situ*. If, instead, one looks at the progression rate in women with Papanicolaou smears of class III or greater, cytologic abnormalities in users of oral contraceptives progress at twice the rate of nonusers. This conflicts with the conclusion reached by these investigators. In short, the results of the four previous studies do not strongly persuade us that oral contraceptive use is unrelated to cervical neoplasia.

We report here our preliminary case–control analyses of the association of premalignant cervical changes (carcinoma *in situ* and dysplasia) and oral contraceptive use. In addition, unlike previous reports, we examine the effect of the variation in diagnosis of cervical neoplasias on the above association. Because the variation is substantial, it is difficult to interpret the biologic meaning of the observed association between premalignant cervical changes and oral contraceptive use.

STUDY SUBJECTS AND METHODS

Selection of Subjects

Study subjects were women who attended a large inner-city family planning clinic during the 6-year period 1967–1972. Since 1967 we have systematically recorded the results of each visit to the family planning clinic, including demographic and reproductive information. In 1965 we began recording the reported results of all cervical cytology and pathology specimens processed by the one hospital associated with this clinic. Both files identify women by hospital number, which allows the linking of records of more than 33,000 women.

This group of women is described in more detail elsewhere (10). Almost all clinic patients are in the low-income bracket; most are black. We restricted this preliminary analysis to black women between the ages of 15 and 44 who used either oral contraceptives or an intrauterine device (IUD). Women who had had hysterectomies or who used injectable dehydromedroxyprogesterone acetate were not included. We further restricted the analysis to women who had had at least three entries in the cytopathology file, of which the first two were normal. Finally, the analysis was limited to women with no abnormal cytopathology entries prior to entry into family planning. The 9,728 women meeting these criteria were then subgrouped into cases and controls.

To qualify, a woman had to have had cervical dysplasia or carcinoma *in situ* first diagnosed during the years 1970–1972. By definition, such women had had at least two normal and no abnormal Papanicolaou smears before their "index" (Papanicolaou) smear—the one by which we classified women as having normal or abnormal cytology. (Normal implies that the cytology or pathology result was not dysplasia or other neoplasia.) Further, we required that the dysplasia or carcinoma *in situ* had been confirmed by biopsy within 365 days of the abnormal index smear. These criteria imply that all cases are incident and biopsy-confirmed.

Of the 9,728 women, 1,175 had an abnormal index smear. Of these, 854 were confirmed by biopsy as dysplasia and 147 as carcinoma *in situ*. Both groups were included in their respective analyses as cases. The remaining 174 women were excluded from the analyses because they did not meet the biopsy criteria.

The 8,553 women who met the criteria for controls had had at least two normal and no abnormal Papanicolaou smears prior to a normal index smear taken during the study period 1970–1972. If a control had had more than one potential index smear, one was chosen at random.

Estimates of oral contraceptive exposure are the sum of the number of cycles of oral contraceptives given each woman at each visit. For example, if a woman made three visits and at each visit received a 6-month supply of contraceptive pills, she was considered to have an 18-month exposure to oral contraceptives. Exposure terminated at the date of the index smear. The clinic prescribed nearly all brands and strengths of oral contraceptives available in the United States. Women who had had an IUD inserted and who had never used any hormonal contraceptives were considered nonusers of oral contraceptives.

Because there appears to be substantial variation in diagnosing histologic sections of the uterine cervix (11,12), we asked two pathologists who are generally accepted as experts in the area of cervical pathology to reread certain of the cervical tissue sections of women in our study. They reviewed 85 sets of slides of carcinoma *in situ;* 26 were from IUD users and 59 from oral contraceptive users of more than 1 year's duration. Fifty-three specimens were obtained by punch biopsy, 28 by cold knife conization, and 4 from hysterectomy. We included 15 additional slides with other diagnoses in order to blind the reviewers to our purpose.

The consultant pathologists independently reviewed the 100 sets of slides in the same order and under similar conditions. They were asked to read the slides according to the criteria they would normally use in their own hospitals. Neither reviewer knew the purpose of our study, and neither was given any clinical information about the slides.

Data Analysis

We compared the duration of oral contraceptive use for cases with controls and estimated the risk of oral contraceptive users developing carcinoma *in situ* relative to the risk of nonusers developing that disease. Such relative risk estimates were computed for yearly increments of oral contraceptive use. Similar analyses were done for dysplasia.

We used two approaches to control for possible confounding by the 10 variables on which we had information (Table 1). First, the crude relative risks were adjusted for the effects of each of the 10 variables by the method of Mantel and Haenszel, which adjusts the variables one at a time or in groups of two or three (13). As a more rigorous approach to controlling confounding, we derived a multivariate score for each subject summarizing (over all 10 variables) her risk of having cervical carcinoma *in situ* (14). The same analysis was done for dysplasia. As expected, subjects with the highest risk tended to have low age at first birth, low educational attainment, and high parity, and to be between the ages of 27 and 34. The *cases* were subgrouped into three strata of equal size on the basis of risk score. Controls were placed into the above-defined tertiles. We computed standardized relative risks over the three strata by the "SRR" method of Miettinen (15). These standardized estimates compared the risk of premalignant cervical changes for oral contraceptive users (of various durations) to the

TABLE 1. *Comparison of women on certain variables by contraceptive method*

Variable	IUD ($N = 2{,}424$)	Oral contraceptives ($N = 7{,}310$)
Age[a]	25.5	23.1
Age at first birth	18.0 (867[b])	18.1 (3,649[b])
Years of education completed[a]	10.7 (1,732[b])	10.9 (6,405[b])
No. smears[c] while in study	2.7	2.4
No. smears prior to study	2.5	2.6
Months in study	28.3	23.6
Total No. pregnancies[a]	3.0 (2,265[b])	2.4 (7,038[b])
Year of entry to family planning (average)	1968.6	1968.8
% Currently using contraceptive method[a]	79.2	60.4
% Currently married[a]	44.9	42.8

[a] At time of index smear.
[b] Number of women for whom information was known for particular variable.
[c] Papanicolaou smears.

risk for nonusers. In both approaches to controlling confounding, Mantel's method was used to compute the chi-square statistic testing relative risk estimates for linear trend (16).

RESULTS

Except for age, number of months in the study, and percent of women currently using a contraceptive method at the date of the index smear, the oral contraceptive users and IUD users were similar (Table 1). Table 2 compares cases of cervical carcinoma *in situ* and dysplasia with controls according to duration of oral contraceptive use. Using stratification by risk score to control confounding, the standardized relative risk of carcinoma *in situ* rises from 1.0 for nonusers of

TABLE 2. *Duration of oral contraceptive use by cervical disease status*

Oral contraceptive use (mo)	Normal controls %	Dysplasia %	Dysplasia SRR[a]	Carcinoma *in situ* %	Carcinoma *in situ* SRR[a]
None	25.6	20.1	1.0	17.1	1.0
1–12	50.1	47.8	1.2	40.8	1.3
13–24	16.0	19.9	1.6	23.8	2.5
25–36	6.2	9.4	1.9	10.9	2.6
37+	2.1	2.8	1.6	6.8	4.7
Total No.	8,553	854		147	

The χ^2_1 testing the SRRs for linear trend in the analysis of dysplasia versus normal $= 22.6$, $p = 2.0 \times 10^{-6}$; for carcinoma *in situ* versus normal χ_1^2 for linear trend $= 29.4$, $p = 5.9 \times 10^{-8}$.

[a] Standardized relative risk—standardized over the three risk strata, with nonusers of oral contraceptives as the standard.

oral contraceptives to 4.7 for women using them for more than 3 years. This trend is significant: X_1^2 for linear trend $= 29.4$, $p = 5.9 \times 10^{-8}$ (two-tail) (13).

Likewise, the standardized relative risk estimate for dysplasia rises from 1.0 for nonusers of oral contraceptives to a maximum of 1.9 for 2- to 3-year oral contraceptive users. However, the relative risk ratio then decreases slightly. This trend is significant: $X^2 = 22.6$, $p = 2.0 \times 10^{-6}$.

The 174 cases with abnormal Papanicolaou smears but no biopsy confirmation of dysplasia or carcinoma *in situ* within the allotted time were dealt with in two ways. First, we made the extreme assumption that they were all cases of carcinoma *in situ*. This resulted in a lowering of all risk estimates to approximately 60% of the estimates shown in Table 2. The trend was still highly significant. Second, we made a more reasonable assumption and classified the 110 cases with subsequent normal examinations as normal; the 24 with dysplasia diagnosed after the allotted time for follow-up were classified as dysplasia; cases having carcinoma *in situ* diagnosed after the allotted follow-up time (3 cases) and those with invasive cancer (4 cases) were both classified as carcinoma *in situ*. The 33 with no recorded follow-up were considered normal. Reanalysis with these cases included showed that relative risk estimates were virtually unchanged from the levels show in Table 2.

Table 3 shows that pathologist A agreed with the hospital diagnosis of carcinoma *in situ* on 6 of the 85 sets of slides (7.1%). Pathologist B agreed with the hospital diagnosis of carcinoma *in situ* in 65 of 85 cases (76.5%). If cases diagnosed as severe dysplasia are combined with those classified as carcinoma *in situ,* pathologist A agreed with the hospital diagnosis in 23.5% of the cases.

We attempted to determine if the size of the tissue specimen in any way affected reproducibility of results. Of the 53 punch biopsy specimens called carcinoma *in situ* at the hospital, pathologist B disagreed with 18 (34%). Of the 32 conization and hysterectomy specimens diagnosed as carcinoma *in situ* at the hospital, pathologist B disagreed in 2 cases (6%). This 5.4-fold difference in agreement according to size of specimen is statistically significant $p \simeq 0.004$.

We also tried to determine if prior use of oral contraceptives in any way

TABLE 3. *Comparison of pathologists' diagnoses*

Pathologist B diagnosis[a]	Carcinoma *in situ*	Severe dysplasia	Moderate dysplasia	Minimum dysplasia	Normal
			Pathologist A		
Total diagnosed	6	14	46	7	12
Carcinoma in situ (65)	6	14	40	1	4
Severe dysplasia (0)	0	0	0	0	0
Moderate dysplasia (12)	0	0	4	3	5
Minimum dysplasia (6)	0	0	2	2	2
Normal (2)	0	0	0	1	1

[a] Numbers in parentheses = total diagnosed.

influences the diagnosis of carcinoma *in situ.* Compared with pathologist B, hospital pathologists diagnosed carcinoma *in situ* 35% more often in the 26 IUD users and 19% more often in the 59 oral contraceptive users ($p = 0.11$). This minor difference persists when the results are standardized for size of specimen. In short, prior contraceptive use does not appear to influence the diagnosis of carcinoma *in situ.*

DISCUSSION

Interpretation of the preceding results is complex. We note that the longer a woman uses oral contraceptives, the greater is her likelihood of developing premalignant cervical changes. However, the variation in diagnosis of such lesions makes the biologic interpretation of the association difficult. Holding the variation issue aside for a moment, we can examine the epidemiologic strengths and weaknesses of our study.

The extremely small *p* values make chance an unlikely explanation of the association between increasing duration of oral contraceptive use and increasing risk of premalignant cervical changes. The question is if oral contraceptive use *causes* this association, or if the association is noncausal and due to bias in collection of information, selection of subjects, or confounding.

We verified that errors in linkage, coding, and transcribing data occurred in less than 2% of the entries and were proportionately distributed between cases and controls (10). Contraceptive exposure histories are systematically computed from data recorded prior to diagnosis. Although there is undoubtedly error in our estimate of oral contraceptive use, there is no reason to suspect that it is disproportionately distributed among cases or controls. The above suggests that our analysis is not biased with respect to data collection or ascertainment of contraception histories. Since all subjects were black and almost all were indigent, race and socioeconomic status probably did not bias our analysis.

Table 1 shows that self-selection of contraceptive method did not result in there being a disproportionate number of women with high-risk attributes (for developing cervical neoplasia) using oral contraceptives. In addition, we showed previously that in women attending this clinic choice of oral contraceptives does not identify a group of women intrinsically at high risk of developing carcinoma *in situ* (10).

None of the variables for which we had information substantially affected our results. By either method of controlling confounding, the crude and standardized relative risks are almost identical. For example, the crude relative risk that carcinoma *in situ* will develop in 1-, 2-, 3-, and over 3-year users of oral contraceptives is 1.2, 2.2, 2.5, and 4.7, respectively. These figures compare closely with those in the last column of Table 2.

Given what we know about our data, defects in epidemiologic methodology does not appear responsible for the association between continued oral contraceptive use and increased risk of developing cervical neoplasia. Selection bias does not appear responsible for the association; however, we have no direct measure of sexual activity, which is probably the single most important predictor of risk of cervical neoplasia (9). If there were different rates of sexual activity between cases and controls, and if this variable were also related to length of oral contraceptive use, our results could be distorted. Not having this information also limits the interpretation of our results.

The association between length of oral contraceptive use and the likelihood of developing what hospital pathologists diagnose as premalignant cervical changes—particularly carcinoma *in situ*—appears statistically and methodologically (epidemiologic) solid. It is possible that because we are studying a population of women with an apparently high risk of developing premalignant cervical lesions (10) we found an association others could not find in lower-risk populations. Alternatively, we may have found an association that others did not because of the criteria used to diagnose premalignant cervical changes in the study institution. For example, if the hospital used pathologist B's criteria, fewer cases of cervical disease would be diagnosed. Under such circumstances there is no way to predict if the association would remain.

In view of this uncertainty we feel it is impossible to assign any biologic meaning to the statistical association between increasing risk of premalignant cervical changes and increasing duration of use of oral contraceptives.

In planning future studies of the effects of drugs on cervical cancer, our results suggest the following: In any multicentered study, all histologic sections must be read in one laboratory. This should help guarantee internal consistency of the study. It will not guarantee data that can be generalized, however, as our results have demonstrated. For generalizable results pathologists should develop and apply standardized criteria for the histologic diagnosis of early cervical neoplasia.

SUMMARY

Hormonal steroids are capable of promoting the development of cervical neoplasia in animals. That steroid-containing contraceptives have a similar effect in women has not been firmly ruled out. The duration of oral contraceptive use was compared in three groups of women: (a) 147 women with newly diagnosed carcinoma *in situ* confirmed by biopsy; (b) 854 women with incident cervical dysplasia confirmed by biopsy; and (c) 8,000 women who were shown by multiple Papanicolaou smears not to have either of these diseases. Study women were drawn from a family planning clinic and used either oral contraception or IUDs as their method of contraception.

In women who used oral contraceptives for 3 years or more, the risk of developing carcinoma *in situ* appeared to be nearly five times that of IUD users. Likewise, the risk of dysplasia rose to a maximum of 1.9 times that of IUD users in women who used oral contraceptives for 2–3 years.

Eighty-five of the 147 cases of carcinoma were submitted for confirmatory histologic interpretation by two pathologists from different institutions. One read approximately 65 of these 85 as carcinoma *in situ;* the other read only 6 as carcinoma *in situ.* The substantial variation in the histologic diagnosis of carcinoma *in situ* of the cervix prevents us from making any firm biologic interpretations of the statistical association of oral contraceptive use and carcinoma *in situ* of the cervix.

REFERENCES

1. Allen, E., and Gardner, W. U. (1941): Cancer of the.cervix of the uterus in hybrid mice following long continued administration of estrogen. *Cancer Res.,* 1:359–366.
2. Dunn, T. B. (1969): Cancer of the uterine cervix in mice fed a liquid diet containing an anti-fertility drug. *J. Natl. Cancer Inst.,* 43:61–692.
3. Murphy, E. D. (1961): Carcinogenesis of the uterine cervix in mice: Effect of diethylstilbestrol after limited application of 3-methylcholanthrene. *J. Natl. Cancer Inst.,* 27:611–653.
4. Kaminetzky, H. A. (1966): Methylcholanthrene induced cervical dysplasia and the sex steroids. *Obstet. Gynecol.,* 27:489–493.
5. Thomas, D. B. (1972): Relationship of oral contraceptives to cervical carcinogenesis. *Obstet. Gynecol.,* 40:508–518.
6. Worth, A. J., and Boyes, D. A. (1972): Case-control study into the possible effect of birth control pills on pre-clinical carcinoma of the cervix. *J. Obstet. Gynaecol. Br. Commonw.,* 79:673–679.
7. Boyce, J. G., Lu, T., Nelson, J. H., et al. (1972): Cervical carcinoma and oral contraception. *Obstet. Gynecol.,* 40:139–146.
8. Fuertes-de la Haba, A., Pelegrena, I., Bangdiwala, I. S., et al. (1973): Changing patterns in cervical cytology among oral and non-oral contraceptive users. *J. Reprod. Med.,* 10:3–10.
9. Barron, B. A., and Richart, R. M. (1971): An epidemiological study of cervical neoplastic disease based on a self-selected sample of 7,000 women in Barbados, West Indies. *Cancer,* 27:978.
10. Ory, H. W., Conger, S. G., Naib, Z., et al. (1975): Non-association of contraceptive choice and cervical dysplasia and carcinoma-in-situ in women entering a family planning clinic. *Am. J. Obstet. Gynecol.,* 123:275–277.
11. Siegler, E. E. (1956): Microdiagnosis of carcinoma-in-situ of the uterine cervix. *Cancer,* 9: 463–469.
12. Holmquist, N. D., McMahan, C. A., and Williams, O. D. (1967): Variability in classification of carcinoma-in-situ of the uterine cervix. *Arch. Pathol.,* 84:334–335.
13. Mantel, N., and Haenszel, W. (1959): Statistical aspects of the analysis of data from retrospective studies of disease. *J. Natl. Cancer Inst.,* 22:719.
14. Jick, H., Miettinen, O. S., Neff, R. K., et al. (1973): Coffee and myocardial infarction. *N. Engl. J. Med.,* 289:63–67.
15. Miettinen, O. S. (1972): Standardization of risk ratios. *Am. J. Epidemiol.,* 96:383–388.
16. Mantel, N. (1963): Chi square tests with one degree of freedom: Extension of the Mantel-Haenszel procedure. *J. Am. Stat. Assoc.,* 58:690–700.

Pharmacology of Steroid Contraceptive Drugs
edited by S. Garattini and H. W. Berendes.
Raven Press, New York © 1977.

Association of Liver Tumors and Cancer of the Endometrium with Oral Contraceptive Use

Heinz W. Berendes

Contraceptive Evaluation Branch, Center for Population Research, National Institute of Child Health and Human Development, National Institutes of Health, Bethesda, Maryland 20014

Concerns about possible health hazards of contraceptive steroids include possible tumorigenic and carcinogenic effects. Recent evidence suggests that two such lesions are related to exposure to contraceptive steroids. These are benign tumors of the liver in women who have used combination oral contraceptives and cancer of the endometrium in women who have used sequential oral contraceptives. This chapter briefly summarizes the evidence currently available in support of this contention.

In 1973 Baum et al. (1) reported seven cases of hepatic adenoma in young women on oral contraceptives and was the first to speculate on the possible association of these lesions with exposure to contraceptive steroids. Since that time, case reports have appeared in increasing numbers (2–13). A recent search on behalf of a subcommittee of the National Cancer Advisory Board of the N.I.H. identified 107 cases of such tumors reported in the medical literature. To this can be added approximately 100–150 additional cases not as yet published which have been collected as part of registries of these tumors maintained by certain investigators.

Synonyms used in describing these pathological lesions include focal nodular hyperplasia, benign hepatoma, liver cell adenoma, and hamartoma. The reported tumors are usually solitary, although multiple lesions have been noted. They may be interspersed with fibrous septa and contain bile duct reduplication. They are almost invariably highly vascular. Blood-filled spaces in the periphery of the nodules may be without endothelial lining, thus resembling peliosis hepatis (2). (The latter condition has been previously described in patients with terminal tuberculosis and after therapy with anabolic steroids.) There may also be proliferation and thickening of the interlobular branches of the afferent veins and arteries (12). Areas of infarction and necrosis may be apparent. Christopherson et al. (7) reported four cases of hepatocellular carcinoma in women on oral contraceptives. In another instance a well-differentiated hepatocellular carcinoma was found in an otherwise histologically benign nodule (14).

The true incidence of these tumors is not known. Berg et al. (5) identified four such tumors during a 3-year period from the Iowa State Cancer Register, where one case was expected. The calculated incidence for women 20–39 years of age was 0.29 per 100,000 per year. A recent summary of 23 cases reveals that 12 women were less than 30 years old, nine more 30–39, and two 40 years and older (9). Forty-two patients recently reported by Edmondson et al. (15) had an age range of 19–54, with most being under 40 years of age. Although most of the reported cases are associated with oral contraceptive steroid exposure, one patient had been pregnant 9 months when the lesion was noted (5), and two women were on Premarin (10). Liver cell adenoma was recently observed in a young male on anabolic steroids (16).

Many of the tumors first came to attention as medical emergencies. Since the tumors are highly vascular, intrahepatic and abdominal hemorrhage with shock were the presenting symptoms. In other instances the diagnosis was made by finding pain in the right upper abdominal quadrant, enlargement of the liver on palpation, and subsequent positive liver scan and arteriogram. In the differential diagnoses of the acute abdominal emergencies, ectopic pregnancies were frequently considered. Several women have died of shock prior to or during surgery or from postoperative complications.

The association between contraceptive steroids and liver tumors is to some extent indirect. Until recently these lesions were thought to be extremely rare, although they have been reported in increasing numbers during the last few years. The best evidence stems from a recent case–control study of benign liver tumors (15). The study included 42 women, with neighbors of similar ages being used as controls; 34 pairs were available for analysis. Twenty-nine of the women reported prior oral contraceptive use compared to 24 of the controls, an insignificant difference. Significantly different, however, was the duration of use of the oral contraceptives. The mean duration of use for the 29 patients with oral contraceptive exposure was 79.7 months, and for the 26 controls 37.8 months. This difference was highly significant at the 0.001 level. Edmondson calculated the relative risk ratio of benign liver tumor by duration of use of oral contraceptives. A risk ratio of 2.5 was found for exposure of 3–5 years. The risk increased sharply above 5 years of use and reached 25 after more than 9 years of use. A strong association was noted between the occurrence of liver tumors and the use of oral contraceptives containing mestranol. This was based on the calculated number of pill months of use for patients and controls who were able to state the brand name. Only 7.4% of the total pill months of use among patients was due to contraceptives containing ethynylestradiol. Among controls, 55.2% of the total months of use was attributed to the use of compounds containing ethynylestradiol. This difference was significant at the 0.0001 level. This preponderance of exposure to mestranol-containing oral contraceptive preparations is also apparent from reported series of other investigators. Whether this apparent association between liver tumors and mestranol-containing oral contraceptive preparations is real remains to be determined. The earlier marketed oral contraceptive preparations largely used mestranol as the synthetic estrogen. It is therefore possible that the apparent association between these tumors and the use of mestranol-containing preparations is due to the also observed increase in risk associated with prolonged exposure.

The natural history of these lesions is not known. Regression of liver tumors after discontinuation of oral contraceptives has been reported by some. On the other hand, cases have been recognized several years after discontinuation of oral contraceptives. The tumors seemed to occur in women who are otherwise healthy and who have no evidence of liver disease or dysfunction in their history or at the time of diagnosis.

The pathogenesis of these lesions is also unknown. Primary hepatocellular carcinomas subsequent to treatment with androgenic steroids have been noted previously in males and females (17). Among these are hepatocellular carcinomas in patients with aplastic anemia or testicular insufficiency who were treated with androgenic steroids.

The reports of several cases of hepatocellular carcinoma among oral contraceptive users render invalid an earlier view, i.e., that androgenic steroids were associated with hepatic carcinoma and estrogenic steroids with benign hepatic adenomas. The apparent association with mestranol-containing preparations requires clarification. If the association proves to be real, one might speculate that the demethylation of mestranol by the liver may account for the increased risk.

A variety of progestational agents were reportedly involved, including norethynodrel, dimethisterone, norgestrel, norethisterone, lynestrenol, ethynodiol, and norethindrone. These are C17-substituted 19 norsteroids, as are the anabolic steroids. Since a case of benign liver adenoma has now been reported in a young man on oxymetholone, it is necessary to suspect also the progestogen component of the contraceptive steroids.

Large doses of progestogens alone or with mestranol have been shown to produce liver cell tumors in rats (18). Progestogens are enzyme inducers and are also cholestatic. Enzyme induction is thought to enhance the carcinogenic effect of some compounds, and cholestasis might also increase the carcinogenic effect of substances excreted in the bile (18).

One must assume that the hitherto reported cases of liver cell adenoma might represent merely the "tip of the iceberg" since clinically inapparent lesions would not be recognized. A detailed postmortem examination of young women dying of accidents or other unrelated causes might clarify this question. Regular examination of the abdomen of women on contraceptive steroids should become routine as part of prudent surveillance for adverse medical effects.

The epidemiology of endometrial cancer has been studied extensively (19). The known risk factors include several which appear to be associated with estrogen stimulation (20). Among young women with endometrial cancer are a relatively high proportion with Stein-Leventhal syndrome, a condition characterized by excess endogenous estrogen production. Moreover, cases of endometrial cancer have been reported among women with gonadal dysgenesis who were treated with diethylstilbestrol (DES) (21). In addition, obesity substantially increases the risk of endometrial cancer. This has been shown to be related to excessive conversion of androstenedione to estrone by adipose tissue in postmenopausal women (22).

There are several recent studies of the relative risk of endometrial cancer in women on postmenopausal estrogen (23–25), and they suggest an increased relative risk of endometrial cancer in these women. Based on these data, it appears that women on chronic estrogen therapy during their postmenopausal years face an annual incidence of endometrial cancer of 4–8/1,000.

The link between endometrial cancer and the use of sequential oral contraceptive preparations was suggested very recently (26). Observation of a few cases of endometrial cancer among young women on oral contraceptives led to the establishment of a registry for endometrial carcinoma in women under 40 who were on oral contraceptive agents. Criteria for acceptance of a case were: age under 40 at time of diagnosis, a documented history of oral contraceptive use, and the diagnosis of endometrial cancer confirmed by the pathologist in charge of the registery. The surprising finding among the reported cases was the high prevalence of use of sequential oral contraceptive preparations. Of 21 patients, 13 were using sequentials, 7 combination pills, and in one the preparation was unknown. This contrasts with market surveys, which suggest that only approximately 8% of women on oral contraceptives are taking sequential preparations. Eight of these patients received oral contraceptive therapy for other than contraceptive purposes. The indications were abnormal bleeding and Stein-Leventhal syndrome. Among 13 women on contraceptive steroids for contraceptive purposes, 11 received sequentials and only 2 combined preparations, an even higher preponderance of sequentials than in the total group. In 10 of these women, Oracon was prescribed. This is a sequential preparation consisting of dimethisterone 25 mg and ethynylestradiol 0.1 mg. Lyon (27) reported four additional cases of adenocarcinoma of the endometrium in young women who were on long-term sequential oral contraceptive therapy; all four also received Oracon. Three more cases of endometrial cancer in women on sequentials were reported by Kelley et al. (28). The preparation(s) involved were not stated.

Combination oral contraceptive therapy characteristically produces a shortened proliferative phase and a subsequent prolonged secretory phase in the cycle, whereas sequentials produce a longer proliferative phase and a shorter period of secretion and regression. It is not known if this difference accounts for the apparent relationship between sequential oral contraceptives and endometrial cancer.

Support for this relationship also can be derived from observations based on endometrial biopsies in women on sequential formulations (29). Endometrial hyperplasia and adenomatous hyperplasia appear to be related to the dose of estrogens used during the priming phase, as well as to the dose of the progestogen and the duration of the progestional phase of the treatment cycle (30). The nature of the data in support of the link between sequentials and endometrial cancer does not permit us to determine if an increased risk of endometrial cancer also exists for women on combination oral contraceptive therapy. The literature is devoid of studies of endometrial cancer in relation to combination oral contraceptives, and this is an area requiring urgent investigation.

Sequential agents have been withdrawn from use in the United States. This action was taken because of the suspicion of a linkage between sequentials and endometrial cancer, in addition to the well-known higher complication rate and lesser efficiency in preventing pregnancies associated with their use and difficulties in defining a group of women who required the use of sequential oral contraceptives rather than combination pills. This discontinuation of use undoubtedly will make it difficult to examine more fully the association between endometrial cancer and this modality of oral contraceptive therapy.

The evidence in support of a role of estrogens in endometrial cancer is compelling, however. Endometrial cancer has been linked to conditions with excessive endogenous estrogen production as occurs in Stein-Leventhal syndrome (20). Nonsteroidal estrogens administered to women with gonadal dysgenesis and, as were recently shown, to patients with breast cancer are associated with an increased risk of endometrial cancer (21,30). Moreover, there is now very strong evidence that the postmenopausal use of conjugated estrogens is followed by an increased incidence of endometrial cancer (23–25). The data regarding sequentials fit the notion that excessive estrogen stimulation unopposed or inadequately opposed by progesterone represents the basic hormonal environment conducive for an increased risk of endometrial cancer. Furthermore, the multiple linkages between nonsteroidal and steroidal forms of estrogen and endometrial cancer suggest that the pathogenetic mechanism is related to the estrogenic effect and not to the chemical configuration of the compounds involved.

REFERENCES

1. Baum, J. K., Bookstein, J. J., Holtz, F., and Klein, E. W. (1973): Possible association between benign hepatomas and oral contraceptives. *Lancet,* Oct. 27: 926–929.
2. Contostavlos, D. L. (1973): Benign hepatomas and oral contraceptives. *Lancet,* Nov. 24:1200.
3. Kelso, D. R. (1974): Benign hepatomas and oral contraceptives. *Lancet,* Feb. 23:315–316.
4. O'Sullivan, J. P., and Wilding, R. P. (1974): Liver hamartomas in patients on oral contraceptives. *Br. Med. J.,* 3:7–10.
5. Berg, J. W., Ketelaar, R. J., Rose, E. F., and Vernon, R. G. (1974): Hepatomas and oral contraceptives. *Lancet,* Aug. 10:349–350.
6. Model, D. G., Fox, J. A., and Jones, R. W. (1975): Multiple hepatic adenomas associated with an oral contraceptive. *Lancet,* Apr. 12:865.
7. Christopherson, W. M., Truman Mays, E., and Barrows, G. H. (1975): Liver tumors in women on contraceptive steroids. *Obstet. Gynecol.,* 46:221–223.
8. Stauffer, J. Q., Lapinski, M. W., Honold, D. J., and Myers, J. K. (1975): Focal nodular hyperplasia of the liver and intrahepatic hemorrhage in young women on oral contraceptives. *Ann. Intern. Med.,* 83:301–306.
9. Nissen, E. D., and Kent, D. R. (1975): Liver tumors and oral contraceptives. *Obstet. Gynecol.,* 24:460–467.
10. Christopherson, W. M. (1975): Liver tumors and the pill. *Br. Med. J.,* Dec. 27:756.
11. Bartok, I., Garas, S., and Szabo, L. (1976): Oral contraceptives and benign liver tumor. *Lancet,* Feb. 28:479–480.
12. Truman Mays, E., Christopherson, W. M., Mahr, M. M., and Williams, H. C. (1976): Hepatic changes in young women ingesting contraceptive steroids. *JAMA,* 235:730–732.
13. Antoniades, K., Campbell, W. N., Hecksher, R. H., Kessler, W. B., and McCarthy, G. E. Liver-cell adenoma and oral contraceptives. *JAMA,* 234:628–629.
14. Davis, M., Portmann, B., Searle, M., Wright, R., and Williams, R. (1975): Histological evidence of carcinoma in a hepatic tumor associated with oral contraceptives. *Br. Med. J.,* 4:496–498.

15. Edmondson, H. A., Henderson, B., and Benton, B. (1976): Liver-cell adenomas associated with use of oral contraceptives. *N. Engl. J. Med.,* Feb. 26:470–472.
16. Lead article. (1975): More on liver tumors and the pill. *Br. Med. J.,* Nov. 29:484–485.
17. Farrall, G. C., Joshua, D. E., Uren, R. F., Barid, P. J., Perkins, K. W., and Kronenberg, H. (1975): Androgen-induced hepatoma. *Lancet,* Feb. 22:430–431.
18. Sherlock, S. (1975): Hepatic adenomas and oral contraceptives. *Gut,* 16:753–756.
19. Wynder, E. L., Escher, G. C., and Mantel, N. (1966); An epidemiological investigation of cancer of the endometrium. *Cancer,* 19:489–520.
20. McMahon, B. (1974): Risk factors for endometrial cancer. *Gynecol. Oncol.* 2:122–129.
21. Cutler, B. S., Forbes, A. P., Ingersoll, F. M., and Scully, R. E. (1972): Endometrial carcinoma after stilbestrol therapy in gonadal dysgenesis. *N. Engl. J. Med.,* 287:628–631.
22. MacDonald, P. C., and Siiteri, P. K. (1974): The relationship between the extraglandular production of estrone and the occurrence of endometrial neoplasia. *Gynecol. Oncol.,* 2:259–263.
23. Zeil, H. K., and Finkle, W. D. (1975): Increased risk of endometrial carcinoma among users of conjugated estrogens. *N. Engl. J. Med.,* 293: 1167–1170.
24. Smith, D. C., Prentice, R., Thompson, D. J., and Herman, W. L. (1975): Association of exogenous estrogen and endometrial carcinoma. *N. Engl. J. Med.,* 293:1164–1167.
25. Mack, T. M., Pike, M. C., Henderson, B. E., Pfeffer, R. I., Gerkins, V. R., Arthur, M., and Brown, S. E. (1976): Estrogens and endometrial cancer in a retirement community. *N. Engl. J. Med.,* 294:1262–1267.
26. Silverberg, S. G., and Makowski, E. L. (1975): Endometrial carcinoma in young women taking oral contraceptive agents. *Obstet. Gynecol.,* 46:503–506.
27. Lyon, F. A. (1975): The development of adenocarcinoma of the endometrium in young women receiving long-term sequential oral contraception. *Am. J. Obstet. Gynecol.,* Oct. 1:299–301.
28. Kelley, H. W., Miles, P. A., Buster, J. B., and Scragg, W. H. (1976): Adenocarcinoma of the endometrium in women taking sequential oral contraceptives. *Obstet. Gynecol.,* 47:200–202.
29. Vanderick G., Beernaert, J., De Mylder, E., and Ferin, J. (1975): Hormonal contraception: Sequential formulations and the endometrium. *Contraception,* 12:655–664.
30. Hoover, R., Everson, R., Fraumeni, J. E., and Myers, M. H. (1976): Cancer of the uterine corpus after hormonal treatment for breast cancer. *Lancet,* Apr. 24:885–887.

Pharmacology of Steroid Contraceptive Drugs
edited by S. Garattini and H. W. Berendes.
Raven Press, New York © 1977.

Association Between Oral Contraceptive Use and Thromboembolism: A New Approach to Its Study

* Anthony P. Fletcher, * Norma K. Alkjaersig, and
†Robert Burstein

*Department of Internal Medicine and †Department of Obstetrics and Gynecology,
Washington University, School of Medicine, and The Jewish Hospital, St. Louis,
Missouri 63110*

Epidemiological evidence strongly suggests that oral contraceptive users exhibit a significant propensity to develop thromboembolic vascular disease complications. Risk estimates calculated from these data indicate that oral contraceptive users are at 4- to 11-fold greater danger of developing deep-vein thrombosis and pulmonary embolism than control unmedicated women, at similar enhanced risk of developing cerebral infarction, and at a lesser but still enhanced risk of developing myocardial infarction. In spite of these significant epidemiological data (1–3), and despite an increase in the use of low-estrogen oral contraceptive agents—hopefully less hazardous than those of high-estrogen content—evidence linking oral contraceptive use with thromboembolism is still appearing (4,5).

Two major problems have hindered the study of the relationship between oral contraceptive use and thromboembolic vascular disease complications. The first results from the notorious inaccuracy of clinical methodology available for the diagnosis of deep-vein thrombosis, and the fact that this disease and other thromboembolic vascular complications are frequently present in clinically silent or minimally symptomatic form. The second problem results from limitations inherent in conventional blood coagulation methodology, for these methods do not provide information about fibrin formation *in vivo* and thus about the presence or absence of thrombosis. However, the development of a new, noninvasive method for the study of fibrinogen catabolism in man, particularly for the study of fibrin formation, at least partially overcomes previous investigative limitations (6–10).

The principle of this approach is shown in Fig. 1. Overall fibrinogen catabolism in man totals 1–2 g/day. Although information on fibrinogen catabolism is incomplete, three distinct catabolic pathways are recognized. Some 70% of fibrinogen is catabolized by poorly defined pathways not resulting in other than subtle changes in fibrinogen structure and configuration during catabolism. However, the other two specific enzymatic catabolic pathways, which induce characteristic changes in the fibrinogen molecule, contribute approximately 30% to total fi-

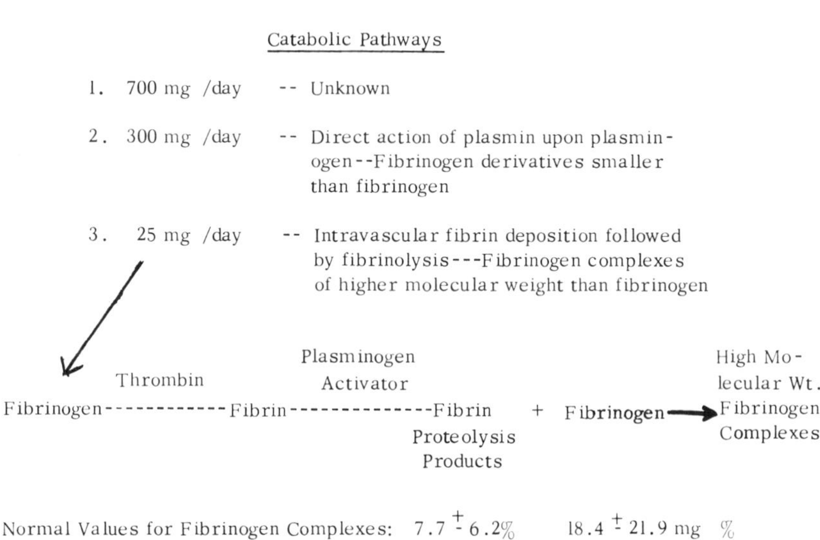

FIG. 1. The three fibrinogen catabolic pathways in man and their relative importance under physiological circumstances. Two of these pathways produce specific catabolic (reaction) products, the assay for which quantifies specific pathway activity.

brinogen catabolism. Between 25% and 30% of overall fibrinogen catabolism results from its degradation by the direct actions of the plasma fibrinolytic enzyme system, with the formation of fibrinogen derivatives of smaller molecular weight than the parent molecule. The activity of this pathway can be quantified by assay for fibrinogen derivatives with lower molecular weight than the parent molecule.

Under physiological conditions only a small fraction of fibrinogen, some 25–50 mg/day, is degraded through intravascular coagulation and subsequent fibrinolysis, a catabolic pathway resulting in the formation of high-molecular-weight fibrin(ogen)/fibrin complexes (HMWFC), mainly by the mechanism shown at the bottom of Fig. 1. The activity of this catabolic pathway is reflected by assay for fibrin(ogen)/fibrin complexes in plasma. Although other mechanisms for the formation of plasma HMWFCs exist, the complex may be regarded as reflecting the direct and remote consequences of thrombin release in the circulation and thus the rate of fibrin formation (11).

The development of thromboembolic vascular disease pathology—specifically intravascular coagulation or the development of a thrombus—results in enchanced fibrinogen catabolism via this normally quantitatively minor catabolic pathway, with an increase in the proportion and concentration of high-molecular-weight fibrinogen complexes. In normal subjects the latter complexes average 7.7% of normal plasma fibrinogen, or 18 mg%. Soluble derivatives of fibrinogen and/or fibrin may be quantified in plasma using plasma fibrinogen chromatography (6–10). Plasma is chromatographed by agarose gel exclusion chromatography, and fibrinogen/fibrin derivatives in the chromatographic effluents are quantified by specific immunological methods using the Technicon immunoprecipitator. A plot of fibrinogen/fibrin antigen concentration against chromatographic volume yields a molecular weight distribution plot of all fibrinogen-derived moieties in plasma; analysis of this plot by chromatographic plate theory (10) determines the relative proportions of plasma HMWFCs, native fibrinogen, and derivatives of fibrinogen smaller than the parent molecule present in the plasma. Enhanced fibrin formation is documented by finding of high-molecular-weight fibrinogen complexes in excess of mean ± 2 SD of normal. Several clinical investigative studies have shown a high correlation between the finding of enhanced plasma HMWFCs and the presence of a thrombus or documented intravascular coagulation (11,12).

Studies in postoperative patients in whom the presence of clinically silent thrombosis was detected by the ^{125}I-labeled fibrinogen scan technique confirmed that values for either the proportion or concentration of plasma HMWFCs exceeding the mean ± 2 SD of normal (i.e., complex proportions exceeding 20% or concentrations of 70 mg%) were significantly ($p < 0.001$) associated with the presence of a thrombus. Similarly, the finding of values for plasma HMWFCs lying within the range of mean ± 2 SD of normal values was significantly ($p < 0.01$) associated with the absence of a detectable thrombus (9).

CLINICAL CONSIDERATIONS

Laboratory findings (presented later) indicative of the high frequency of minimally symptomatic or clinically silent thrombotic disease in oral contraceptive users must be interpreted within a clinically relevant context. The most frequent thromboembolic pathology associated with oral contraceptive use is deep venous thrombosis (DVT) of the legs, often of the clinically silent type. Such venous pathology may spontaneously resolve, undergo local extension, or embolize to the lung. The prognosis of clinically silent DVT is greatly influenced by the patient's clinical status at the time of lesion development. In the surgically treated patient in whom a DVT is detected using the ^{125}I-labeled fibrinogen scan method, Kakkar's survey (14) indicates that pulmonary embolism will be detected in 8% of those afflicted, and in 3% pulmonary embolism will be of the severe type. In this situation circumstances favor disease extension: The patient suffered from a disease necessitating surgery, which may have predisposed to the development of thromboembolic vascular complications; an operation itself is a strong thrombogenic stimulus; and the patient is frequently in the older age group and is also partially immobilized during the postoperative period.

On the other hand, the average oral contraceptive user who develops clinically silent or minimally symptomatic DVT is young, healthy, and mobile. In these circumstances the prognosis for disease resolution is excellent. It can be estimated that in these favorable circumstances disease expression as pulmonary embolism will occur in only 0.1–0.01% of such instances, compared with an incidence of 8% in the postoperative surgical patient.

RATIONALE FOR PRESENT STUDY

On each occasion an oral contraceptive user develops a small deep venous thrombosis, she is at limited risk of developing disease extension and expression at the clinical level. Conversely, if fibrin formation in the oral contraceptive user is within physiological limits, she is not, at that time, at risk of developing thromboembolic vascular pathology.

Evidence that oral contraceptive drugs predispose to thromboembolism has been derived from epidemiological studies. Such studies involving the enumeration of episodes of clinically overt, but not always precisely diagnosed, thromboembolic vascular disease requires the study of very large patient populations for prolonged time periods, since clinically overt disease represents "only the tip of the iceberg" in the spectrum of thromboembolic vascular disease.

In this study we tested the hypothesis that drug thrombogenicity can be assessed by an approach based on the relative frequencies with which oral contraceptive users and control subjects are determined to be "at risk" of developing thromboembolic vascular disease, i.e., on the basis of the relative frequencies with which each group develops an elevated plasma HMWFC level in excess of the mean ± 2 SD of normal values (13).

CLINICAL STUDIES

We used serial plasma fibrinogen chromatography in longitudinal and cross-sectional studies of women receiving oral contraceptive agents. For the longitudinal population studies (Fig. 2) we followed new contraceptive users treated either with Ovulen (an oral contraceptive containing 100 μg mestranol) or Demulen (an oral contraceptive containing 50 μg ethinylestradiol). Sixty-six Ovulen-treated women and 57 Demulen-treated women were studied. The abscissa in Fig. 2 shows the percentage of plasma samples in which the HMWFC level exceeded the mean ± 2 SD of normal values at each time period prior to the use and following the start of oral contraceptives. These two groups of contraceptive-treated women were examined prior to the use of oral contraceptive therapy and were then followed by serial plasma fibrinogen chromatography after 1 and 3 months and thereafter at 3-month intervals.

Prior to commencing oral contraceptive therapy, the incidence of abnormal plasma fibrinogen chromatographic findings in this group of women was 6.3%. Following the institution of therapy, the percentage of samples showing chromatographic abnormality increased significantly to 25% at the end of 1

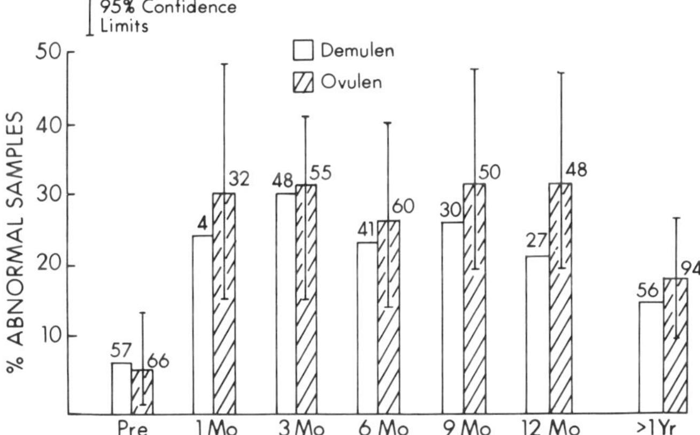

FIG. 2. Data from the new user oral contraceptive longitudinal study, plotted as percentage of samples showing plasma HMWFCs in excess of the mean ± 2 SD of normal values. The abscissa is time after commencing oral contraceptive medication. The number of samples examined at this time period are indicated at the top of each bar. One month after commencing oral contraceptive therapy, the percentage of subjects showing abnormal plasma fibrinogen chromatographic findings had risen from 6.3% (the value obtained prior to starting medication) to 29%. Similarly, statistically significant changes over control values are shown for each subsequent sampling period over the first year ($p < 0.001$). (From Alkjaersig et al., ref. 13.)

month; the percentage of abnormality in samples remained at approximately this figure for other time periods during the first year of therapy. These differences between plasma fibrinogen chromatographic findings in control, unmedicated women and the oral contraceptive users were highly statistically significant ($p < 0.001$). Although there was an apparent fall in the incidence of abnormal plasma fibrinogen chromatographic findings during the second year of oral contraceptive therapy, the difference is not statistically significant, a finding that may relate to loss of study patients (in some cases because of the development of adverse symptomatology). It may be noted that in each patient group studied, those on Demulen had a lower incidence of abnormal plasma fibrinogen chromatographic patterns than did the patients on Ovulen, the latter containing a higher daily content of estrogen. This apparent difference did not reach statistical significance; but when all the data from our studies are combined, there was a definite trend ($p < 0.1$) suggesting that oral contraceptive agents containing 50 μg ethynylestradiol induced a lesser degree of plasma fibrinogen chromatographic abnormality in users than did preparations containing a greater amount of estrogen.

Figure 3 shows data from the cross-sectional study on women receiving oral contraceptive agents for periods varying from 3 months to more than 8 years. The data are plotted in a similar fashion to those shown in Fig. 2. This was a relatively large-scale study involving 194 age-matched unmedicated, control women and 193 women receiving oral contraceptive medication of various types from whom 1,350 blood samples were analyzed by plasma fibrinogen chromatog-

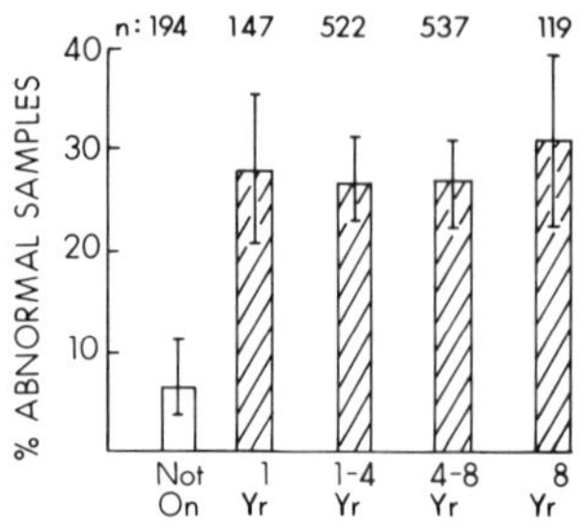

FIG. 3. This is similar in format to Fig. 2 but shows the results of the cross-sectional trial. Again, the unmedicated control women showed 6.3% incidence of abnormal plasma fibrinogen chromatographic findings, whereas the oral contraceptive users sampled at < 1, 1–4, 4–8, and > 8 years showed percentage abnormalities that ranged from 27.5% to 30.5%. All results of the oral contraceptive users at each sampling period differ significantly from the control value ($p < 0.001$). (From Alkjaersig et al., ref. 13.)

raphy. The control, unmedicated age-matched women had a 6.3% incidence of abnormal plasma fibrinogen chromatographic findings, whereas those who had received oral contraceptive medication for the periods shown in Fig. 2 demonstrated 25%–32% of abnormal plasma fibrinogen chromatographic patterns. It is to be noted that the percentage of plasma fibrinogen chromatographic abnormality in these patients did not increase with the duration of oral contraceptive use, a finding confirming the data of epidemiological studies, which rather surprisingly indicate that the risk of developing thromboembolic vascular disease pathology does not increase with increased duration of oral contraceptive therapy. Differences between control women and oral contraceptive users, shown in Fig. 2, are statistically highly significant ($p < 0.001$) and again show that patients receiving oral contraceptive therapy exhibit a significantly increased incidence of abnormal plasma fibrinogen chromatographic findings compared with unmedicated women. These data from the cross-sectional study are in excellent conformity with those obtained from the longitudinal study. Both studies demonstrate that women receiving oral contraceptive medication show a four- to five-fold[1] greater incidence of abnormal plasma fibrinogen chromatographic findings than do the unmedicated control women, an increase presumably attributable to the development of mainly clinically silent thrombotic pathology. This estimate of thromboembolic disease risk derived from our laboratory data is of similar magnitude to that derived by epidemiological study.

DURATION OF COAGULOPATHY

Patients who develop abnormal plasma fibrinogen chromatographic patterns characteristically do so in an episodic fashion. Abnormal plasma fibrinogen chromatographic findings usually persist for 1–6 weeks and then terminate in a plasma fibrinogen chromatographic pattern recognized as that of thrombus resolution. This pattern is defined as a fall in the percentage of plasma HMWFCs, together with a concomitant increase in the proportion of fibrinogen first deriva-

---

[1] Theoretically, the definition of chromatographic abnormality as values exceeding the mean ± 2 SD of normal implies that 2.5% of patients classed as abnormal should have been classed as normal. If correction is made for this "statistical artifact," the "risk factor" for oral contraceptive users is approximately sevenfold greater than that for unmedicated women.

tive, a moiety of lesser molecular weight than fibrinogen itself, the presence of which is indicative of enhanced plasma fibrinolytic activity and fibrinolysis.

The episodic nature of these plasma fibrinogen chromatographic findings is documented by data obtained in 73 subjects who were examined 1, 2, and 3 months after detection of abnormal plasma fibrinogen chromatographic findings. After 1 month 50% of the patients showed normal plasma fibrinogen chromatographic findings; after 2 months chromatographic findings were normal in 85%; and after 3 months in more than 90%. Since only three plasma samples were drawn during the 3-month study period after detection of abnormal plasma fibrinogen chromatographic findings, abnormal findings probably persisted for a shorter period of time than suggested by these data. These findings are consistent with the view that patients on oral contraceptive agents develop usually transient and resolving thromboembolic pathology at four- to fivefold greater frequency than do unmedicated controls.

However, some initially clinically silent thrombotic lesions, detected by plasma fibrinogen chromatography, undergo extension and are expressed as clinically overt disease. This series of events is shown in Fig. 4, where the first clinically silent thrombotic episode observed spontaneously resolved, whereas the second was expressed as clinically overt disease. Plasma fibrinogen chromatographic findings were initially normal in this subject, who had been on oral contraceptive agents for the previous 5 years. Shortly after the patient was first observed, plasma

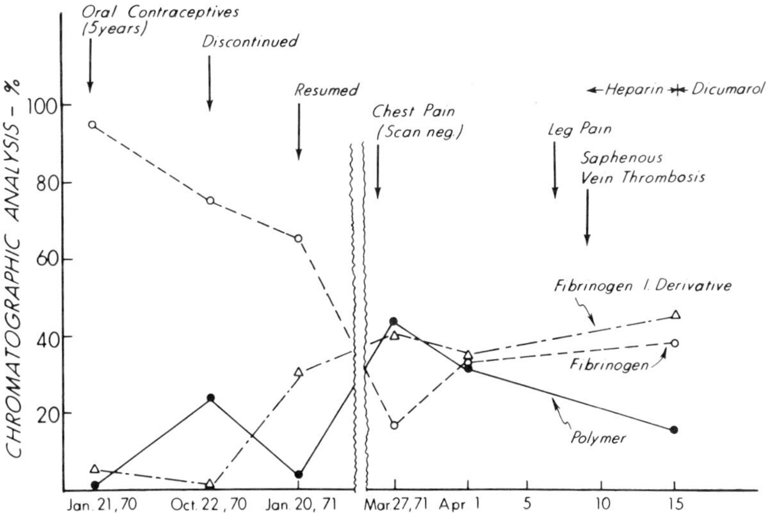

FIG. 4. Serial plasma fibrinogen chromatographic studies in a patient previously on oral contraceptive therapy for 5 years. Plasma HMWFCs percent (●——●); fibrinogen first derivative percent (△---△), and native fibrinogen percent (○---○). Plasma HMWFCs exceeded 20% on two occasions; the first time the patient was asymptomatic, but the second time there was clinical expression in the form of acute ileofemoral thrombosis (see text for details). (From Fletcher et al., ref. 1.)

fibrinogen chromatographic findings became abnormal; and although she was asymptomatic, medication was discontinued at her request. After plasma fibrinogen chromatographic findings spontaneously reverted to normal, the patient resumed the use of contraceptive medication but later developed an abnormal plasma fibrinogen chromatographic pattern with the amount of plasma HMWFCs exceeding 40% of the total, together with chest pain, suggestive of pulmonary embolism. At this time an isotopic chest scan was negative, but it was elected to discontinue oral contraceptive agents. Finally, 14 days later the patient developed clinically overt ileofemoral thrombosis and was successfully treated with heparin and Dicumarol therapy.

SUSCEPTIBILITY OF PATIENTS TO ORAL CONTRACEPTIVE MEDICATION

It is pertinent to question whether all or only a proportion of the patients using oral contraceptive agents are at increased risk of developing thromboembolic vascular disease complications. This problem can be approached by examining the frequency distribution of abnormal plasma fibrinogen chromatographic findings in our population. If all subjects examined are at equal risk of developing such complications, the frequency distribution of abnormal chromatographic findings in the population should be normal, i.e., of the gaussian type. On the other hand, if only a proportion of those receiving oral contraceptive medication were at risk of developing the complications, this frequency distribution would deviate significantly from gaussian characteristics.

The frequency distribution shown in Fig. 5 was calculated from a study of 165 oral contraceptive users who had been followed for 1 year or longer and whose plasma had been examined on at least five occasions; the average frequency was seven and the range five to nine. The abscissa shows the percentage of samples with > 20% HMWFCs observed in each set of patient samples, and the ordinate

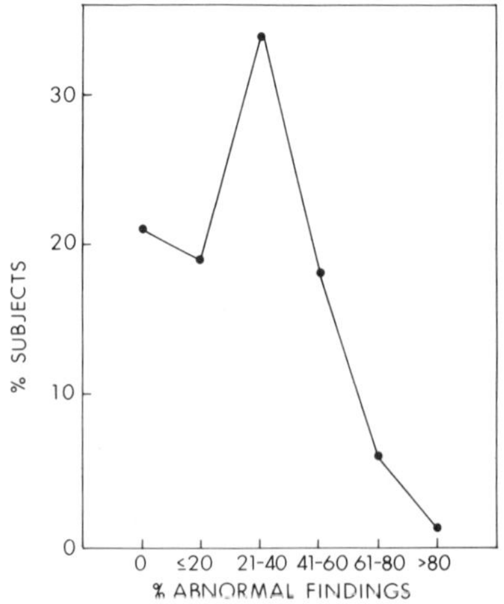

FIG. 5. Percentage of abnormal plasma fibrinogen chromatographic readings in each patient's assays (average of seven per patient) plotted against the percentage of the population. This frequency distribution is abnormal in shape, containing an obvious excess of patients with zero abnormal chromatographic findings. Statistical testing shows that this distribution is abnormal ($p <$ 0.001). (From Alkjaersig et al, ref. 13.)

is the percentage of patients with these sample frequencies. Figure 5 shows, for example, that 21% of the subjects had no abnormal plasma fibrinogen chromatographic findings during the study period, and there appears to be an apparent excess number of these patients with a zero incidence of abnormal plasma fibrinogen chromatographic findings. Calculation of expected frequencies on the basis of a binomial distribution and test by χ^2 of this distribution against the observed frequencies shows that this apparent anomaly was statistically significant ($p <$ 0.001). This finding suggests that some other factor besides the use of oral contraceptive agents influences the frequency of abnormal plasma fibrinogen chromatographic findings in the individual patient and suggests that the population is composed of individuals who reacted differently to oral contraceptive administration.

PATIENT SYMPTOMATOLOGY

Ethical and practical considerations precluded confirmation of the diagnoses of clinically silent thrombosis by specialized techniques such as venography or ^{125}I-labeled fibrinogen scan methodology. However, since patient symptomatology and physical signs were recorded, an indirect approach to the relationship between laboratory findings and the presence of clinical disease was undertaken.

The diagnosis of minimally symptomatic deep vein thrombosis is notoriously inaccurate, but symptoms and signs of this disease may be regarded as offering suggestive evidence of its presence. Consequently, if abnormal plasma fibrinogen chromatographic findings detect the presence of minimal thrombotic disease, it would be expected that symptoms suggestive but not diagnostic of these disorders would show a significant association with abnormal plasma fibrinogen chromatographic findings.

This hypothesis was investigated by comparing the percentage of abnormal plasma fibrinogen chromatographic findings in the group with symptoms suggestive of thromboembolic vascular disease (leg pain, chest pain, and transient cerebral ischemic attacks) and those with symptoms not apparently related to thromboembolic vascular disease (gynecological symptoms, water retention, easy bruisability, etc.). Abnormal plasma fibrinogen chromatographic findings ($> 20\%$ HMWFCs) were present in 42% of the first group but in only 20% of the second group ($p < 0.02$). Also, the incidence of abnormal plasma fibrinogen chromatographic findings in the thrombotic vascular disease "symptomatic" group was significantly greater ($p < 0.001$) than that observed in the total series (13). Thus a significant correlation is demonstrable between abnormal plasma fibrinogen chromatographic findings and symptoms suggestive of thromboembolic vascular disease.

DISCUSSION

Our studies demonstrate that abnormality of the plasma fibrinogen chromatogram with an increase in the proportion of high-molecular-weight fibrinogen complexes to $> 20\%$ occurs four- to fivefold more frequently in women receiving oral contraceptive agents than in unmedicated controls. These data provide a new link in the chain of evidence linking oral contraceptive use with a propensity to develop thromboembolic vascular disease complications. The risk factor for oral contraceptive usage and thromboembolic vascular disease complications, calculated from our data, corresponds to that estimated by epidemiological studies. Consequently it may be inferred that predisposition of women receiving oral contraceptive agents to develop clinically overt thromboembolic vascular disease results from the higher incidence of minor thrombotic episodes, each carrying a very small but definite risk of producing clinically evident disease, rather than because thrombotic episodes carry a poor prognosis for those on medication.

Although it may reasonably be held that the medical and social benefits of oral contraceptive use substantially outweigh the hazard inherent in their propensity to predispose to thromboembolic vascular disease complications, there is a need to develop oral contraceptive formulations or other birth control methods devoid of this danger. Thus the requirement to devise methods for testing the *in vivo* thrombogenicity of various oral contraceptive formulations and/or devices using small subject groups is one of priority. Our methods appear to meet the criteria for reasonably rapid testing of drug *in vivo* thrombogenicity using small subject groups followed for a short period of time, in contrast with large-scale epidemiological studies necessitating the observation of very large populations over several years. For example, new oral contraceptive formulations containing as little as 30 μg ethynylestradiol have recently been marketed in the hope of reducing user predisposition to thromboembolism. Using the current epidemiological approach, years will pass before this supposition can be adequately tested. In contrast, it is likely that the study of as few as 200 subjects for a year, using serial plasma fibrinogen chromatography, could provide very useful screening data as to whether this or another approach to reduce drug thrombogenic risk should be pursued.

Our new methods are also helpful in clinical practice, for in many patients on oral contraceptive medication suspicion of thromboembolic vascular disease necessitates hospitalization. In most cases signs or symptoms are suggestive but not diagnostic of thromboembolic vascular disease, and screening procedures such as the lung scan frequently produce equivocal results. In such instances the presence of significant thromboembolic vascular disease complications can be excluded by normal plasma fibrinogen chromatographic findings. This is a conclusion most reassuring to both patient and physician, and justifying the continuance of a therapy of unsurpassed effectiveness in preventing unwanted pregnancy.

ACKNOWLEDGEMENTS

This study was supported by the National Institute of Child Health and Human Development (NICHHD 71–2302).

REFERENCES

1. Fletcher, A., Alkjaersig, N., and Burstein, R. (1973): Effects of contraceptives on vascular system. In: *Human Reproduction: Conception and Contraception,* edited by E. S. Hafez and T. N. Evans, pp. 539–558. Harper & Row, New York.
2. Vessey, M. (1973): The epidemiology of venous thromboembolism. In: *Recent Advances in Thrombosis,* edited by L. Poller, pp. 39–58. Churchill-Livingstone, London.
3. Collaborative Group for the Study of Stroke in Young Women (1973): *N. Engl. J. Med.,* 288:871.
4. Boston Collaborative Drug Surveillance Program (1973): *Lancet,* 1:1399.
5. Stolley, P., et al. (1975): Thrombosis with low estrogen oral contraceptives. *Am. J. Epidemiol.,* 102:197–208.
6. Fletcher, A., et al. (1970): Blood hypercoagulability and thrombosis. *Trans. Am. Assoc. Physicians,* 83:159–167.
7. Fletcher, A., and Alkjaersig, N. (1972): Blood hypercoagulability, intravascular coagulation and thrombosis: New diagnostic concepts. *Thromb. Diath. Hemorrh. (Supp 1.),* 45:389–394.
8. Fletcher, A., et. al. (1973): Early detection of blood hypercoagulable states and early thromboembolic lesions in man. In: *Advances in Automated Analysis,* Vol. 4, edited by M. Erdrich, pp. 31–38. Mediaid, New York.
9. Fletcher, A., Alkjaersig, N., and O'Brien, J. (1972): Blood screening methods for the diagnosis of thromboembolism. In: *Bethesda Conference on Venous Thromboembolism,* Vol. 50, edited by S. Wessler, pp. 170–189. Millbank Memorial Fund Quarterly, New York.
10. Alkjaersig, N., et al. (1973): Analysis of gel exclusion chromatographic data by chromatographic plate theory analysis: Application to plasma fibrinogen chromatography. *Thromb. Res.,* 4:525–544.
11. Fletcher, A., and Alkjaersig, N. (1977): Physiological and pathophysiological study of blood coagulation system function by plasma fibrinogen chromatography. In: *Automated Immunoanalysis,* edited by R. Ritchie, Marcel Dekker, New York *(in press).*
12. Fletcher, A., and Alkjaersig, N. (1973): Laboratory diagnosis of intravascular coagulation. In: *Recent Advances in Thrombosis,* edited by L. Poller, pp. 87–111. Churchill-Livingstone, London.
13. Alkjaersig, N., Fletcher, A., and Burstein, R. (1975): Association between oral contraceptive use and thromboembolism: A new approach to its investigation based on plasma fibrinogen chromatography. *Am. J. Obstet. Gynecol.,* 122:199–209.
14. Kakkar, V. (1975): Deep vein thrombosis: Detection and prevention. *Circulation,* 51:8–19.

Pharmacology of Steroid Contraceptive Drugs
edited by S. Garattini and H. W. Berendes.
Raven Press, New York © 1977.

Experimental Studies on the Effects of Steroid Contraceptive Drugs on Lipid Metabolism

A. Bizzi, A. M. Tacconi, E. Veneroni, and S. Garattini

Istituto de Ricerche Farmacologiche "Mario Negri," 20157 Milan, Italy

It is well known that the use of oral steroid contraceptive drugs (SCD) leads in a number of cases to hyperlipemia characterized by a mild rise in plasma triglycerides (30–40 mg%) (1,23,24); this is sometimes particularly severe (7,26) and increases in relation to the length of time SCDs are used (15). Several investigations were carried out to elucidate the mechanism of hypertriglyceridemia in SCD users, but the picture is still unclear. It has been reported, for instance, that women under SCD treatment showed enhanced plasma triglyceride turnover (15, 16); other studies indicated reduced postheparin lipolytic activity (PHLA) (18), which might be due to a form of resistance to heparin (8,14). According to others, PHLA depression should be ascribed to hepatic lipase (present in PHLA but not responsible for triglyceride clearance) rather than to lipoprotein lipase (13). On the other hand, the hypothesis that induced hypertriglyceridemia is due to stimulation of endogenous triglyceride synthesis is now supported by a number of authors (10,15,16). This effect might be due to impaired pancreatic glucagon secretion and consequent alteration of the glucagon/insulin ratio (2).

In view of the difficulties in understanding the mechanism(s) by which plasma triglycerides increase under SCD treatment, we thought it useful to investigate the effects of SCDs in small laboratory animals in order to find models resembling the human situation. This chapter summarizes results obtained with three animal species—rats, mice, and guinea pigs—giving details of some of the results obtained with rats in order to establish similarities and dissimilarities between rat and human hypertriglyceridemia induced by SCDs.

MATERIALS AND METHODS

The effects of SCDs on lipid metabolism were studied in: (a) adult female Charles River rats (CD), body weight approximately 180 g; (b) adult female Swiss mice (CD-1-COBS), body weight approximately 33 g; and (c) adult female guinea pigs (Albino New England), body weight approximately 530 g.

The combinations of SCDs used throughout these experiments were: (a) lynestrenol + mestranol 17:1; (b) norethindrone + mestranol 20:1; and (c) norethynodrel + mestranol 65:1. The dosage was the minimal antifertility dose for each strain of animals. In some instances estrogen and progestins were given separately.

The treatment schedule was as follows: The progestin-estrogen combinations were dissolved in corn oil. Rats and mice received the doses in 0.1 ml per animal; guinea pigs received 0.5 ml/kg; and controls received only corn oil. The compounds were administered orally at 3 P.M. each day for 30 consecutive days. Animals were usually killed 18 hr after the last treatment. Triton WR 1339 (TWR 1339) was injected into the femoral vein at the dose of 600 mg/kg, and blood was collected at various intervals thereafter.

Chemical Determinations

Lipids were extracted from plasma and tissues with chloroform/methanol 2:1 according to the procedure of Carlson (4). The chloroform phase was divided into two aliquots. One was used for phospholipid determinations, according to Svanborg and Svennerholm (21); and the other was shaken with silicic acid and used for triglyceride and cholesterol determinations, according to van Handel et al. (11) and by the Lieberman-Burchard reaction, respectively.

Lipoproteins: Serum chylomicrons (Chyl) were separated by ultracentrifugation at 87,000g for 15 min; very low density lipoproteins (VLDL), low density lipoproteins (LDL), and high density lipoproteins (HDL) were separated according to Havel et al. (12).

Lipoprotein lipase activity: This was measured in adipose tissues of rats treated with SCDs, essentially as described by Cherkes and Gordon (5).

PHLA: Rats were injected with heparin (5–10 mg/kg i.v.) and exsanguinated 3 and 10 min later. Plasma 0.5 ml was incubated with an Ediol-fresh serum mixture (1:1) at 37°C for 15 min. Free fatty acids released in the medium were measured by the method of Trout et al. (22).

RESULTS

Effect of SCDs on Plasma and Tissue Lipids in the Mouse, Guinea Pig, and Rat

Table 1 summarizes the effect of chronic administration of the progestin-estrogen combinations lynestrenol-mestranol, norethindrone-mestranol, and norethynodrel-mestranol on plasma and liver lipids of mice. These compounds were given at the lowest doses required to cause 100% sterility in mice. As shown, regardless of the compound administered, the effects were confined to a marked decrease in liver triglycerides, and no alterations were observed in plasma lipids. When mestranol and lynestrenol were given singly, only mestranol was able to deplete liver triglycerides (controls 789 ± 69 mg/100 g, mestranol 452 ± 41 mg/-100 g tissue), suggesting that estrogen was the active compound. In this experi-

TABLE 1. *Effect of chronic SCD treatment on plasma and liver lipids in mice*

Treatment (mg/kg/day p.o. X 30 days)	Plasma (mg/100 ml ± SE)			Liver(mg/100 g±SE)
	TG	Chol	P	TG
Controls	97 ± 7	100 ± 7	6.7 ± 0.3	1,201 ± 147
Lynestrenol (5)+ mestranol (0.3)	103 ± 2	126 ± 8	7.1 ± 0.2	603 ± 45[a]
Controls	118 ± 10	119 ± 4	6.5 ± 0.1	1,254 ± 110
Norethynodrel (0.5) + mestranol (0.0075)	111 ± 20	125 ± 12	7.0 ± 0.8	615 ± 44[a]
Controls	133 ± 10	107 ± 5	7.8 ± 0.1	1,567 ± 145
Norethindrone (4) + mestranol (0.2)	96 ± 5	97 ± 5	7.0 ± 0.3	777 ± 62[a]

TG, triglycerides. Chol, cholesterol. P, phosphorus content in phospholipids.
Each figure is the average of five animals.
[a] $p < 0.01$ against controls (Student's *t*-test).

TABLE 2. *Effect of chronic SCD treatment on plasma lipids in guinea pigs*

Treatment (mg/kg/day p.o. × 30 days)	Plasma (mg/100 ml ± SE)		
	TG	Chol	P
Controls	53 ± 4	68 ± 6	1.6 ± 0.1
Lynestrenol (1.25)+ mestranol (0.075)	38 ± 5[a]	51 ± 3[b]	1.0 ± 0.2
Norethynodrel (1)+ mestranol (0.015)	31 ± 5[a]	55 ± 4	1.3 ± 0.1
Norethindrone (4)+ mestranol (0.2)	27 ± 2	38 ± 1	1.0 ± 0.1
Controls	60 ± 5	44 ± 4	1.1 ± 0.1
Lynestrenol (5)+ mestranol (0.3)	25 ± 5	34 ± 5	0.7 ± 0.1
Norethynodrel (4)+ mestranol (0.06)	32 ± 2[a]	33 ± 2	1.0 ± 0.5
Controls	51 ± 7	45 ± 3	1.4 ± 0.1
— Mestranol (0.075)	24 ± 2[a]	27 ± 4[a]	0.9 ± 0.1
— Mestranol (0.3)	24 ± 3[a]	26 ± 2[a]	0.8 ± 0.1
— Lynestrenol (1.25)	48 ± 7	37 ± 4	1.2 ± 0.1
— Lynestrenol (5)	36 ± 4[b]	32 ± 3	1.1 ± 0.1

TG, triglycerides. Chol, cholesterol. P, Phosphorus content in phospholipids.
Each figure is the average of five animals.
[a] $p \leqslant 0.01$. [b] $p \leqslant 0.05$ (Student's *t*-test).

ment adrenal cholesterol was not affected by the estrogen, the progestin, or the combination.

The picture was different when the progestin-estrogen combinations were given to the guinea pig. Table 2 shows that when the SCD combinations were given either at minimal doses causing 100% sterility or at much higher doses there was only a slight decrease in plasma lipids. When the compounds were given singly, each caused a decrease in plasma lipids although estrogen was effective at a lower dose.

When adult female rats received the above-mentioned SCD combinations (at minimal doses causing 100% sterility), the results were as expected (Table 3): increased plasma triglycerides, decreased liver triglycerides, decreased plasma and adrenal cholesterol. As shown with the lynestrenol-mestranol combination, the effects were not dose-related and still appeared when only 1/80 of the minimal dose which inhibited conception 100% was given.

When the effect of progestins and estrogen given singly at the doses present in each combination were investigated, at least in our experimental conditions, the estrogen and the progestin had the same effect on lipid levels in plasma and tissues (Table 3). However, data not reported here in detail indicate that a different progestin, *d*-norgestrel, given at doses up to 3 mg/kg/day p.o. for 1 month, did not affect plasma, liver, or adrenal lipids and did not antagonize the effect of mestranol.

Effect of SCDs on Lipid Metabolism in Rats

An investigation was carried out to characterize the effect of SCDs on triglyceride metabolism in rats. First it was observed that when chronic treatment was

TABLE 3. Effect of chronic treatment with different SCDs and with their single components on plasma and tissue lipids in the female rat.

Treatment (mg/kg/day p.o. × 30 days)		Plasma (mg/100 ml ± SE)			Liver TG (mg/100 g ± SE)	Adrenals Chol (mg/100 g ± SE)
Progestin	Estrogen	TG	Chol	P		
Controls		82 ± 10	78 ± 10	5.5 ± 0.4	473 ± 33	4,044 ± 392
Lynestrenol 5 +	Mestranol 0.3	161 ± 13[a]	47 ± 3[a]	5.3 ± 0.3	237 ± 7	1,748 ± 262[a]
Norethynodrel 4 +	Mestranol 0.06	157 ± 23[a]	54 ± 4[a]	4.4 ± 0.3	264 ± 24	2,219 ± 170[a]
Norethindrone 4 +	Mestranol 0.2	186 ± 4[a]	59 ± 7[a]	5.1 ± 0.6	226 ± 13	2,075 ± 604[a]
Lynestrenol 2.5 +	Mestranol 0.15	139 ± 13[a]	53 ± 3[a]	6.5 ± 0.6	265 ± 9	1,622 ± 162[a]
Lynestrenol 0.62 +	Mestranol 0.037	121 ± 13[a]	49 ± 3[a]	5.2 ± 0.2	432 ± 49	2,790 ± 250[a]
Lynestrenol 2.5	—	154 ± 23	43 ± 2	4.8 ± 0.8	346 ± 27	2,898 ± 578[a]
—	Mestranol 0.15	146 ± 6	43 ± 2	4.4 ± 0.1	290 ± 8	2,915 ± 491[a]
Norethynodrel 4	—	148 ± 13	43 ± 3	4.2 ± 0.3	278 ± 9	2,017 ± 174[a]
—	Mestranol 0.06	160 ± 16	52 ± 3	5.1 ± 0.2	237 ± 3	2,739 ± 215[a]
Norethindrone 4	—	113 ± 12	45 ± 3	3.7 ± 0.3	231 ± 33	2,181 ± 23
—	Mestranol 0.2	171 ± 21	52 ± 5	4.9 ± 0.2	205 ± 28	2,169 ± 372

Each figure represents the average of five animals.
TG, triglycerides. Chol, cholesterol. P, phosphorus content in phospholipids.
[a] $p \leq 0.01$ against controls (New Duncan multiple test).

withdrawn plasma and tissue lipid levels returned to normal within 3–4 days in fed rats (Table 4). Data in Table 5 indicate the marked difference in the extent of the plasma triglyceride rise in SCD-treated rats caused by the presence or absence of food; in the fasted rats the before and after treatment differences were still significant, but the extent of this increase was considerably less than in fed rats. An additional dose of these compounds (which were effective in fed rats) to fasted rats did not further increase plasma triglycerides. These results suggest that the hypertriglyceridemia might be partially related to the nutritional status of the animals. To define better the lipid alterations which occur after chronic administration of lynestrenol plus mestranol, lipids were measured in individual lipoprotein fractions (chylomicrons, VLDL, LDL, HDL). Table 6 summarizes the results. Triglycerides were higher in VLDL and chylomicrons; cholesterol was lower in HDL, which in rats carry the bulk of cholesterol; and a considerable portion of phospholipids shifted from HDL to LDL. Qualitatively similar results were obtained in the fasted rats.

Since the increase in plasma triglycerides might be related to increased intestinal absorption, as well as to increased hepatic secretion or lower plasma clearance, we decided to check these points. When rats pretreated for 30 days with lynestrenol plus mestranol (5 + 0.3 mg/kg) received an oral load of olive oil (20 ml/day), their plasma triglyceride levels were higher than those in the controls given the oil but not pretreated (Table 7).

To establish whether the rise in plasma triglycerides was due to increased intestinal absorption or slower clearance, an attempt was made to determine the lymphatic triglycerides in rats with the thoracic ductus cannulated (3). In spite of broad variations in both flow and triglyceride concentrations, the values in controls and SCD-treated rats were in the same range. It must be borne in mind, however, that the rats underwent anesthesia and surgery, so the conditions of this experiment were different from the previous ones. On the other hand, if the animal is allowed to recover completely from the stress of surgery, the prolonged lymph deprivation could result in some metabolic alterations.

The possibility that plasma clearance might be affected was investigated by injecting intravenously a suspension of chylomicrons obtained from donor rats and then measuring chylomicron clearance from plasma. Table 8 shows that plasma triglyceride levels remained higher in lynestrenol-mestranol-treated rats than in controls.

The most likely factor in plasma triglyceride clearance is lipoprotein lipase activity. However, PHLA measured in the serum of lynestrenol-mestranol-treated rats was not significantly different from that in control sera (Table 9).

Since in humans it has been postulated that the use of oral contraceptives may affect the hepatic secretion of triglycerides, the effect of pretreatment with oral steroid contraceptives was challenged against TWR 1339. TWR 1339 is a surfactant which, when given by the parenteral route, causes hyperlipemia by changing the physicochemical properties of lipids in such a way that they are no longer available to lipoprotein lipase (17,20).

TABLE 4. *Duration of the effects of chronic SCD treatment on plasma and adrenal lipids*

Treatment (mg/kg/day × 30 days)	Withdrawal duration	Plasma (mg/100 ml ± SE)			Adrenal Chol (mg/100 ml ± SE)
		TG	Chol	P	
Controls	18 hr	55 ± 4	88 ± 4	4.9 ± 0.2	3,642 ± 432
Lynestrenol (5) + mestranol (0.3)	18 hr	188 ± 11[a]	55 ± 6[a]	5.3 ± 0.6	1,757 ± 343[a]
Controls	2 days	80 ± 15	89 ± 5	4.9 ± 0.2	4,618 ± 142
Lynestrenol (5) + mestranol (0.3)	2 days	135 ± 17[a]	71 ± 6	5.6 ± 0.4	8,482 ± 199[a]
Controls	4 days	62 ± 7	125 ± 7	6.2 ± 0.1	4,395 ± 458
Lynestrenol (5) + mestranol (0.3)	4 days	77 ± 4	100 ± 4	5.7 ± 0.2	4,330 ± 109

TG, triglycerides. Chol, cholesterol. P, phosphorus content in phospholipids.
The rats had free access to food until they were killed.
[a] $p \leqslant 0.01$ against respective controls (Student's t-test).

TABLE 5. *Interaction of nutritional conditions with the effect of SCDs on lipid metabolism*

Physiological conditions[a]	Treatment[b] (mg/kg/day p.o. × 30 days)	Time between last treatment and killing (hr)	Plasma (mg/100 ml ± SE)		
			TG	Chol	P
Fed	Controls	—	70 ± 4	94 ± 6	4.0 ± 0.2
Fasted	Controls	—	51 ± 8	89 ± 7	4.2 ± 0.2
Fed	L + M (5 + 0.3)	18	165 ± 14^{c}	47 ± 3^{c}	4.3 ± 0.3
Fasted	L + M (5 + 0.3)	18	92 ± 5^{c}	46 ± 2^{c}	3.9 ± 0.3
Fasted	L + M (5 + 0.3)	2	89 ± 7^{c}	40	$3.3 + 0.2$

[a] Fed means that rats had food available until they were killed. Fasted means rats fasted overnight before being killed. Each figure represents the average of five animals.
TG, triglycerides. Chol, cholesterol. P, phosphorus content in phospholipids.
[b] L, lynestrenol. M, mestranol.
[c] $p \leqslant 0.01$ against controls (Student's *t*-test).

TABLE 6. *Lipid composition in lipoproteins from serum of rats treated with SCDs*

Lipoprotein fractions[a]	Fed			Fasted		
	Chol	TG	P	Chol	TG	P
L + M treatment[b]						
Chylomicrons	78	878	4.4	26	481	1.7
VLDL	87	687	5.4	50	256	2.9
LDL	117	70	9.5	128	60	8.5
HDL	187	31	12.0	214	28	8.5
Control						
Chylomicrons	32	310	2.2	8	213	2.4
VLDL	37	306	2.5	15	103	0.4
LDL	96	98	1.9	85	94	1.7
HDL	651	70	19.0	694	74	20.0

CHOL = Cholesterol; TG = triglycerides; P = phosphorus content in phospholipids.

[a] VLDL, very low density lipoproteins. LDL, low density lipoproteins. HDL, high density lipoproteins.

[b] L + M = lynestrenol + mestranol (5 + 0.3 mg/kg/day X 30 days). Each figure represents a pool of five rats.

TABLE 7. *Effect of chronic SCD treatment on hypertriglyceridemia induced by an olive oil load*

Chronic treatment (mg/kg/day X 23 days)	Olive oil load, 20 mg/kg (2 hr)	Plasma triglycerides (mg/100 ml ± SE)	Δ
Controls	—	60 ± 10	
Controls	+	239 ± 27[a]	179
Lynestrenol 5 + mestranol 0.3	—	166 ± 21	
Lynestrenol 5 + mestranol 0.3	+	562 ± 36[b]	396

The last SCD administration was given 18 hr and the olive oil 2 hr before blood sampling. $p < 0.01$ against controls,[a] and controls plus olive oil.[b]

TABLE 8. *Effect of pretreatment with SCDs on disappearance of exogenous chylomicrons from plasma*

Acute treatment (mg/kg i.v.)	Min	Plasma triglycerides (mg/100 ml ± SE)	
		Controls	L + M
—	0	61 ± 4	104 ± 26
Saline	2	55 ± 3	108 ± 12
Chyl-TG (33)	1	853 ± 39	908 ± 4
Chyl-TG (33)	2	800 ± 25	800 ± 50
Chyl-TG (33)	4	382 ± 56	625 ± 41[a]
Chyl-TG (33)	8	183 ± 29	397 ± 40[a]

Lymph chylomicrons (Chyl) suspended in saline (triglyceride content 6.6 mg/ml) were injected into fed rats (15 ml/kg). Min, the time between injection and killing. L + M, lynestrenol + mestranol (5 + 0.3 mg) daily for 30 days. Last treatment was given 18 hr before the chylomicron injection.

[a] $p \leqslant 0.01$ against respective controls (Student's *t*-test).

TABLE 9. *Effect of chronic SCD treatment on PHLA*

Heparin (mg/kg i.v.)	Duration[a] (min)	PHLA (FFA, μEq/ml $\pm$ SE)[b]	
		Controls	Treated
—	—	0.18 ± 0.04	0.52 ± 0.09
5	3	1.8 ± 0.06	2.27 ± 0.18
5	10	1.77 ± 0.11	1.51 ± 0.19
10	3	1.70 ± 0.08	2.02 ± 0.29
10	10	1.62 ± 0.07	1.33 ± 0.27

Treated rats received lynestrenol + mestranol (5 + 0.3 mg/kg p.o.) daily for 30 days.

[a] Time between heparin injection and blood collection.

[b] FFA, free fatty acids.

In fasted animals TWR 1339-induced hyperlipemia is generally considered to be an index of hepatic secretion. Preliminary results from rats pretreated with SCDs and fasted the night before the experiment indicated that the degree of hyperlipemia induced by TWR 1339 was similar to that in the controls. Since fasting limited the hypertriglyceridemia induced by contraceptive steroids, however, we decided to study the effect of TWR 1339 on lynestrenol-mestranol-treated rats which had had food available until the beginning of the experiment. The results (Table 10) show that even in these experimental conditions a comparable rise in plasma triglycerides occurred in both groups.

CONCLUSIONS

Findings presented in this chapter show that the administration of SCDs caused alterations in lipids, differing according to the animal species used (mouse, guinea pig, rat). Adult female rats treated with SCDs showed a rise in plasma triglycerides which might resemble that observed in humans. This hypertriglyceridemia was accompained by a decrease in liver triglycerides and in plasma and adrenal cholesterol. Plasma triglycerides increased in chylomicrons and VLDL, whether the animals had free access to food or were fasted overnight. The fall in plasma triglycerides induced by fasting was much greater in SCD-treated rats than in controls.

The fall of triglycerides during fasting and the low hepatic triglyceride levels might be due to reduced synthesis in the liver endoplasmic reticulum, as postulated by Young, with estradiol (25). In contrast with this view, however, administration of TWR 1339 raised plasma triglycerides at a comparable rate in controls and SCD-treated rats, suggesting that hepatic secretion of triglycerides was not affected by SCDs. However, it must be also considered that TWR 1339 has other effects in addition to its well-known inhibition of lipoprotein lipase (9). Although lipoprotein lipase from parametrical adipose tissue and PHLA seemed normal, the reduced rate of clearance of exogenous triglycerides and the higher levels of

TABLE 10. *Effect of SCDs on TWR 1339 hypertriglyceridemia*

Treatment		Plasma triglycerides (mg/100 ml ± SE) at 1–6 hr after TWR 1339			
Days 1–30	Day 31	1 hr	2 hr	4 hr	6 hr
—	—				
—	TWR 1339 (600 mg/kg i.v.)	329 ± 16	965 ± 64	1,893 ± 81	2,235 ± 94
—	—				
Lynestrenol + mestranol (5 + 0.3 mg/kg p.o.)	TWR 1339 (600 mg/kg i.v.)	402 ± 25	1,095 ± 108	2,048 ± 128	2,235 ± 136

Rats had food available until the beginning of the experiment.
Basal values for controls were 81 ± 5 mg/100 ml, and 126 ± 18 mg/100 ml for lynestrenol + mestranol.

plasma but not lymphatic triglycerides in SCD-treated rats after an oral triglyceride load might be indirect evidence of decreased plasma triglyceride clearance
during SCD treatment. This effect might be due to altered lipoprotein lipase
activation. In fact, the phospholipid shift from HDL to LDL might have caused
an alteration or deficiency in HDL apoproteins, which are known to be important
for lipoprotein lipase activation (6,19). The overall picture gained from this data,
rather than clarifiying the mechanism of action of SCDs on the lipid metabolism,
suggests that SCDs may elicit more than one effect.

REFERENCES

1. Aurell, M., Cramér, K., and Rybo, G. (1966): Serum lipids and lipoproteins during long-term administration of an oral contraceptive. *Lancet,* 1:291–293.
2. Beck, P., Eaton, R. P., Arnett, D. M., and Alsever, R. N. (1975): Effect of contraceptive steroids on arginine-stimulated glucagon and insulin secretion in women. I. Lipid physiology. *Metabolism,* 24:1055–1065.
3. Bollman, J. L., Cain, J. C., and Grindlay, J. H. (1948): Techniques for the collection of lymph from the liver, the small intestine and the thoracic duct of the rat. *J. Lab. Clin. Med.,* 33:-1349–1352.
4. Carlson, L. A. (1963): Determination of serum triglycerides. *J. Atheroscler. Res.,* 3:334–336.
5. Cherkes, A., and Gordon, R. S., Jr. (1959): The liberation of lipoprotein lipase by heparin from adipose tissue incubated "in vitro." *J. Lipid Res.,* 1:97–101.
6. Chung, J., Scanu, A. M., and Reman, F. (1973): Effects of phospholipids on lipoprotein lipase activation "in vitro." *Biochim. Biophys. Acta,* 296:116–123.
7. Davidoff, F., Tishler, S., and Rosoff, C. (1973): Marked hyperlipidemia and pancreatitis associated with oral contraceptive therapy. *N. Engl. J. Med.,* 289:552–555.
8. Ence, T. J., Wilson, D. E., Flowers, C. M., Chen, A. L., Glad, B. W., and Hershgold, E. J. (1976): Heparin metabolism and heparin-released lipase activity during long-term estrogen-progestin treatment. *Metabolism,* 25:139–145.
9. Garattini, S., Paoletti, P., and Paoletti, R. (1959): The effect of Triton and diphenylethylacetic acid on cholesterol and fatty acid biosynthesis in isolated perfused liver. *Experientia,* 15:33–34.
10. Glueck, C. J., Fallat, R. W., and Scheel, D. (1975): Effects of estrogenic compounds on triglyceride kinetics. *Metabolism,* 24:537–545.
11. Handel, E. Van, Zilversmit, D. B., and Bowman, K. (1957): Micromethod for the direct determination of serum triglycerides. *J. Lab. Clin. Med.,* 50:152–157.
12. Havel, R. J., Eder, H. A., and Bragdon, J. H. (1955): The distribution and chemical composition of ultracentrifugally separated lipoproteins in human serum. *J. Clin. Invest.,* 34:1345–1353.
13. Hazzard, W. R., Brunzell, J. D., Applebaum, D. M., Goldberg, A. P., Gagne, C., Albers, J. J., Wahl, P. W., and Hoover, J. J. (1976): Steroid contraceptives and human lipoprotein metabolism: Effects and mechanisms. This volume.
14. Hazzard, W. R., Notter, D. T., Spiger, M. J., and Bierman, E. L. (1972): Oral contraceptives and triglyceride transport: Acquired heparin resistance as the mechanism for impaired post-heparin lipolytic activity. *J. Clin. Endocrinol. Metab.,* 35:425–437.
15. Kekki, M., and Nikkilä, E. A. (1971): Plasma triglyceride turnover during use of oral contraceptives. *Metabolism,* 20:878–889.
16. Kissebah, A. H., Harrigan, P., and Wynn, V. (1973): Mechanism of hypertriglyceridaemia associated with contraceptive steroids. *Horm. Metab. Res.,* 5:184–190.
17. Otway, S., and Robinson, D. S. (1967): The effect of a non-ionic detergent (Triton WR 1339) on the removal of triglyceride fatty acids from the blood of the rat. *J. Physiol. (Lond.),* 190:-309–319.
18. Rössner, S., Larsson-Cohn, U., Carlson, L. A., and Boberg, J. (1971): Effects of an oral contraceptive agent on plasma lipids, plasma lipoproteins, the intravenous fat tolerance and the post-heparin lipoprotein lipase activity. *Acta Med. Scand.,* 190:301–305.
19. Scanu, A. (1967): Binding of human serum high density lipoprotein, apoprotein with aqueous dispersions of phospholipids. *J. Biol. Chem.,* 242:711–719.

20. Schotz, M. C., Scanu, A., and Page, I. H. (1957): Effect of Triton on lipoprotein lipase of rat plasma. *Am. J. Physiol.,* 188: 399–402.
21. Svanborg, A., and Svennerholm, L. (1961): Plasma total lipid, cholesterol, triglycerides, phospholipids and free fatty acids in a healthy Scandinavian population. *Acta Med. Scand.,* 169:43–49.
22. Trout, D. L., Estes, E. H., Jr., and Friedberg, S. J. (1960): Titration of free fatty acids of plasma: A study of current methods and a new modification. *J. Lipid Res.,* 1:199–202.
23. Wynn, V., Doar, J. W. H., and Mills, G. L. (1966): Some effects of oral contraceptives on serum-lipid and lipoprotein levels. *Lancet,* 2:720–723.
24. Wynn, V., Doar, J. W. H., Mills, G. L., and Stokes, T. (1969): Fasting serum triglyceride, cholesterol, and lipoprotein levels during oral-contraceptive therapy. *Lancet,* 2:756–760.
25. Young, D. L. (1971): Estradiol- and testosterone-induced alterations in phosphatidylcholine and triglyceride synthesis in hepatic endoplasmic reticulum. *J. Lipid Res.,* 12:590–595.
26. Zorrilla, E., Hulse, M., Hernandez, A., and Gershberg, H. (1968): Severe endogenous hypertriglyceridemia during treatment with estrogen and oral contraceptives. *J. Clin. Endocrinol. Metab.,* 28:1793–1796.

Pharmacology of Steroid Contraceptive Drugs
edited by S. Garattini and H. W. Berendes.
Raven Press, New York © 1977.

Steroid Contraceptives and Human Lipoprotein Metabolism: Effects and Mechanisms

William R. Hazzard, John D. Brunzell, Deborah M. Applebaum, Andrew P. Goldberg, Claude Gagne, John J. Albers, Patricia W. Wahl, and J. Joanne Hoover

University of Washington Schools of Medicine and Public Health; and Veterans Administration Hospital, Division of Metabolism, Seattle, Washington

The side effects of chronic medications may affect the incidence and course of the chronic, age-related diseases so prevalent in economically developed nations. Shortly after the introduction of steroid contraceptive hormones some 15 years ago, several side effects were reported with implications for the incidence of ischemic cardiovascular disease: thromboembolism and changes in the homeostasis of blood coagulation, increased blood pressure, carbohydrate intolerance and hyperinsulinism, and increased plasma lipid levels. The dramatic increase in the use of these hormones during the ensuing years has greatly magnified these implications, so that a review of current advances and knowledge regarding these phenomena is timely.

This chapter is confined to the increased lipid levels. However, the reader will do well to bear in mind the interactive nature of the risk factors to ischemic disease and the potential synergism between hyperlipidemia and other risk factors induced by the steroid contraceptives. This communication reviews the following: (a) the prevalence and types of hyperlipidemia induced by steroid contraceptives, with new information contrasting the changes associated with combination contraceptives versus those with postmenopausal estrogen replacement; (b) the changes in plasma apolipoproteins which accompany (and possibly control) the altered blood lipid levels; (c) changes in the levels of lipolytic enzymes induced by these steroids; (d) the balance between plasma triglyceride (TG) input and removal during contraceptive steroid therapy in normo- and hyperlipidemic persons; and (e) special insights into the control of normal and abnormal lipid metabolism which proceed from the unique and paradoxical hypolipidemic response of subjects with type III hyperlipoproteinemia (broad-β disease) to estrogen therapy.

HYPERLIPIDEMIA INDUCED BY STEROID CONTRACEPTIVES

Increased plasma TG levels during steroid contraceptive therapy were predicted by the known effects of estrogens on plasma lipid levels (1). The frequency of such increases was well demonstrated by Wynn and Doar in cross-sectional (2) and longitudinal (3) studies. Under the auspices of the Lipid Research Clinics Program of the National Heart & Lung Institute, we have recently been participating in a collaborative, comprehensive epidemiological survey of the determinants of plasma lipid levels in several populations of widely differing demographic characteristics in four nations. Since a sizable number of adult participants were women, many consuming steroid contraceptives or estrogen supplements, this has afforded us an opportunity to assess the effects of these medications on plasma lipoproteins qualitatively and quantitatively.

A preliminary analysis of the national collaborative data (4) served to underscore the potential impact of the contraceptives on hypertriglyceridemia and hypercholesterolemia in women of childbearing age. In those under age 40, contraceptive steroid use was associated with an 8–16 mg% increase in cholesterol (CH), resulting in values exceeding those in men of comparable age. TG levels were 30–40 mg% higher in contraceptive users. Since the proportion of users was high (over 40%, for example, in the 20–29 age group) and the magnitude of the shifts in distribution of both lipids was adequate to raise many subjects above NHLI cut-off points, calculation of the population-attributable risk suggested that approximately half the instances of hyperlipidemia were related to hormone use. Moreover, among subjects aged 20–29, the ratio of hyperlipidemia among users versus nonusers exceeded 2.0 for hypercholesterolemia alone, 3.0 for hypertriglyceridemia alone, and 4.0 for the combination of hypercholesterolemia and hypertriglyceridemia. Of note, however, is that the association between hyperlipidemia and hormone use declined with age such that no dramatic effect on the prevalence of hyperlipidemia was attributable to postmenopausal estrogen replacement.

APOLIPOPROTEIN CHANGES

Since lipids are by definition insoluble in an aqueous medium and must be complexed with proteins for plasma transport, recent research has focused on these apolipoproteins, especially in studies of the genetically determined hyperlipidemias. To date, however, only limied studies measuring apolipoproteins during steroid contraceptive and estrogen therapy have been performed. Regarding apolipoprotein B, the major structural protein in VLDL and LDL, only inferential data are available. Kane (5) found no change in the proportion of this tetramethylurea (TMU)-insoluble apolipoprotein (6) in the very low density lipoproteins (VLDL) of women taking combination oral contraceptives. Since VLDL and low density lipoproteins (LDL) are increased by these agents, so must be the total plasma apolipoprotein B levels [confirmed by us in pilot studies of young women before and during estrogen treatment (see below)]. Kane reported a slight decrease in the percent of TMU-soluble apolipoproteins represented by apo-C-II (the major apolipoprotein activator of lipoprotein lipase): from 9.7 in control women of childbearing age to 7.9–7.0% in women of comparable age taking anovulatory steroids.

No reports have yet appeared of LDL apoprotein levels in women taking either oral contraceptives or estrogen alone. To date, greater emphasis has been placed on the changes in high density lipoprotein (HDL) apoproteins induced by these hormones. Following the development and validation of a radial immunodiffusion assay for plasma apo A-I (measuring the level of the major HDL apoprotein), we compared the levels of this apoprotein in a sample of men and women drawn from a survey of the determinants of hyperlipidemia among employees of the Pacific Northwest Bell Telephone Company and, among the latter, in those using and not using contraceptive steroids and estrogens (7).

These studies revealed higher levels of plasma A-I in women not taking gonadal steroids than in men (129± 25 versus 120 ± 20 mg%, mean ± SD). Taking gonadal hormones further increased the A-I levels (mean 141 mg%) (Fig. 1). Significantly higher levels were recorded among those taking estrogens alone (mean 149%). Thus combination contraceptives raise the A-I but not the cholesterol content

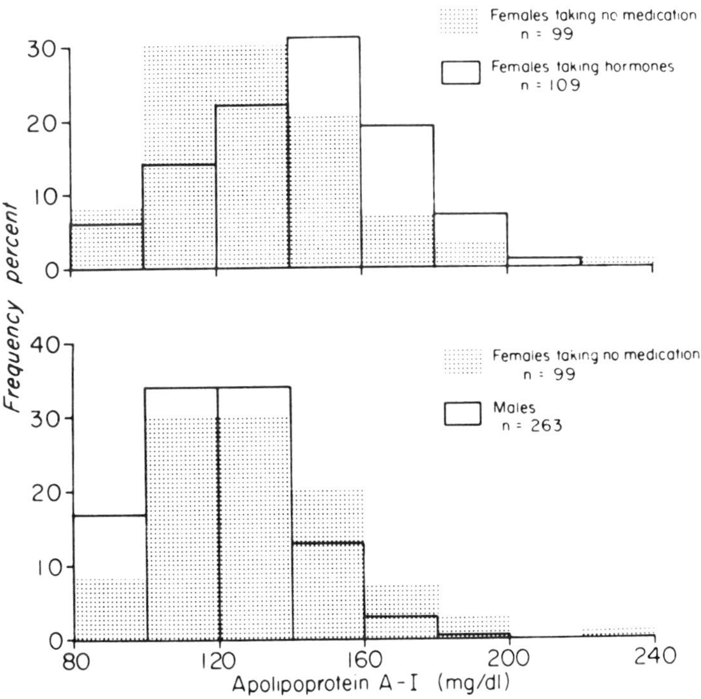

FIG. 1. Distribution of plasma apolipoprotein A-I in males, females taking no medication, and females taking hormones (oral contraceptives, estrogen for hot flashes, or estrogen to regulate menses).

of HDL, whereas estrogen alone increases both (although A-I to a greater degree than cholesterol). This was confirmed in paired studies of 14 normolipidemic women before and during short-term ethynylestradiol therapy (1 μg/kg/day) (see below): Estrogen increased apo A-I levels in 12 of 14 by a group mean of 25%, whereas HDL-CH increased by only 19%.

EFFECTS ON LIPOLYTIC ENZYMES

Early attempts to determine the mechanism of hypertriglyceridemia induced by oral contraceptives (8) focused on the major and consistent depression of postheparin lipolytic activity (PHLA) associated with their use. This was logical since PHLA—an indirect index of TG removal capacity dependent on the release of lipoprotein lipase (LPL) from capillary endothelial binding sites by heparin— had been shown to be depressed in genetic lipoprotein lipase deficiency [type I hyperlipoproteinemia (9)] and diabetic lipemia (10).

However, it was noted that the depression in PHLA associated with oral contraceptive use, often to the levels recorded in these other states of massive hyperlipemia, was far out of proportion to the minor, relative hypertriglyceridemia induced by these agents. Furthermore, oral (11) and intravenous (6) fat tolerance remained unchanged during oral contraceptive treatment in normal young women. Hence subsequent research has been directed to providing alternative explanations for the decrease in PHLA. One possibility lay in an acquired resistance to the release of lipoprotein lipase by heparin induced by oral contraceptives. This was tested (11) in paired studies of the PHLA response of three women before and during therapy with a wide range of heparin dosage. These dose-response studies suggested a lesser sensitivity to the release of lipolytic activity by heparin during oral contraceptive therapy, which could be overcome, at least in part, by administering larger doses. They also suggested that this resistance to heparin did not extend to its anticoagulant properties. This finding has since been confirmed by Ence et al. (12), who extended it to the demonstration of normal kinetics of heparin and PHLA disappearance during oral contraceptive therapy.

However, the development of additional techniques for the quantification of postheparin lipolytic enzymes has led to further studies of the effects of estrogen. Thus postheparin plasma was recently demonstrated to contain at least two enzymes capable of hydrolyzing TG (13,14): One, of hepatic origin, is resistant to inhibition by protamine and NaCl, and is not activated by apo C-II. The other, of extrahepatic (principally adipose tissue) origin, is the classic LPL; it is inhibited by both protamine and NaCl, and is activated by apo C-II. These activities can be separated by heparin-Sepharose affinity column chromatography into two peaks elutable by NaCl at approximately 0.72 M (peak I, hepatic TG lipase) and 1.2 M (peak II, extrahepatic LPL) (15). Moreover, the isolation of these two enzymes has permitted the raising of antibodies which specifically inhibit the corresponding enzyme and quantification of the remaining activity against the artificial TG substrate (16).

We recently employed two techniques for the quantification of postheparin lipolytic enzymes plus direct analysis of LPL activity in buttock adipose biopsies in paired studies of 13 normal young women performed on day 5 of their menstrual cycles and again 2 weeks later after the daily ingestion of ethynylestradiol (1 μg/kg/day). Blood samples collected on each occasion 10 min after intravenous injection of heparin (380 units/meter^2) were analyzed for total PHLA, hepatic TG lipase as peak I and following antibody inhibition of LPL, and extrahepatic LPL as peak II and following antibody inhibition of TG lipase. Adipose biopsy specimens were analyzed for their LPL content in extracts of acetone-ether powders (considered total LPL) and following elution with heparin (considered the activated form of LPL) (17).

Estrogen produced a selective decline in peak I (Fig. 2). This decline in TG lipase as measured by both techniques was closely correlated with and sufficient to account totally for the decrease in PHLA (Fig. 3). Extrahepatic LPL, on the other hand, varied widely, with no substantial change for the group as a whole. Moreover, adipose tissue LPL similarly varied widely with no mean change (Fig. 4). The change in TG lipase showed no correlation with the change in VLDL-TG, whereas despite the lack of a group change in extrahepatic LPL there was a weak but suggestive correlation with the change in VLDL-TG ($r = -.560$; $p < 0.05$). These studies complemented those of Ehnholm et al. (16), who reported the selective increase in hepatic TG lipase by the antibody technique in subjects

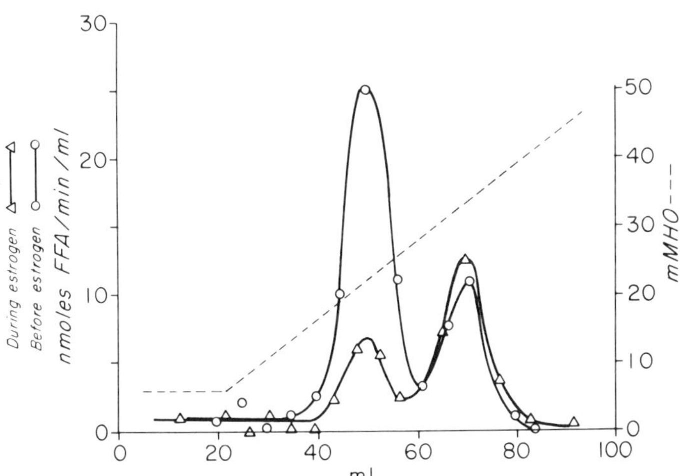

FIG. 2. Elution patterns of triglyceride lipolytic activity following heparin-Sepharose chromatography of postheparin plasma from subject 10 before and during estrogen. The NaCl gradients were measured by conductivity in mMHO.

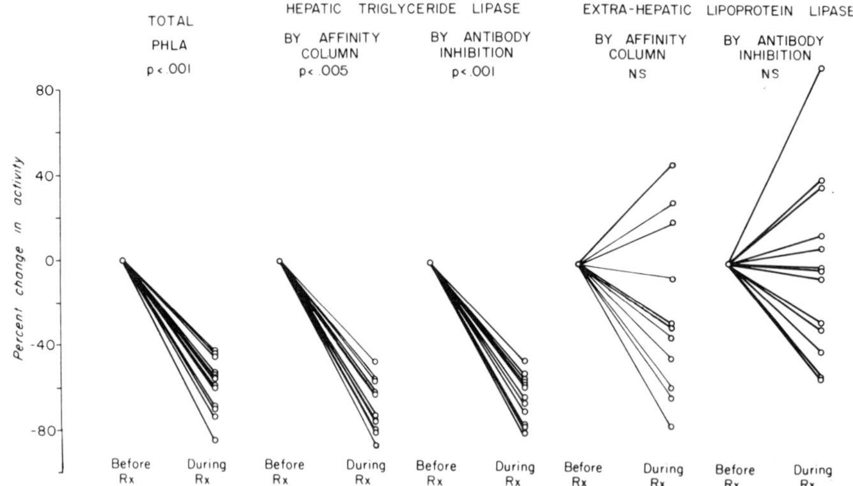

FIG. 3. Percent change in plasma postheparin lipolytic activities during estrogen: PHLA, triglyceride lipase (as peak I and by antibody inhibition), and lipoprotein lipase (as peak II and by antibody inhibition).

taking the anabolic-androgenic steroid oxandrolone, which has been shown to increase PHLA (18).

Low-high heparin dose-response studies in two of three women indicated that the relative resistance to the release of lipolytic enzymes by heparin induced by the estrogen was equivalent for both TG lipase and extrahepatic LPL. Thus estrogens induce a selective decline in postheparin TG lipase but do not appear to affect consistently postheparin or adipose LPL in humans. These studies go far toward resolving the paradox of normal TG removal in the face of greatly diminished PHLA in women using estrogenic contraceptives, and they point toward changes in TG production as the predominant mechanism whereby estrogens and steroid contraceptives increase plasma TG levels.

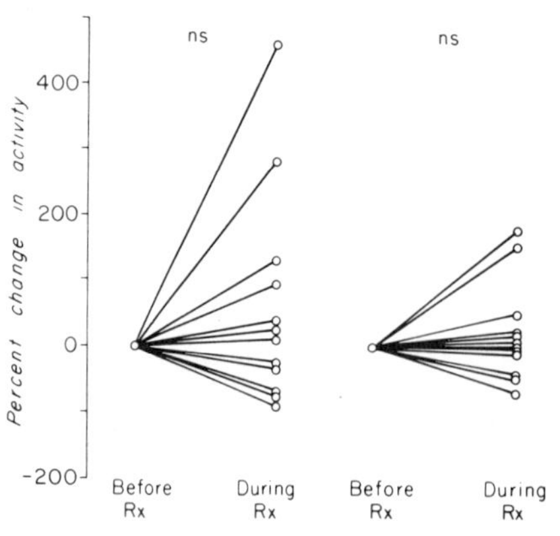

FIG. 4. Percent change in adipose tissue LPL during estrogen: heparin-elutable LPL **(left)** and the LPL extracted from acetone-ether powders **(right).**

TRIGLYCERIDE TURNOVER DURING ESTROGEN AND STEROID CONTRACEPTIVE TREATMENT

Changes in the balance between TG production and removal induced by steroid contraceptives can best be evaluated by studies of TG turnover. Reports of several such studies have appeared in the literature, yet inconsistencies in experimental design, methods, and results preclude definitive conclusions at this time. Furthermore, preliminary analysis of our own data suggest substantive differences from previous reports from this (19) and other laboratories. A portion of these differences undoubtedly stems from the imprecision of the measurement of TG turnover in human subjects. Of the several techniques developed, the validity of none is universally accepted, and three methods have been applied to measuring the effect of estrogens and steroid contraceptives on TG turnover.

A critical discussion of the relative merits of the various methods of assessing TG turnover is beyond the scope of this review, nor would such an analysis permit more definitive statements to be made. Therefore this discussion reviews the extant literature on this topic, presents our accumulated data from paried studies in subjects with endogenous hypertriglyceridemia, and reports the unique response to estrogen of subjects with type III hyperlipoproteinemia. Finally, we present a hypothesis whereby these disparate results may be rationalized through an effect of estrogen on non-LPL-related chylomicron and VLDL remnant removal.

The first reported study, by Kekki and Nikkilä (20), employed the technique developed by Farquhar et al. (21). This entails injecting ^{3}H-glycerol and then quantifying its disappearance from VLDL-TG. During the maintenance of steady-state TG levels, the half-life, fractional catabolic rate, and TG production rate are calculated. These workers compared the TG levels and production rates in 13 women on oral contraceptives with those from 17 control women. They recorded an increase of 1.9-fold in the TG production rate among the contraceptive-taking group, exceeding their 1.5-fold increase in TG concentration. Hence oral contraceptives appeared to increase TG production and TG removal. Analysis of their data according to the principles of Michaelis-Menten kinetics suggested that TG removal was potentiated by more efficient enzyme-substrate interaction (i.e., a reduced apparent K_m), whereas maximal removal (V_{max}) was unaffected. Because progestational agents had been reported to increase PHLA (and decrease TG) in hyperlipidemic women (22), these workers suggested that the increased TG removal in their subjects taking combination contraceptives was probably attributable to the progestational component and that the estrogen accounted for the increase in TG production.

A similar conclusion was reached by Kissebah et al. (23) following their study of 35 healthy premenopausal women (15 controls and 11 taking estrogen-progestin combination steroids, 5 estrogen alone, and 7 either progesterone or megestrol alone). TG turnover was calculated from the slope of the specific activity disappearance curve of TG labeled endogenously following the intravenous infusion of ^{14}C-palmitate. The estrogen-progestin and estrogen-alone groups had a TG production rate twice that of the control group, whereas the progestin alone did not affect this parameter. From kinetic plots they concluded that contraceptive steroids do not alter the V_{max} of TG removal, whereas, as suggested by Kekki and Nikkilä, K_m is reduced. Since this reduction was also noted in the group taking only the progestin but was not apparent in those taking estrogen alone, Kissebah et al. concluded that the improvement in TG removal efficiency recorded among those taking the combination oral contraceptives was attributable to the progestational component.

An additional point made by these authors was the close correlation between the TG turnover rate in the women on the combination oral contraceptives and their peak plasma immunoreactive insulin levels during an oral glucose tolerance test ($r = .869$), lending credence to the earlier suggestion (13) that compensatory hyperinsulinism might be the mechanism whereby oral contraceptives stimulate TG production. A more recent contribution to this concept was provided by Beck et al. (24), who demonstrated an even greater depression of pancreatic immunoreactive glucagon levels during oral contraceptive therapy (with consequent elevation of the insulin/glucagon ratio, proposed by this group to be a critical determinant of TG production rates).

Against these relatively consonant reports from studies of normal women must be set the less-secure findings from studies of the effect of estrogens on TG turnover in hypertriglyceridemic women. These studies have received special impetus from reports of occasional massive hypertriglyceridemia (25) and even hyperlipemic pancreatitis (26,27) induced by oral contraceptives and estrogens. Glueck et al. (28) studied eight such women on and off postmenopausal estrogen. Six had a familial form of hypertriglyceridemia and so remained hyperlipidemic (albeit to a lesser degree) after the cessation of estrogen. The two least hypertriglyceridemic women had no hyperlipidemic family members and became normolipidemic after estrogen withdrawal. Paired studies of TG turnover were performed by the ^{3}H-glycerol technique during and approximately 14 days following the withdrawal of estrogen (conjugated equine estrogens, 1.25 mg/day) while the subjects were consuming diets of constant composition, containing 40% fat, 35% carbohydrate, and 15% protein.

The results of these estrogen-withdrawal studies were highly variable. Nevertheless, as a group the subjects experienced a decline in VLDL-TG (from 555 to 349 mg%) and VLDL-TG turnover (from 30 to 18 mg/kg/hr). In contrast with the previous studies, however, estrogen appeared to affect the apparent V_{max} and K_m, approximately doubling each (i.e., decreasing the efficiency but increasing the maximal removal of plasma TG). These authors were unable to resolve their findings with those of Kekki and Nikkilä (20) and Kissebah et al. (23), noting the differences in the kinds of subject under study, techniques of measurement, and study design.

Rather different and surprising results have emerged from our studies of hypertriglyceridemic subjects. These studies employed the nonisotopic heparin infusion technique of measuring TG turnover developed by Porte and Bierman (29), as extended by Brunzell et al. (30). All such studies were performed in subjects with primary hypertriglyceridemia of varying genetic classification (31) who were maintained on isocaloric, 0% fat, 85% carbohydrate, liquid formula diets. Paired measurements were made after 10–14 days on the fat-free diet and again approximately 14 days later following 2 weeks on estrogen (usually ethynylestradiol, 1 μg/kg/day). During each TG turnover study heparin is injected in a dose demonstrated to release essentially peak levels of PHLA, then maintained by infusion at a constant level for 4–6 hr. The rate of hydrolysis of endogenous substrate is measured *in vitro* at physiological pH and temperature, and a whole-body LPL-related TG lipolytic rate is projected from estimates of total plasma volume. The rate calculated late during the heparin infusion, when TG levels have declined to a new steady state, is plotted relative to the antecedent TG concentration (Fig. 5). The hyperbolic solid line in Fig. 5 is that calculated as the best fit by least squares analysis after Woolf linear transformation of data points derived from measurements in multiple subjects with classic endogenous hypertriglyceridemia studied before and after caloric manipulation on the fat-free diet. This line describes a system which obeys saturation kinetics.

It is important, however, to emphasize the differences between this system and the relationship between TG turnover and TG concentration evident from measurements made by the ^{3}H-glycerol technique, which also follows saturation kinetics. Whereas the heparin technique estimates TG removal mediated by LPL, the glycerol method estimates total TG turnover. Thus if non-LPL-related forms of TG removal are quantitatively important, a decrease in LPL-related removal might imply either a decrease in total TG removal (and a decline in TG production at steady-state TG levels) or diversion to a non-LPL-related removal pathway. This point is central to our hypothesis regarding the mechanism of the

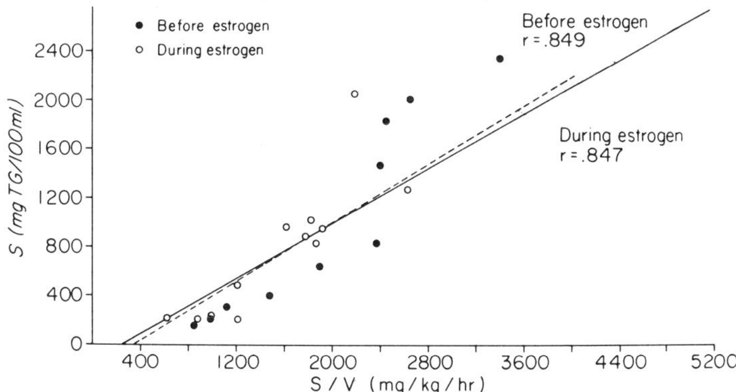

FIG. 5. Woolf linear transformation of the relationship between TG level (S) and TG level/LPL-related TG hydrolysis (S/V) in subjects with primary endogenous hypertriglyceridemia (non-type III) before and during estrogen [or combination oral contraceptive ($N = 1$)] therapy.

hypolipidemic response to estrogen observed in several of our hypertriglyceridemic subjects and all of those with type III hyperlipoproteinemia.

Thus in paired studies of the short-term effects of estrogen in 12 subjects with hyperlipidemia other than type III, 8 experienced a decline in TG levels during estrogen treatment on the fat-free diet (Fig. 6). In general, the greatest decreases occurred in the most hyperlipidemic subjects, but declines were noted at all levels. Heterogeneity in response is clearly evident, but most of the changes occurred in parallel to the saturation line. Preliminary analysis of these data according to the principles of Michaelis-Menten kinetics revealed no group change during estrogen in either V_{max} (0.556 mg/kg/hr before estrogen; 0.590 mg/kg/hr during estrogen) or K_m (122 mg% before estrogen; 162 mg% during estrogen), with equal, highly significant correlation coefficients before and during estrogen between S and S/V in the plot of the Woolf transformation (Fig. 5). Hence these studies would be consistent with either a reduction in TG production or an increase in non-LPL-related TG removal induced by estrogen in these hyperlipidemic subjects.

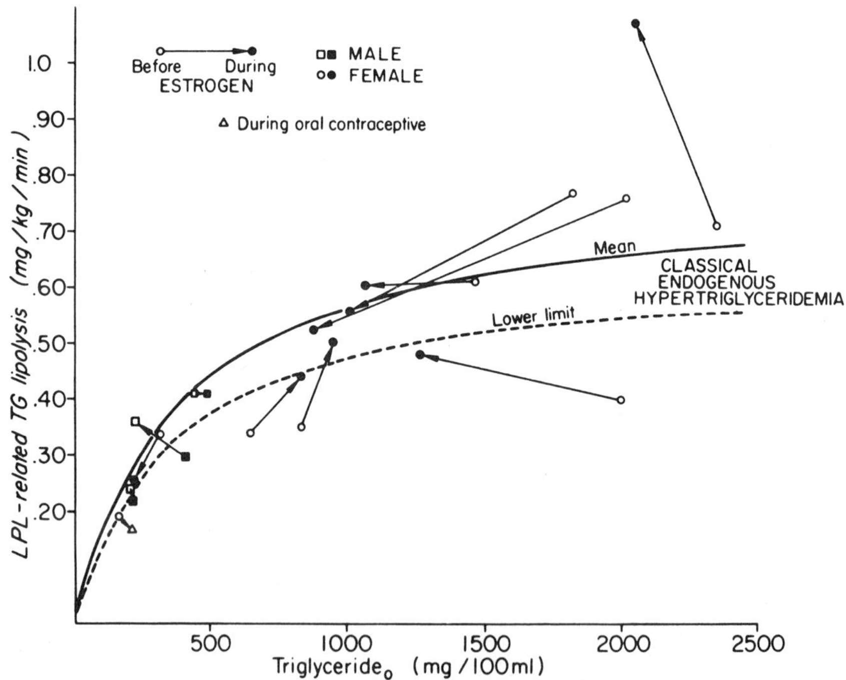

FIG. 6. Changes in the relationship between TG levels and LPL-related TG hydrolysis before and during estrogen (or combination oral contraceptive) treatment on a fat-free, high-carbohydrate diet in subjects with primary endogenous hypertriglyceridemia (non-type III). The solid hyperbolic line is that calculated as best fit by least-squares analysis after Woolf linear transformation of data describing this relationship in multiple subjects studied before and after caloric manipulation (29).

HYPOLIPIDEMIC RESPONSE TO ESTROGEN IN TYPE III HYPERLIPOPROTEINEMIA

The latter possibility is germane to an understanding of the unanticipated hypolipidemic response of a subject with type III hyperlipoproteinemia to estrogen. Type III is an uncommon, hereditary form of hyperlipidemia characterized by hypercholesterolemia and hypertriglyceridemia. These elevations reflect the accumulation in fasting plasma of VLDL abnormal in lipid composition (CH-rich and TG-poor) and electrophoretic mobility (β instead of pre-β) (14). Chylomicrons also often persist after an overnight fast and are similarly enriched in CH (32). Dietary manipulations have suggested that the endogenous VLDL (33) and the exogenous chylomicrons (32,34) are normal when first formed but become abnormal during the course of their catabolism to form LDL. Hence these abnormal chylomicrons and VLDL appear to represent "remnants" which persist in subjects with type III by virtue of a defect in their conversion to LDL (33) or, alternatively, the saturation of a normal remnant conversion capacity through greatly increased VLDL production (34).

According to either alternative hypothesis, forces which increase VLDL production should aggravate the hyperlipidemia of type III. Such is clearly the case with high-carbohydrate (Fig. 7) and hypercaloric (Fig. 8) feeding. For that reason we predicted that estrogen would exaggerate type III hyperlipidemia, and we undertook a trial of estrogen in a surgically postmenopausal, 50-year-old woman with type III hyperlipidemia (subject T.S.) on a fat-free diet, when hyperlipemic pancreatitis would not supervene (Fig. 7). Following the expected carbohydrate induction, however, institution of the estrogen produced a dramatic decline in TG levels. CH levels fell more slowly but to a greater relative extent, in parallel with the correction of the abnormal VLDL lipid composition and electrophoretic mobility characteristic of this disorder. She was left with a type IV lipoprotein pattern (i.e., moderately increased levels of normal VLDL). Studies of her VLDL apoprotein composition revealed that estrogen also corrected the abnormal enrichment in the content of the arginine-rich peptide characteristic of this disorder (35). When estrogen was withdrawn, the classic findings of type III returned. Subsequent monthly cycling of estrogens over a 2-year period confirmed this sequence of events in each cycle. Similar studies of four other subjects with type III (three females and one male) produced similar although less dramatic results. Hence the paradoxical hypolipidemic response to estrogen, together with conversion to a type IV pattern, appears to be typical of type III hyperlipoproteinemia.

What are the implications of this response for the mechanism of the effect of estrogen on TG metabolism? While far from definitive, serial measurements of TG turnover by the heparin infusion technique in subject T.S. are instructive in several ways (Fig. 9). First, all seven studies suggest that the relationship between TG level and LPL-related TG hydrolysis is normal, i.e., obeys the saturation kinetics derived from studies in subjects with classic endogenous hypertriglyceridemia. Second, this is confirmed by paired studies performed during ca-

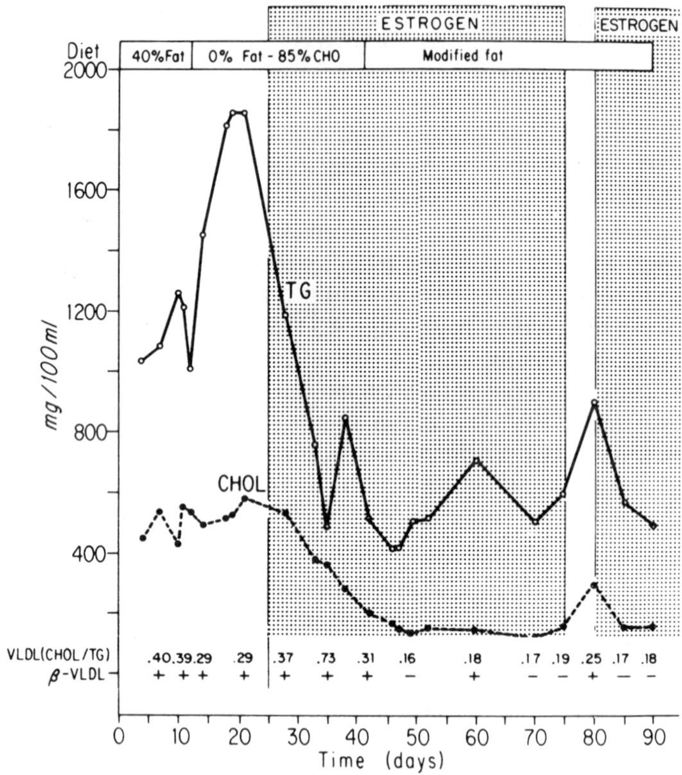

FIG. 7. Initial response of subject T.S. to estrogen (ethynylestradiol 1 μg/kg/day) during Clinical Research Center study (on isocaloric liquid formula diets composed either of 40% fat + 45% carbohydrate + 15% protein, or 0% fat + 85% carbohydrate + 15% protein) and outpatient follow-up on a diet low in saturated fat and cholesterol. TG, triglyceride. CHOL, cholesterol. VLDL, very low density lipoprotein. β-VLDL, β-migrating VLDL on agarose electrophoresis.

loric manipulation: overfeeding increased and underfeeding decreased TG levels along the hyperbolic line. Third, estrogen institution and withdrawal produced TG changes which mimicked those of under- and overfeeding, respectively. Similar studies in three other subjects with type III hyperlipidemia produced similar decrements in TG level—in two, clearly parallel to the hyperbolic line.

Do these studies suggest that estrogen decreases TG production in subjects with type III disease? This seems unlikely in view of the uniform conclusion from other studies using different techniques of estimating TG turnover that estrogens increase TG production. Furthermore, suppression of TG production in subject T.S. by hypocaloric feeding did not normalize VLDL composition and electrophoretic mobility. Hence even were estrogens paradoxically to depress TG production in subjects with type III, a second effect would have to be postulated to account for the conversion to a type IV pattern.

It therefore seems preferable to choose the alternative interpretation of these

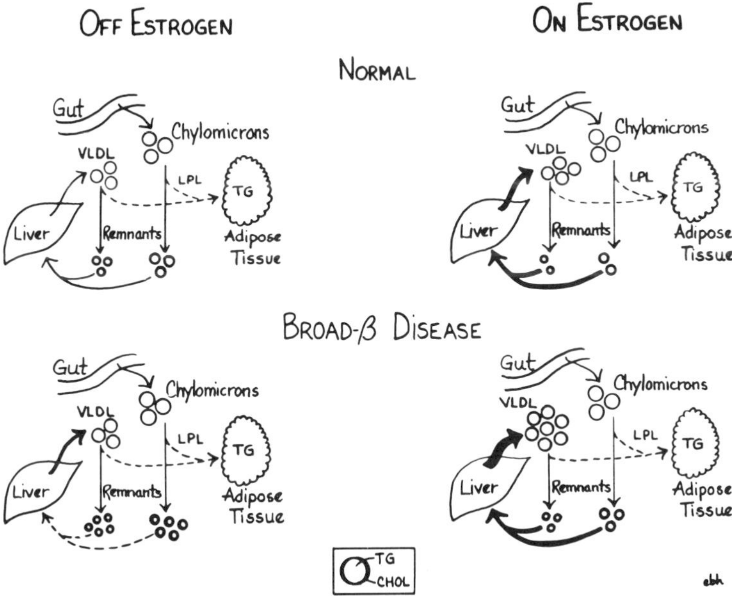

FIG. 8. Hypothesis proposed for the effect of estrogen on VLDL metabolism in normal persons and those with broad-β disease (type III hyperlipoproteinemia). See text for details.

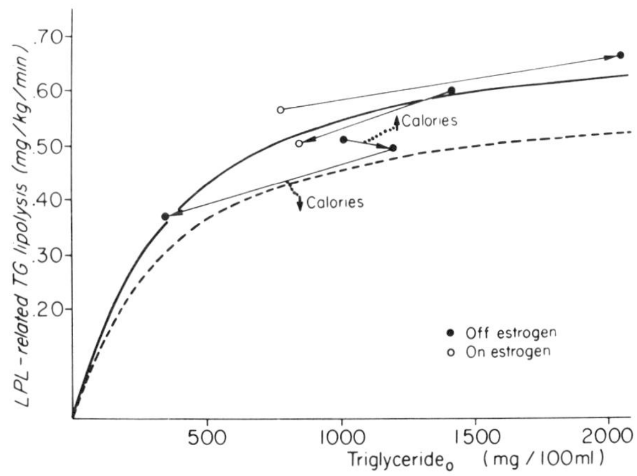

FIG. 9. Relationship between TG level and LPL-related TG hydrolysis in subject T.S. with type III hyperlipoproteinemia during isocaloric, hypercaloric (↑ calories) and hypocaloric (↓ calories) fat-free feeding prior to estrogen therapy and isocaloric fat-free feeding before and during estrogen (1 μg/kg/day ethynylestradiol) and following its withdrawal. The derivation of the hyperbolic line is described in the legend to Fig. 5.

results, i.e., that estrogens promote TG removal via a pathway independent of LPL, diverting it from LPL-related lipolysis. Confirmation of this possibility must come from studies comparing the effect of estrogen on total TG turnover (as estimated by, for example, the glycerol technique) and LPL-related TG removal by the heparin technique. A single such study performed to date suggested that total TG turnover was greatly increased by estrogen in a subject with type III, whereas LPL-related TG hydrolysis was less obviously affected (35). The normalization of VLDL composition by estrogen in subjects with type III suggests that the non-LPL-related pathway might involve facilitation of remnant removal.

Hence the following hypothesis of the effect of estrogens on VLDL metabolism (Fig. 8):

1. Estrogens stimulate TG synthesis and VLDL production in normal and hyperlipidemic subjects.
2. Estrogens facilitate chylomicron and VLDL remnant removal.
3. The net effect of both changes varies among individuals.
   a. In normal persons the VLDL level increases.
   b. In subjects with type III, who have limited remnant removal, abnormal VLDL declines or disappears, leaving an increased level of normal VLDL in a type IV pattern.
   c. In subjects with hyperlipidemia of varieties other than type III, the net effect depends on their individual susceptibility to further stimulation of VLDL synthesis versus their relative saturation of remnant removal. If their remnant removal is saturated prior to estrogen therapy and VLDL synthesis does not dramatically increase during estrogen, they (like subjects with type III) may experience a paradoxical, hypolipidemic response.

ACKNOWLEDGMENTS

This investigation was supported in part by NIH Contract NHLI-71–2157 (Northwest Lipid Research Clinic); HL 18291–01 (Estrogen Effects); and NIH AM 06670. Portions of this work were conducted through the University of Washington Clinical Research Center at University Hospital (NIH Grant FR-37) and Harborview Medical Center (NIH Grant RR-133). Dr. William R. Hazzard is an Investigator for Howard Hughes Medical Institute.

REFERENCES

1. Furman, R. H., Howard, R. P., Lakshmi, K., and Norcia, L. N. (1961): The serum lipids and lipoproteins in normal and hyperlipidemic subjects as determined by preparative ultracentrifugation. *Am. J. Clin. Nutr.,* 9:73–102.
2. Wynn, V., Doar, J. W. H., and Mills, G. L. (1966): Some effects of oral contraceptives on serum lipid and lipoprotein levels. *Lancet,* 2:720–723.

3. Wynn, V., Mills, A. L., Doar, J. W. H., and Stokes, T. (1969): Fasting serum triglyceride, cholesterol, and lipoprotein levels during oral contraceptive therapy. *Lancet,* 2:756–760.
4. Hoover, J. J., Tyroler, H. A., et al. (1975): Epidemiologic studies of the LRC program. Report prepared by the LRC Prevalence Committee. Presented at American Public Health Association Meeting, Chicago, Nov. 19.
5. Kane, J. P. (1975): The effect of ovarian hormones and synthetic anovulatory steroids on the content of the R-glutamic polypeptide in human serum very low density lipoprotein. *Circulation (Suppl. II),* 52:40.
6. Kane, J. P., Sata, T., Hamilton, R. L., and Havel, R. J. (1975): Apoprotein composition of very low density lipoproteins of human serum. *J. Clin. Invest.,* 56:1622–1634.
7. Albers, J. J., Wahl, P. W., Cabana, V. G., Hazzard, W. R., and Hoover, J. J. (1976): Quantitation of apolipoprotein A-I of human plasma high density lipoprotein. *Metabolism,* 25:633–644.
8. Hazzard, W. R., Spiger, M. J., Bagdade, J. D., and Bierman, E. L. (1969): Studies on the mechanism of increased plasma triglyceride levels induced by oral contraceptives. *N. Engl. J. Med.,* 280:471–474
9. Fredrickson, D. S., and Levy, R. L. (1972): Familial hyperlipoproteinemia. In: *The Metabolic Basis of Inherited Disease,* 3rd ed., edited by J. B. Stanbury, J. B. Wyngaarden, and D. S. Fredrickson, pp. 595–614. McGraw-Hill, New York.
10. Bagdade, J. D., Porte, D., Jr., and Bierman, E. L. (1967): Diabetic lipemia: A form of acquired fat-induced lipemia. *N. Engl. J. Med.,* 276:427–433.
11. Hazzard, W. R., Notter, D. T., Spiger, M. J., and Bierman, E. L. (1972): Oral contraceptives and triglyceride transport: Acquired heparin resistance as the mechanism for impaired post-heparin lipolytic activity. *J. Clin. Endocrinol. Metab.,* 35:425–437.
12. Ence, T. J., Wilson, E. D., Flowers, C. M., Chen, A. J., Glad, B. W., and Hershgold, E. J. (1976): Heparin metabolism and heparin-released lipase activity during long-term estrogen-progestin treatment. *Metabolism,* 25:139–145.
13. LaRosa, J. C., Levy, R. I., Windmueller, H. G., and Fredrickson, D. S. (1972): Comparison of the triglyceride lipase of liver, adipose tissue, and postheparin plasma. *J. Lipid Res.,* 13:356–362.
14. Krauss, R. M., Levy, R. I., and Fredrickson, D. S. (1974): Selective measurement of two lipase activities in postheparin plasma from normal subjects and patients with hyperlipoproteinemia. *J. Clin. Invest.,* 54:1107–1124.
15. Boberg, J., Augustin, J., Baginsky, M., Tejada, P., and Brown, W. V. (1974): Quantitative determination of hepatic and lipoprotein lipase activities from human post-heparin plasma. *Circulation [Suppl. III],* 49–50:21.
16. Ehnholm, C., Huttinen, J. K., Kinnunen, P. J., Miettinen, T. A., and Nikkilä, E. A. (1975): Effect of oxandrolone treatment on the activity of lipoprotein lipase, hepatic lipase and phospholipase A_1 of human postheparin plasma. *N. Engl. J. Med.,* 292:1314–1317.
17. Pykalisto, O. J., Smith, P. J., and Brunzell, J. D. (1975): Human adipose tissue lipoprotein lipase: Comparison of assay methods and expressions of activity. *Proc. Soc. Exp. Biol. Med.,* 148: 297–300.
18. Glueck, C. J., Ford, S., Jr., Steiner, P., and Fallat, R. (1973): Triglyceride removal efficiency and lipoprotein lipases: Effects of oxandrolone. *Metabolism,* 22:807–814.
19. Hazzard, W. R., Brunzell, J. D., Notter, D. T., Spiger, M. J., and Bierman, E. L. (1973): Estrogens and triglyceride transport: increased endogenous production as the mechanism for the hypertriglyceridemia of oral contraceptive therapy. In: *Endocrinology,* pp. 1006–1012. Excerpta Medica, Amsterdam.
20. Kekki, M., and Nikkilä, E. A. (1971): Plasma triglyceride turnover during use of oral contraceptives. *Metabolism,* 20:878–889.
21. Farquhar, J. W., Gross, R. C., Wagner, R. M., and Reaven, H. M. (1965): Validation of an incompletely coupled two-compartment nonrecycling catenary model for turnover of liver and plasma triglyceride in man. *J. Lipid Res.,* 6:119–134.
22. Glueck, C. J., Brown, W. V., Levy, R. I., Greten, H., and Fredrickson, D. S. (1969): Amelioration of hypertriglyceridemia by progestational drugs in familial type V hyperlipoproteinemia. *Lancet,* 1:1290–1291.
23. Kissebah, A. H., Harrigan, P., and Wynn, V. (1973): Mechanism of hypertriglyceridemia associated with contraceptive steroids. *Horm. Metab. Res.,* 5:184–190.
24. Beck, P., Eaton, R. P., Arnett, D. M., and Alsever, R. N. (1975): Effect of contraceptive steroids on arginine-stimulated glucagon and insulin secretion in women. I. Lipid physiology. *Metabolism,* 24:1055–1065.

25. Zorilla, E., Hulse, M., Hernandez, A., and Gershberg, H. (1968): Severe endogenous hypertriglyceridemia during treatment with estrogen and oral contraceptives. *J. Clin. Endocrinol. Metab.,* 28:1793–1796.
26. Glueck, C. J., Scheel, D., Fishback, J., and Steiner, P. (1972): Estrogen induced pancreatitis in patients with previously covert familial type V hyperlipoproteinemia. *Metabolism,* 21:657–666.
27. Davidoff, F., Tishler, S., and Rosoff, C. (1973): Marked hyperlipidemia and pancreatitis associated with oral contraceptive therapy. *N. Engl. J. Med.,* 289:552–555.
28. Glueck, C. J., Fallat, R. W., and Scheel, D. (1975): Effects of estrogenic compounds on triglyceride kinetics. *Metabolism,* 24:537–546.
29. Porte, D., Jr., and Bierman, E. L. (1969): The effect of heparin infusion on plasma triglyceride *in vivo* and *in vitro* with a method for calculating triglyceride turnover. *J. Lab. Clin. Med.,* 73:631–648.
30. Brunzell, J. D., Hazzard, W. R., Porte, D., Jr., and Bierman, E. L. (1973): Evidence for a common, saturable, triglyceride removal mechanism for chylomicrons and very low density lipoproteins in man. *J. Clin. Invest.,* 52:1577–1585.
31. Goldstein, J. L., Hazzard, W. R., Schrott, H. G., Bierman, E. L., and Motulsky, A. G. (1973): Hyperlipidemia in coronary heart disease. II. Genetic analysis of lipid levels in 176 families and delineation of a new inherited disorder: combined hyperlipidemia. *J. Clin. Invest.,* 52:1544–1568.
32. Hazzard, W. R., Porte, D., Jr., and Bierman, E. L. (1970): Abnormal lipid composition of chylomicrons in broad-β disease (type III hyperlipoproteinemia). *J. Clin. Invest.,* 49:1853–1858.
33. Hazzard, W. R., and Bierman, E. L. (1975): Broad-β disease vs. endogenous hypertriglyceridemia: Levels and lipid composition of chylomicrons and very low density lipoproteins during fat-free feeding and alimentary lipemia. *Metabolism,* 24:817–828.
34. Hall, M. H., III, Bilheimer, D. W., Phair, R. D., Levy, R. I., and Berman, M. (1974): A mathematical model for apoprotein kinetics in normal and hyperlipemic patients. *Circulation* [*Suppl. III*], 49–50:114.
35. Gagne, C., Kushwaha, R., Albers, J., Brunzell, J., and Hazzard, W. (1975): Type III hyperlipidemia: Implications of paradoxical hypolipidemic response to estrogen. *Circulation* [*Suppl. II*], 52:149.

Pharmacology of Steroid Contraceptive Drugs
edited by S. Garattini and H. W. Berendes.
Raven Press, New York © 1977.

Experimental Analysis of the Effects of Oral Contraceptives on the Function of the Lymphoid System

F. Spreafico, A. Vecchi, A. Anaclerio, M. L. Moras, A. Tagliabue, C. Barale, A. Mantovani, M. Sironi, and N. Polentarutti

Istituto di Ricerche Farmacologiche "Mario Negri," 20157 Milan, Italy

During the last few years increasing attention has been given to the side effects of steroid contraceptive drugs (SCD), but their possible effects on immunological responses has so far received comparatively little attention. This is somewhat surprising considering, for instance, the continuing debate on the alleged tumor-promoting capacity of chronic treatment with SCDs. Data suggesting that SCDs may have possible immunodepressive activity in humans are available (2,4, 10,11,22), but clinical results are still limited and in some respects contradictory; at the experimental level (8,18) information is still only preliminary. Against this background it was considered of interest to investigate if steroid contraceptives significantly affect immune responsiveness in rodents in a series of experimental conditions. This chapter summarizes the initial data obtained, using three widely employed estroprogestagen combinations.

EFFECTS ON HUMORAL ANTIBODY PRODUCTION

The three SCD combinations, composed of a standard estrogen (mestranol) in different doses together with three progestagens (lynestrenol, norethindrone, or norethynodrel), were administered orally to rats and mice in the minimal doses that exert full contraceptive effects in both species after 4 days of treatment. The first type of experimental immune reaction on which the effects of these contraceptives were investigated was a classic one, i.e., the primary response of rodents to an injection of sheep erythrocytes (SRBC) evaluated by means of Jerne's technique (9), detailed elsewhere (20).

Table 1 presents the results obtained in CD_1 female mice after a 30-day treatment, withdrawing the drugs 24 hr before assay. Only two combinations (mestranol-norethindrone and mestranol-norethynodrel) induced a clear, although not very marked, decrease in the number of hemolytic plaque-forming cells (PFC) in the spleen, where the majority of antibody-producing cells are present in these conditions. These results refer to the evaluation of the immune response at its peak (i.e., day 4) in normal mice.

TABLE 1. *Effect of SCDs on the primary immune response to sheep erythrocytes*

Experimental group	Daily dose (mg/kg)	Day of treatment	PFCs/spleen
Control	—	—	39,840 (34,500–46,630)
Lynestrenol + mestranol	5 0.3	−27 to +3	35,020 (30,800–41,380)
Norethindrone + mestranol	4 0.2	−27 to +3	20,850[a] (19,100–25,930)
Norethynodrel + mestranol	4 0.06	−27 to +3	21,110[a] (20,690–24,730)

Eight mice per group were injected i.p. with SRBCs on day 0; assay was performed on day +4.

Results are geometric means ± 1 SE (in parentheses) after logarithmic transformation of the data.

[a] $p < 0.05$.

To establish more firmly that these agents do indeed depress this response and not merely delay the appearance of its peak, the kinetics of the response were also followed. Table 2 shows that in these animals the anti-SRBC response was lowered throughout, not only the peak; furthermore, the depression appears to be balanced, since production of both immunoglobulin M (IgM) and IgG antibodies is reduced in the same proportion. Table 2 refers to treatment with norethindrone-mestranol for only 8 days. When the effects of the length of SCD treatment on this immune reactivity were investigated, it was observed that this was the shortest treatment with this SCD combination capable of significantly depressing PFC numbers; administration for only 4 days, either before antigen injection or ending 24 hr before assay, was ineffective. At variance with the other combination active on this system (norethynodrel-mestranol), treatment with the minimal contraceptive doses for less than 30 days was not significantly immunodepressive. Although a formal dose-response curve is not available, when both these SCD combinations were given at half the dose for 30 days the mouse anti-SRBC response was unaffected.

Tests were also conducted to evaluate whether the estrogenic or progestagenic component of the SCD was responsible for PFC depression. When the single components were administered for 30 days at the dosages active in the combinations, no significant immunodepression was observed (Table 3).

The effects of the same three SCDs on this type of immune response was also evaluated in female rats. None of the treatments which were immunodepressive in the mouse significantly reduced the anti-SRBC response in the rat.

In view of clinical reports of possible improvement in patients with autoimmune conditions under treatment with the pill (3), we investigated if SCD treatment influenced the production of antierythrocyte autoantibodies in C57B1/6 mice. The autoimmune condition was induced by repeated injection of cross-

TABLE 2. *Effect of SCDs on the immune response at different times after antigenic stimulation*

Experimental group	Daily dose (mg/kg)	Days of treatment	PFC/spleen				
			Day 4 IgM	Day 7		Day 10	
				IgM	IgG	IgM	IgG
Control	—	—	29,650 (25,070–31,060)	1,550 (1,372–1,889)	2,315 (2,084–2,647)	1,078 (890–1,240)	2,588 (2,240–2,710)
Norethindrone+ mestranol	4 0.2	−4 to +3	13,210[a] (10,780–16,460)	605[a] (540–700)	995[a] (890–1,040)	425[a] (320–520)	647[a] (581–789)

Eight mice per group were injected i.p. with SRBCs on day 0.
Results are geometric means ± 1 SE (in parentheses) after logarithmic transformation of the data.
[a] $p < 0.05$.

TABLE 3. *Effect of estrogen or progestagen treatment on immune response to sheep erythrocytes*

Experimental groups	Daily dose (mg/kg)	Day of treatment	PFC/spleen
Control	—	—	51,800 (47,890–53,500)
Norethindrone	4	−27 to +3	49,450 (46,700–54,810)
Norethynodrel	4	−27 to +3	53,300 (50,620–56,000)
Mestranol	0.3	−27 to +3	52,250 (48,700–55,440)

Eight mice per group were injected i.p. with SRBCs on day 0; assay was performed on day +4.

Results are geometric means ± 1 SE (in parentheses) after logarithmic transformation of the data.

TABLE 4. *Effect of SCDs on the formation of antimouse erythrocyte autoantibodies*

Experimental group	Daily dose (mg/kg)	Days of treatment	Mean $\log_2$ DCT titer	% DCT-positive mice
Control	—	—	12.5 ± 0.8	100
Lynestrenol + mestranol	5 0.3	−4 to +26	14.0 ± 0.9	100
Norethindrone + mestranol	4 0.2	−4 to +26	7.5 ± 1.2[a]	60
Norethynodrel + mestranol	4 0.06	−4 to +26	11.8 ± 1.3	100

Sixteen $C_{57}B1/6$ mice per group were injected i.p. with 10^8 rat erythrocytes on days 0, 7, 14, and 21; antimouse erythrocyte autoantibodies were measured on day 34 by the direct Coombs test (DCT).

[a] $p < 0.05$.

reacting rat red blood cells as described by Playfair and Marshall-Clarke (16). As shown in Table 4, neither the incidence of animals with circulating antiery-throcyte autoantibodies nor their titers evaluated by a direct Coombs test were significantly modified after 30-day treatments with either lynestrenol-mestranol or norethynodrel-mestranol. On the other hand, significant effects on both these parameters were seen 8 days after discontinuation of 1 month's treatment with norethindrone-mestranol, given again at the minimal doses having 100% con-traceptive effect.

EFFECTS ON CELL-MEDIATED RESPONSIVENESS

As a first model of a cell-mediated immunological reactivity on which to investigate the effects of SCDs, we selected experimental allergic encephalomyeli-tis (EAE), a condition which is inducible and whose severity can be evaluated with relative ease. Disease induction and evaluation are described elsewhere (20). All three SCD combinations were active in these experimental conditions when

TABLE 5. *Effect of SCDs on allergic encephalomyelitis in rats*

Experimental group	Daily dose (mg/kg)	Days of treatment	No. of rats showing disease[a]			Mean value of the angle in the inclined plane test
			0	+	++	
Normal control	—	—	10	—	—	48.3 ± 1.9
EAE control	—	—	0	4	6	39.1 ± 1.6
EAE + lynestrenol + mestranol	5 0.3	−15 to +15	7	2	1	46.4 ± 1.2[b]
EAE + norethindrone + mestranol	4 0.2	−15 to +15	8	1	1	47.8 ± 0.9[b]
EAE + norethynodrel + mestranol	4 0.06	−15 to +15	6	2	2	46.9 ± 1.8[b]

Rats were immunized with cord tissue on day 0. Results refer to day +16.
[a] 0, normal motility. +, frank muscular weakness and/or unilateral paralysis. ++, bilateral hind limb paralysis.
[b] $p < 0.05$.

administered at the standard dose for a total of 30 days beginning 15 days before disease induction (Table 5). This protective effect is revealed by the lower percentage of diseased animals compared with positive controls, by the clinical scoring of the disease in affected animals, and by the angle values measured in an "inclined plane" test for quantitative evaluation of the functional capacity of the hind limbs in these animals. In these conditions, practically only the hind limbs are affected. The return to normal mobility was also more rapid in treated than in normal animals, the three combinations being equally active in this respect too. We also checked if shorter treatments gave any significant protection against this disease, but 15-day treatments administered either entirely before or subsequent to immunization with cord tissue were totally ineffective.

To date, the only cell-mediated response on which we investigated the effects of SCD in the mouse is tumor-allograft rejection. In C_3H (H-2^k) mice transplanted with 10^7 cells of the L 1210 leukemia, syngeneic in DBA/2 (H-2^d) mice, 30-day pretreatment with any of the three SCD combinations had no significant immunodepressive effect as revealed by the fact that all transplanted animals totally rejected this tumor graft. This is perhaps not surprising in view of the very strong antigenic stimulus at play in these conditions and the fact that the immunodepressive activity of these SCDs appears relatively moderate, at least employing the treatments considered in this study.

ATTEMPTS AT DEFINING THE TARGET OF SCD IMMUNODEPRESSION

In analyzing the target of SCD immunodepression, it was considered of interest to obtain at least preliminary indications of whether the immunodepressive activity of these agents was selective for thymus-derived (T) or bone marrow-derived (B) lymphocytes. To this end, mice were injected with an optimal immunizing dose of the T-independent pneumococcal polysaccharide S-III (7). No significant depression of the primary immune response to this antigen was observed when CD_1 mice were given SCD treatments capable of depressing the response to SRBCs (Table 6), the latter requiring the collaboration of both T- and B-cells.

These results led us to hypothesize that T-lymphocytes are at least an important target of SCD immunodepression, this contention being supported by the depression observed of EAE and anti-RBC autoantibody formation, which are both T-cell-dependent reactions (11,16). More direct data also favor this tentative conclusion. Table 7 shows that 8 days' treatment with norethindrone-mestranol, a schedule which suppresses the anti-SRBC response in the mouse, does not significantly reduce spleen cellularity but significantly lowers the percentage of T-lymphocytes (evaluated here by their sensitivity to cytotoxic antiserum directed against their specific membrane marker, theta antigen). At the same time, cells capable of forming rosettes with sensitized erythrocytes (EA-RFC), a measure of non-T-elements, are unchanged by this treatment in both proportion and total

TABLE 6. *Effect of SCDs on the immune response to the pneumococcal polysaccharide SIII*

Experimental group	Daily dose (mg/kg)	Days of treatment	PFC/spleen
Control	—	—	12,400 (10,050–19,600)
Lynestrenol + mestranol	5 0.3	−27 to +4	13,520 (9,870–18,520)
Norethindrone + mestranol	4 0.2	−27 to +4	11,970 (8,790–19,010)
Norethynodrel + mestranol	4 0.06	−27 to +4	12,570 (10,820–17,450)

Eight mice per group were injected i.p. with 0.5 μg SIII on day 0; assay was performed on day +5.

TABLE 7. *Effect of norethindrone-mestranol combination on spleen lymphoid cell subpopulations*

Experimental group	Daily dose (mg/kg)	Days of treatment	Total No. ($\times 10^6$) splenocytes	% Theta + splenocytes	% EA-RFC
Control	—	—	78.6 ± 13.5	19.5 ± 0.9	55.6 ± 4.9
Norethindrone + mestranol	4 0.2	0 to +8	80.1 ± 5.4	11.7 ± 1.4[a]	51.8 ± 5.1

[a] $p < 0.05$.

TABLE 8. *Effect of SCDs on splenocyte reactivity to mitogens*

Experimental group	Daily dose (mg/kg)	Days of treatment	Stimulant	Stimulation index
Control	—	—	LPS 50 μg/ml	7.2
Norethindrone + mestranol	4 0.2	0 to +8	LPS 50 μg/ml	7.6
Lynestrenol + mestranol	5 0.3	0 to +8	LPS 50 μg/ml	10.5
Control	—	—	LPS 10 μg/ml	3.0
Norethindrone + mestranol	4 0.2	0 to +8	LPS 10 μg/ml	3.7
Lynestrenol + mestranol	5 0.3	0 to +8	LPS 10 μg/ml	4.1
Control	—	—	ConA 1 μg/ml	2.2
Norethindrone + mestranol	4 0.2	0 to +8	ConA 1 μg/ml	0.6[a]
Lynestrenol + mestranol	5 0.3	0 to +8	ConA 1 μg/ml	2.9

[a] $p < 0.05$.

numbers. Splenocytes from animals given an immunodepressive SCD regimen had an altered *in vivo* response to selective lymphocyte stimulants. In fact, when spleen cells treated for 8 days with norethindrone-mestranol were cultivated in the presence of *E. coli* lipopolysaccharide, a specific B-cell stimulant, a normal reaction was observed (Table 8). The stimulation index (i.e., the ratio of tritiated thymidine uptake in cultures exposed to the stimulant over that of nonstimulated cells) was not significantly different in mice given a nonimmunodepressive treatment with lynestrenol-mestranol. In contrast, reduced reactivity was found when concanavallin A (Con A), a specific T-cell stimulant (21), was employed in the same conditions.

CONCLUSION

The frequently employed contraceptive estrogen-progestagen combinations described herein can exert a clear, although not marked, immunodepressive effect on both cell-mediated and humoral responses in rodents. Since the lynestrenol-mestranol combination was active only in EAE, and considering that at least some SCDs possess corticoid-stimulating activity (5), the protective capacity of this combination in this system might have been the consequence of anti-inflammatory activity. The reasons, however, for believing that this SCD combination also has immunodepressive potential have been discussed elsewhere (24).

That SCDs could be immunodepressants was previously suggested by others employing different estroprogestinic combinations (8,12,17,23). However, no formal conclusion could be reached on this point since the previous studies had investigated only high doses not correlated with the contraceptive effect, given in short-term treatment exploiting a limited range of experimental testing conditions. From our studies, evident differences emerged in the overall immunodepressive activity of SCDs; norethindrone-mestranol proved to be the most active combination since it was the only one capable of reducing anti-RBC autoantibody formation in the mouse and of decreasing mouse anti-SRBC reactivity after shorter treatments. Whether this holds true and has biological significance after more prolonged treatment is impossible to assess at present.

The differences in sensitivity to these agents observed even in closely related species (e.g., the differential susceptibility of the primary anti-SRBC response to the same SCD in mice and rats) is a further warning against direct extrapolation of these results from one species to another and, more important, to man. However, data suggesting that oral contraceptives may have an immunodepressive effect in humans have been reported, including a decrease in lymphocytic PHA responsiveness (2,4), changes in immunoglobulin and autoantibody levels (6,14), the response to standard vaccine injections (10), and improvements in patients with autoimmune conditions (3,22). This aspect is considered in more detail elsewhere in this volume.

A question of considerable practical relevance is the relative role of the estrogenic and progestinic components of SCD in this immunodepressive effect. Unfortunately this cannot yet be answered. In animals the results are complex since, as discussed elsewhere (24), both types of hormones have given positive and negative results, comparisons between the various studies being impossible in view of the broad differences in conditions. In addition, a major criticism against most of the past studies is that these hormones have been used in nonphysiological conditions, e.g., high doses in acute treatments. Our own data add no new information on this point since the single components of immunodepressive combinations were inactive in our conditions; the only conclusion possible is that there may be some additive effect. The scant clinical data available also shed no light on this point; although the higher incidence of chickenpox injections in chronic oral contraceptive users appeared to be positively correlated with the estrogen content of the SCD preparation used (19), it should be noted that progestinic contraceptives have also been reported to decrease antibody production (13,23).

Our findings appear clearly to indicate that thymus-derived lymphocytes are a primary target of the immunodepressive effect of SCDs; these elements play a pivotal role in immunological reactivity at both the antigen-recognition and effector phases. This conclusion, based on a series of direct and indirect data, does not, however, exclude that SCD may also affect other cells involved in immune responses (e.g., macrophages), as suggested by some indirect results (15). In addition, it is possible that not all SCDs share the same mechanism(s) of action.

The clinical significance of the immunodepressive activity of SCDs is still a matter of debate; if confirmed by more systematic analysis, it could provide a basis for explaining the higher incidence of some viral infections observed in chronic oral contraceptive users (19). This may be of special relevance in populations with low nutritional status and where certain infectious diseases are endemic. In this connection, T-lymphocytes are more important in the defense against viral injections, whereas B-cells are considered more important in protection against bacterial infections (1).

ACKNOWLEDGMENTS

This work was supported by Contract NIH-NICHD-72-2733.

REFERENCES

1. Allison, A. C. (1973): Interactions of T- and B-lymphocytes and macrophages in recovery from virus infections. *Proc. R. Soc. Med.,* 66:1151–1154.
2. Barnes, E. W., McCuish, A. C., Loudon, N. B., Jordan, J., and Irvine, W. J. (1974): Phytohaemagglutinin-induced lymphocyte transformation and circulating autoantibodies in women taking oral contraceptives. *Lancet,* 1:898–900.
3. Demers, R., Blais, J. A., and Pretty, H. (1966): Arthrite rhumatoide traitée par noréthynodrel associée à mestranol: Aspects cliniques et tests de laboratoire. *Can. Med. Assoc. J.,* 95:350–358.
4. Hagen, C., and Frøland, A. (1972): Depressed lymphocyte response to P.H.A. in women taking oral contraceptives. *Lancet,* 1:1185.
5. Haller, J. (1970): A review of the long-term effects of hormonal contraceptives. *Contraception,* 1:233.

6. Horne, C. H. W., Howie, P. W., Weir, R. J., and Goudie, R. B. (1970): Effect of combined oestrogen-progestogen oral contraceptives on serum-levels of α_2-macroglobulin, transferrin, albumin, and IgG. *Lancet,* 1:49–50.
7. Howard, J. G., Christie, G. H., Courtenay, B. M., Leuchars, E., and Davies, A. J. S. (1971): Studies on immunological paralysis. VI. Independence of tolerance and immunity to type III pneumococcal polysaccharides. *Cell. Immunol.,* 2:614–626.
8. Hulka, J. K., Mohr, K., and Liebermann, M. W. (1965): Effect of synthetic progestational agents on allograft rejection and circulating antibody production. *Endocrinology,* 77:897–901.
9. Jerne, N. K., and Nordin, A. A. (1963): Plaque formation in agar by single antibody-producing cells. *Science,* 140:405.
10. Joshi, U. M., Rao, S. S., Kora, S. J., Dikshit, S. S., and Virkar, K. D. (1971): Effect of steroidal contraceptives on antibody formation in the human female. *Contraception,* 3:327–333.
11. Lennon, V. A., and Byrd, W. J. (1973): Role of T lymphocytes in the pathogenesis of experimental auto-immune encephalomyelitis. *Eur. J. Immunol.,* 3:243–245.
12. Mueller, M. N., and Kappas, A. (1964): Estrogen pharmacology. II. Suppression of experimental immune polyarthritis. *Proc. Soc. Exp. Biol. Med.,* 117:845–847.
13. Munroe, J. S. (1971): Progesteroids as immunosuppressive agents. *J. Reticuloendothel. Soc.,* 9:361–375.
14. Musa, B. U., Doe, R. P., and Seal, U. S. (1967): Serum protein alterations produced in women by synthetic estrogens. *J. Clin. Endocrinol. Metab.,* 27:1463–1469.
15. Nicol, T., Vernon-Roberts, B., and Ruautock, D.C. (1965): The influence of various hormones on the reticulo-endothelial system: Endocrine control of body defence. *J. Endocrinol.,* 33:365–383.
16. Playfair, J. H. L., and Marshall-Clarke, S. (1973): Induction of red cell autoantibodies in normal mice. *Nature [New Biol.],* 243:213–214.
17. Rangnekar, K. N., Yoshi, U. M., and Rao, S. S. (1972): Diminution in humoral antibodies to tetanus toxoid after ovulen therapy in mice. *Contraception,* 5:53–56.
18. Rao, S. S., and Yoshi, U. M. (1971): Primary immune response of rats and rabbits treated with Enovid. *J. Reprod. Fertil.,* 27:310.
19. Royal College of General Practitioners (1974): *A Report from Oral Contraception Study.* Pitman Medical Publications, London.
20. Spreafico, F., Vecchi, A., Mantovani, A., Poggi, A., Franchi, G., Anaclerio, A., and Garattini, S. (1975): Characterization of the immunostimulants levamisole and tetramisole. *Eur. J. Cancer,* 11:555–563.
21. Stobo, J. D., Rosenthal, A. S., and Paul, W. E. (1972): Functional heterogeneity of murine lymphoid cells. I. Responsiveness to and surface binding of concanavalin A and phytohemagglutinin. *J. Immunol.,* 108:1–17.
22. Tarzy, B. J., Garcia, C. R., Wallach, E. E., Zweiman, B., and Myers, A. R. (1972): Rheumatic disease, abnormal serology, and oral contraceptives. *Lancet,* 2:501–503.
23. Turcotte, J. G., Haines, R. F., Brody, G. L., Meyer, T. J., and Schwartz, S. A. (1968): Immunosuppression with medroxyprogesterone acetate. *Transplantation,* 6:248–260.
24. Vecchi, A., Tagliabue, A., Mantovani, A., Anaclerio, A., Barale, C., and Spreafico, F. (1976): Steroid contraceptive agents and immunological reactivity in experimental animals. *Biomedicine* 24:231–237.

Pharmacology of Steroid Contraceptive Drugs
edited by S. Garattini and H. W. Berendes.
Raven Press, New York © 1977.

Incidence of Hypertension in the Walnut Creek Contraceptive Drug Study Cohort

Savitri Ramcharan, Eric Peritz, Frederick A. Pellegrin, and
Winfield T. Williams

Kaiser-Permanente Medical Center, Walnut Creek, California 94596

Numerous reports have appeared indicating that oral contraceptive drugs (OCs) have produced hypertension in women. Mackay et al. (5) published a review in 1973, and since then additional reports based on larger or longer studies have confirmed the relationship between OCs and hypertension (1,2,4,7–9). Because of differences in study design, sample size and selection, follow-up methods, diagnostic criteria, etc., estimates of the risk of developing hypertension to which OC users are exposed have varied widely among the various studies. The Walnut Creek Contraceptive Drug Study (CDS) is an ongoing prospective study of the noncontraceptive effects of OCs and includes as a major part of its effort a follow-up study on hypertension (6).

The following is therefore a report of work in progress concerning one aspect of a single disease and forming part of a more comprehensive set of investigations that cover a variety of OC effects related not only to the cardiovascular system but to other body systems as well. The aim of this chapter is to bring up to date the published information about hypertension from the Walnut Creek CDS. It deals specifically with the incidence of hypertension in the CDS cohort and the relative risk associated with OC use. It encompasses certain areas not covered in a previous report (7): (a) It computes incidence rates by person-months of follow-up; (b) it controls for associated factors by appropriate multivariate analyses; and (c) it includes cases of labile hypertension.

MATERIALS AND METHODS

Study Population

The data used here are derived from the cohort of 17,932 women 18–54 years of age, a full description of which was published elsewhere (6). These women were mostly white and middle class, living in suburban communities of the San Francisco Bay area of northern California in the United States. At entry into the study all of the women were members of the Kaiser Foundation Health Plan, which is a prepaid comprehensive medical care program, including among its benefits an annual general physical examination. Women became study subjects by having a medical or gynecological checkup examination during the period December 1968 through February 1972 in an automated multitest laboratory (AML) especially designed for the purpose at the Kaiser-Permanente Medical Center in Walnut Creek, California. They came for the examination either by self-referral or physician referral and were not selected on the basis of contraceptive use or because of requests for contraception.

Study Sample

The present report is based on a subgroup from this cohort, consisting of the 15,256 white women who were 20–54 years of age and not pregnant at entry into the study. Of this number, 1,167 were found to have hypertension at their entry into the study. The group at risk was therefore reduced to 14,089. This group of women was observed for a total of 557,230 person-months or, on the average, 39.6 months per woman. The averages were 41.0 for women who had never used OCs, 37.5 for past users, and 39.9 for current users. (The age distributions of women, person-months, and incident cases are given in Tables 1 and 2.)

Oral Contraceptive Use

Based on information obtained at the first AML examination, the women could be placed into groups according to OC use as follows:

1. Never users were those who had never used OCs.

2. Past users were those who had taken OCs prior to their initial examination but were no longer taking them.

3. Current users were those who were taking OCs at the time of their initial examination.

4. Estrogen users were those who were taking estrogenic hormones (primarily conjugated estrogens) at the time of their initial examination or during the preceding year, whatever their use of OCs (never, past, or current).

Examination Procedures and Follow-up

The medical examination consisted of comprehensive, self-administered medical, psychological, and social history questionnaires which included detailed questions on OC use; a battery of physiological and biochemical measurements; a pelvic and breast examination by a gynecologist; and a general medical examination by an internist. Blood pressure measurements were made in a systematic manner at the AML examination by means of an automated machine (Godart BP apparatus, Godart N. V., Bilthoven, Holland) (6). Blood pressure measurements in the clinics were taken by the usual manual method with a mercury manometer.

Follow-up information about the health of the women and their use of OCs was obtained through interim questionnaires administered by mail or telephone, by repeat AML examinations, and from the patients' clinic and hospital records

TABLE 1. *Women at risk, person-months, and incident cases by OC use status and age at entry*

OC use status and age (years)	No. of women at risk	No. of person-months	Incident cases	
			Essential only	Essential and labile
Never users	4,479	183,609	78	128
20–29	533	17,894	2	5
30–34	596	24,477	2	9
35–39	903	37,339	11	17
40–44	1,049	43,980	19	37
45–54	1,398	59,919	44	60
Past users	4,441	166,334	49	86
20–29	1,676	58,098	4	14
30–34	1,015	37,415	10	17
35–39	773	30,420	11	18
40–44	560	22,823	12	21
45–54	417	17,578	12	16
Current users	3,815	151,986	43	99
20–29	1,862	67,337	5	21
30–34	699	28,728	6	16
35–39	485	21,401	8	17
40–44	410	18,135	12	20
45–54	359	16,385	12	25
Estrogen users	1,354	55,301	43	74
20–29	48	1,596	—	1
30–34	52	1,810	—	—
35–39	81	3,335	2	4
40–44	225	8,551	6	10
45–54	948	40,009	35	59
Total	14,089	557,230	213	387
20–29	4,119	144,925	11	41
30–34	2,362	92,430	18	42
35–39	2,242	92,495	32	56
40–44	2,244	93,489	49	88
45–54	3,122	133,891	103	160

at the Kaiser-Permanente Medical Center in Walnut Creek. The data on the questionnaires and on the AML records were precoded for keypunching onto cards. Abstracts of the medical charts were made manually by trained chart readers. This was a time-consuming process which resulted in a time gap between a subject's most recent visit and her abstract date. In computing the length of the follow-up period for each woman, her abstract date was used if it preceded her termination from the study.

Ascertainment of Cases and Definition of Hypertension

As a first screening, abstracts of the clinic charts were set aside for further consideration if they showed at least one of the following: (a) mention of hypertension, hypertensive disease, or some related term; or (b) record of a diastolic

TABLE 2. *Women at risk, person-months, and incident cases; current and past OC users by length of use and age at entry*

OC use status and age (years)	No. of women at risk	No. of person-months	Incident cases	
			Essential only	Essential and labile
Past users	4,441	166,334	49	86
Less than 1 year	1,675	64,619	21	38
20–29	488	17,172	1	6
30–34	352	12,991	5	7
35–39	331	13,482	6	8
40–44	293	11,883	5	10
45–54	211	9,091	4	7
One to four years	1,982	73,903	21	35
20–29	915	31,792	2	5
30–34	442	16,632	4	6
35–39	283	11,082	3	8
40–44	193	8,079	7	10
45–54	149	6,318	5	6
More than 4 years	784	27,812	7	13
20–29	273	9,134	1	3
30–34	221	7,792	1	4
35–39	159	5,856	2	2
40–44	74	2,861	—	1
45–54	57	2,169	3	3
Current users	3,815	152,166	43	99
Less than 1 year	269	10,142	2	4
20–29	174	5,820	—	—
30–34	30	1,239	—	—
35–39	17	868	—	—
40–44	30	1,389	1	3
45–54	18	826	1	1
One to four years	1,822	72,285	19	52
20–29	1,054	37,903	2	14
30–34	239	10,108	4	10
35–39	193	8,832	2	7
40–44	150	6,721	6	7
45–54	186	8,721	5	14
More than 4 years	1,724	69,739	22	43
20–29	634	23,614	3	7
30–34	430	17,381	2	6
35–39	275	11,594	6	10
40–44	230	10,312	5	10
45–54	155	6,838	6	10

blood pressure of at least 100 mm Hg. To the cases thus obtained, the following definitions were applied:

1. A woman was considered to have *essential hypertension* from the time of the first "high" blood pressure reading that fulfilled the following criteria: (a) it was followed by at least one more "high" reading; (b) it was followed by *no* intervening normal blood pressure reading while the woman was not under

treatment. A woman was also called hypertensive from her first "high" blood pressure reading if treatment started immediately subsequent to it.

2. A woman was considered to have *labile hypertension* from the time of her first "high" blood pressure reading, provided it was followed at some time by a normal blood pressure reading while the patient was not under treatment.

3. The term "high" blood pressure as used above means a systolic blood pressure of 140 mm Hg or more, or a diastolic blood pressure of 90 mm Hg or more. The term "treatment" means the prescription of antihypertensive drugs or diuretics; the latter are ignored if prescribed only for short-term or occasional use.

It should be emphasized that these definitions allow for a case to become first labile and then essential hypertension. Any woman who, by these definitions, had either labile or essential hypertension at entry into the study was considered a prevalent case. Also considered as prevalent cases were women in whose medical charts the attending physicians had recorded a diagnosis of essential or labile hypertension at entry into the study. All other cases were considered incident cases. When computing incidence rates all prevalent cases were excluded from the sample.

Methods of Analysis

The first step in the analysis was the computation of age-specific (per 1,000 person-years) and age-adjusted incidence rates according to the main variable under study: OC use status at entry into the study, which was classified into four categories: never, past, current, and estrogen user. As a second step, the past and current users were subclassified according to their total length of use of OCs at time of entry into the study. Three categories were used in this analysis: less than 1 year, 1–4 years, 4 years or more. Again, age-adjusted rates were computed. In both of these analyses the standard population for age adjustment comprised the total person-years under study.

As a complement to the incidence rates, age-adjusted prevalence rates at entry into the study were calculated. Here the standard population comprised all women at entry into the study.

In order to control for other variables, as well as age, a procedure developed for these studies was used (3). Its essence is as follows: It is assumed that at each point in time a woman was subjected to a given risk of developing an incident case of hypertension. This risk is assumed to be the product of two factors: One expressing the effect of OC use status and length of use, and one representing the joint effects of all the other covariates. Applying this model to the data, one can obtain maximum likelihood estimates of the effects of OC use status and length of use measured against the standard of the never-user group. These estimates (called relative risk estimates in the present report) can be visualized as ratios of the "pure" incidence rate for a given OC use and length-of-use group to the incidence rate for the never users. The group of women taking estrogens was excluded from this analysis because of their small number and skewed age distribution.

The covariates included in this analysis are, in addition to age:

1. Number of liveborn children at entry, in three categories: no children, 1–3 children, 4 or more children.

2. Family history of hypertension as stated by the subject at entry, in two categories: father and/or mother hypertensive, otherwise.

3. Relative weight at entry, in two categories: more than two standard deviations above the mean weight of the woman's age and height group, otherwise.

4. "Utilization of medical services" index. This variable was introduced to adjust for the fact that a woman who has a high frequency of contact with the medical clinics stands a better chance of having hypertension detected than a woman of low-frequency contact. In this study the utilization index of a woman was defined as her mean number of clinic and hospital contacts per month.[1] The mean utilization index in the study group was roughly 0.4. This variable was therefore dichotomized into two categories: less than 0.4, 0.4 or more.

The distribution of the covariates in the study population is given in Table 3.

TABLE 3. *Women at risk by OC use status, weight status, parity, family history of hypertension, and utilization index*

		Oral contraceptive use status			
Covariate	Total	Never users	Past users	Current users	Other Estrogen users
Weight status					
Overweight	1,520	598	470	315	137
Not overweight	12,572	3,881	3,975	3,499	1,217
Parity					
No live births	2,425	757	734	763	171
1–3 Live births	8,863	2,579	2,884	2,497	903
4+ Live births	2,804	1,143	827	554	280
Family history					
Hypertension	2,615	821	932	571	291
No hypertension	11,477	3,658	3,513	3,243	1,063
Utilization index					
Index < 0.4	8,633	3,067	2,616	2,282	668
Index ≥ 0.4	5,459	1,412	1,829	1,532	686
Total	14,092	4,479	4,445	3,814	1,354

Among current users as compared to never users, there were fewer overweight women, fewer with high parity and with a family history of hypertension, and more with a high utilization index for medical services.

Since OC use status, length of use, age, and three of the other covariates were

---

[1] For incident cases only the period previous to onset is used in this calculation.

measured at entry into the study, one might ask if the results could not have been affected by subsequent changes in these variables. To answer this question, relative risk was also estimated for a shorter period of time, during which no substantial changes in the variables were likely to have occurred. This shorter period extended from the women's entry into the study to July 1, 1972. Another advantage of this analysis based on the earlier period is that it would be less likely to be biased by physicians' awareness of the possibility of an association between blood pressure and OC use.

RESULTS

The age-adjusted rates (Table 4) were higher for the current users and women on estrogens than for the other two groups—at least for the combined rate of essential and labile hypertension. There was virtually no difference between past and never users. From Table 5 it seems that length of use had little impact on the incidence rates, but the number involved was too small to permit any firm conclusion. The prevalence rates of Table 6 show again higher values for the current users and estrogen-taking women, and almost no difference between past and never users.

Relative risks of Table 7 are more informative. The relative risks for the current users were considerable, and significantly above one. The value was particularly higher for the shorter observation period terminating July 1, 1972; it was lower and statistically not significant for essential hypertension alone.

There was no clear interaction between length of use and the relative risk

TABLE 4. *Age-specific and age-adjusted[a] incidence rates[b]* for hypertensive women

Age (years)	Never	Past	Current	Estrogen	Total
	\multicolumn{5}{c}{Oral contraceptive use status}				
Essential hypertension					
20–29	1.3	0.8	0.9	—	0.9
30–34	1.0	3.2	2.5	—	2.3
35–39	3.5	4.3	4.5	7.2	4.2
40–44	5.2	6.3	7.9	8.4	6.3
45–54	8.8	8.2	8.8	10.5	9.2
Age-adjusted	4.1	4.5	4.8	5.1	4.6
Essential and labile hypertension					
20–29	3.4	2.9	3.7	7.5	3.4
30–34	4.4	5.5	6.7	—	5.5
35–39	5.5	7.1	9.5	14.4	7.3
40–44	10.1	11.0	13.2	14.0	11.3
45–54	12.0	10.9	18.3	17.7	14.3
Age-adjusted	7.1	7.3	10.3	11.0	8.3

[a] Standard population = distribution of total person-months by age.
[b] Per 1,000 person-years.

TABLE 5. *Age-adjusted*[a] incidence rates[b] by OC use status and length of use at entry

Length of use at entry	Essential hypertension		Essential and labile hypertension	
	Past	Current	Past	Current
Less than 1 year	4.0	4.9[c]	7.3	7.9[c]
1–4 years	5.2	4.9	7.9	11.4
4 Years or more	1.6	5.2	3.8	9.5

[a] Standard population = distribution of total person-months by age.
[b] Per 1,000 person-years.
[c] Based on fewer than 1,000 person-years.

TABLE 6. *Age-adjusted*[a] prevalence rates[b] by OC use status

OC use status	Total	Essential hypertension	Labile hypertension
Never	67.6	47.6	20.0
Past	75.3	47.7	27.6
Current	97.8	61.8	36.1
Estrogen	91.0	64.7	26.3
All	76.5	51.7	24.8

[a] Standard population = distribution of all women at risk by age.
[b] Per 1,000 women.

TABLE 7. *Relative risk estimates by OC use status* [a]

Risk	OC use status	
	Past	Current
Essential and labile hypertension		
Relative risk estimates	1.06	1.57[b]
95% Confidence interval	0.79–1.41	1.18–2.08
Essential and labile hypertension (shorter period)[c]		
Relative risk estimates	1.02	1.82[b]
95% Confidence interval	0.71–1.46	1.28–2.57
Essential hypertension		
Relative risk estimates	1.12	1.31
95% Confidence interval	0.77–1.64	0.89–1.93

[a] Controlled for covariates, never users = 1.
[b] Departure from unity significant at $p < 0.001$. The difference between "current" and "past" users is significant at $p < 0.001$.
[c] From entry to July 1, 1972.

TABLE 8. *Relative risk estimates* [a] by OC use status and length of use at entry

Hypertension	Less than 1 year	1–4 Years	4 Years or more
Essential and labile hypertension			
Past	1.04	1.10	1.01
Current	0.83[b]	1.80	1.42
Essential and labile hypertension (shorter period)[c]			
Past	0.67	1.36	0.96
Current	0.89[b]	2.17	1.55
Essential hypertension			
Past	1.02	1.28	1.01
Current	0.88[b]	1.34	1.34

[a] Controlled for covariates, never users = 1.
[b] Based on less than 1,000 person-years.
[c] From entry to July 1, 1972.

(Table 8). The relative risk associated with 4 years or more of use was slightly lower than that for 1–4 years, but the difference is far from significant.

COMMENTS

There were several conditions in the data which would tend to underestimate the effect of OCs on hypertension.

1. Those related to changes in OC status following entry. There has been a trend toward discontinuance of OC use among study women who were current users at entry. Assuming that the increase in relative risk with OC use is real, this trend will lead to its underestimation. Similarly, cases of OC-induced hypertension occurring among past or never users who later started taking OCs would falsely inflate the hypertension rates within the past or never user groups. Both of these effects would reduce the relative risk for hypertension among current users as computed in this study. Some indication that this effect did obtain in this study is apparent from the fact that the relative risk as determined for the earlier follow-up period is higher than that for the later period.

2. Elimination of prevalent cases of labile hypertension. Most cases of OC-induced hypertension are known to be reversible on discontinuance of OCs. It is reasonable to assume therefore that many, if not the majority, of cases would have a clinical course such that in the initial phases they would tend to be called labile hypertension. Exclusion of all prevalent cases of labile hypertension from the data would then preclude from the analysis any cases that might develop into a persistent form of hypertension. The effect of this would be to reduce the measured relative risk for OC-induced hypertension. Further analysis of the data is in progress, and the plan is to determine how many prevalent labile cases progressed to fixed hypertension and what effect, if any, they had on the relative risk. It should therefore be emphasized that the relative risk reported here (ap-

proximately twofold) does not reflect the total risk of hypertension that may be attributed to OCs but may be considered as the minimum. On the other hand, the sixfold relative risk of hypertension in OC users previously reported by the authors (7) appears rather high in comparison. There are marked differences in the procedures used for ascertainment of cases and criteria for diagnosis between the two reports. Cases of labile hypertension were not analyzed in the earlier report; only reported diagnoses by physicians were used; and most importantly, the date on which the physician recorded the diagnosis was used as the date of onset. This procedure would tend to label already existing cases as newly occurring ones and would therefore increase the relative risk. It is therefore not unreasonable to assume that the actual increase in risk lies somewhere between two- and sixfold.

Since in this study the diagnosis of hypertension is not an all-or-none process and its certainty is to a large extent determined by the clinical course, it was frequently necessary to label a case in retrospect. The procedure followed in this study was to assign as the date of onset the date of the first recorded elevated blood pressure. The effect of this on those patients with labile hypertension who had high blood pressure measurements on entry was to assign their date of onset to their date of entry. This made them prevalent cases of labile hypertension and thus eliminated them from further consideration, even with respect to the analysis of essential hypertension.

The question frequently arises as to the effect of the secular trend of increased awareness of the relationship of OCs to hypertension on the measures of risk obtained in studies. The risk estimates presented here did not show a higher rate for the later as compared to the earlier time period. However, it must be noted that in these data there is a confounding effect of changes in OC use over that time period, which makes the results inconclusive.

The Royal College of General Practitioners (8) reported an increase in the incidence of hypertension with duration of OC use; and Weir et al. (9) showed a rising rate of increase in systolic and diastolic pressures with length of time on OCs. The data presented here provide no evidence of such a trend; but confounding the effect of duration of use in the present study is the possibility that discontinuance of OCs after entry into the study might be related to duration of use at entry. Such a possibility might explain the lower incidence rate in the group with the longest duration of use. More of these women would presumably be likely to stop OC use. The data are being examined for these effects.

The relationship of labile hypertension to fixed hypertension has been and remains unclear. Even more unclear is the relationship of labile hypertension to OC-induced hypertension. It is hoped that a more detailed examination of the data provided by this prospective study will yield information about the natural history of labile hypertension, which in turn would make it possible to determine if a history of labile hypertension is of value in predicting the development of essential hypertension in response to OC use.

Of considerable interest, even though tangential to the main thrust of the present study, is the observed parallel effect of conjugated estrogens. The incidence rates for hypertension are even higher in the group of women who were taking estrogens or had been taking them during the past year than among current OC users. Because of the confounding effect of OC use by some of the women in the estrogen-use group, the difference between estrogen users and never users cannot be ascribed to estrogens alone. However, since the use of estrogens (as the only sex hormone used) predominated in this group, much of the effect seen was very likely associated with estrogen use.

Work is currently in progress to include in the analysis changes in OC use following entry into the study. Certain other aspects not covered here are also under further study. One concerns the severity of OC-induced hypertension. Is OC-related hypertension only a mild form of the disease, or is there a small group of women who are specially prone to a malignant form of OC-induced hypertension (10)? Other areas under investigation are concerned with the assessment of possible predisposing and predictive factors (e.g., family history of hypertension, obesity, smoking) in their relationship to the effect of OC use. The question of dosage and type of OC is also being considered, insofar as the data will allow. Subsequent reports from CDS are expected to incorporate the results obtained after considering the factors mentioned above.

ACKNOWLEDGMENTS

The authors wish to express their thanks to Natalie Lloyd and her staff for abstracting medical charts; Bruce Brainard, Roberta Heintz, and Sylvia Huang for programming and data processing; Jess Frank for developing statistical procedures; and Dr. Irwin R. Fisch for his suggestions. This study was supported by contract NO1-HD-3-2710 with the Center for Population Research, National Institute of Child Health and Human Development.

REFERENCES

1. Clezy, T. M., Foy, B. N., Hodge, R. L., and Lumbers, E. R. (1972): Oral contraceptives and hypertension: An epidemiological survey. *Br. Heart J.,* 34:1238–1243.
2. Fisch, I. R., Freedman, S. H., and Myatt, A. V. (1972): Oral contraceptives, pregnancy, and blood pressure. *JAMA,* 222:1507–1510.
3. Frank, J. (1977): Survival analysis with time-dependent covariates. U.C. Berkeley, *unpublished Ph.D. thesis.*
4. Greenblatt, D. J., and Koch-Weser, J. (1974): Oral contraceptives and hypertension: A report from the Boston Collaborative Drug Surveillance Program. *Obstet. Gynecol.,* 44:412–417.
5. Mackay, E. V., Khoo, S. K., and Shah, N. A. (1973): Reproductive steroids and the circulatory system with particular reference to hypertension: A review. *Obstet. Gynecol. Surv.,* 28:155–165.
6. Ramcharan, S., editor (1974): *The Walnut Creek Contraceptive Drug Study: A Prospective Study of the Side Effects of Oral Contraceptives, Vol. 1.* D.H.E.W. Publication No. (N.I.H.) 74–562.
7. Ramcharan, S., Pellegrin, F. A., and Hoag, E. (1974): The occurrence and course of hypertensive disease in users and nonusers of oral contraceptive drugs. In: *Oral Contraceptives and High Blood Pressure,* edited by M. J. Fregley and M. S. Fregley, pp. 1–16. Dolphin Press, Gainesville, Florida.
8. Royal College of General Practitioners (1974): Hypertension. In: *Oral Contraceptives and Health,* pp. 37–42. Pitman, New York.

 9. Weir, R. J., Briggs, E., Mack, A., Naismith, L., Taylor, L., and Wilson, E. (1974): Blood pressure in women taking oral contraceptives. *Br. Med. J.,* 1:533–535.
10. Zech, P., Rifle, G., Lindner, A., Sassard, J., Blanc-Brunat, N., and Traeger, J. (1975): Malignant hypertension with irreversible renal failure due to oral contraceptives. *Br. Med. J.,* 4:326–327.

Pharmacology of Steroid Contraceptive Drugs
edited by S. Garattini and H. W. Berendes.
Raven Press, New York © 1977.

Oral Contraceptives and Myocardial Infarction in Young Women

J. I. Mann

*Department of Social and Community Medicine, Oxford University,
Oxford, OX1 3QN, England*

Subsequent to 1963 there have been no fewer than 12 series of case reports in which small numbers of patients were described who developed myocardial infarction while using oral contraceptives (1,2). Oliver (3) alone has reported on an appreciable number of patients under the age of 45 years; and of the patients admitted to the hospital during the years 1964–1974 (during which time use of oral contraceptives had become widespread), 52% were taking these preparations. This proportion was thought to be greater than might have been expected; but because there was no difference in the prevalence of major risk factors for ischemic heart disease in those women taking oral contraceptives compared with those who were not, Oliver concluded that the preparations increased the risk of myocardial infarction only in the presence of one of the major risk factors. In the absence of control data, no definite conclusions can be drawn from the results of such studies.

In their study of deaths from thromboembolic disease, Inman and Vessey (4) found that women who died from coronary thrombosis in the absence of predisposing causes had been using oral contraceptives more frequently than would have been expected from the experience of the control group, but statistically significant differences between the infarction patients and controls were apparent only when patients with obesity were excluded. A Danish study (5) of fatal myocardial infarction suggested that oral contraceptive use before death from this cause was not different from that of the general population in the same age group, and other studies failed to provide conclusive answers (6,7). The studies described in this chapter were undertaken to determine if an association does exist between oral contraceptives and myocardial infarction.

STUDIES OF FATAL MYOCARDIAL INFARCTION

Procedure

In 1973 Inman and I (8) obtained transcripts of all death certificates relating to women under age 50 who died in England and Wales, and whose records had been coded to rubric 410 according to the eighth revision of the International

Classification of Diseases (myocardial infarction and synonymous terms). Initially we investigated all the deaths of women under 40 years of age and a random sample of those in the older age groups (40–49 years). Information concerning drug use was obtained chiefly from the patients' general practitioners, who were also asked to provide control information by selecting at random from their files women who matched each fatal case with regard to age and marital status. Twenty-one percent of the patients selected for study could not be investigated because their physicians could not be traced, their records had been lost, or the physician could not be interviewed. The data presented in this chapter are based on those cases in whom the diagnosis was substantiated by postmortem findings or by a history of chest pain together with electrocardiographic or enzymatic confirmation as defined by the World Health Organization (9).

Results

The frequency of use of oral contraceptives during the month before death (current users) was significantly higher in the group with infarction than during the same month in the control group (Table 1); the average duration of use was also longer. It is apparent from Table 1 that the relative and attributable risks

TABLE 1. *Oral contraceptive practice and mortality from myocardial infarction*

	Mortality from myocardial infarction per 100,000 Women[a]	
Measurement	Aged 30–39 years	Aged 40–44 years
Women currently using oral contraceptives	5.4	54.7
Women not currently using oral contraceptives	1.9	11.7
Mortality attributable to oral contraceptives	3.5	43.0

[a] These estimates were based on the data given below and published by Mann and Inman (8), as well as on information concerning the structure of the female population of England and Wales and the total number of deaths from myocardial infarction during 1973, derived from the Registrar General's Report.

	Aged < 40 years		Aged 40–44 years	
Oral contraceptive practice	MI patients	Controls	MI patients	Controls
First study				
Current users	21 (44.7%)	17 (22.4%)	8 (15.4%)	2 (3.8%)
Not current users	26 (55.3%)	59 (77.6%)	44 (84.6%)	50 (96.2%)

Comparison between current users and women not currently using oral contraceptives:

$$X_1^2 = 5.78 \qquad p = 0.05 \text{ (Fisher's exact test)}$$
$$0.01 < p < 0.02$$
$$\text{Relative risk estimate} = 2.8 \qquad \text{Relative risk estimate} = 4.7$$

were strikingly greater in the 40–44 age group than in women under age 40.

Partly on the basis of these data, the Food and Drug Administration of the United States issued during the summer of 1975 a bulletin recommending that patients over 40 years of age be made thoroughly aware of the increased risks of oral contraceptives and be urged to utilize other methods of contraception.

Very few women in the infarction and control groups aged 40–44 years had been current users of oral contraceptives, and we therefore considered it desirable to study a larger number of deaths in order to make a more reliable estimate of the risk in older women using these preparations. We did this by attempting to investigate all the deaths in this age group not previously selected for study and we now have information concerning 108 of the 227 deaths certified as due to myocardial infarction in 1973. The remainder could not be studied, either because their medical records could not be found (20 deaths), their physicians were unable to help or could not be traced (39 deaths), or owing to administrative difficulties the death certificate could not be retrieved (35 deaths). Twenty-five deaths were excluded from the study because investigation suggested that the cause of death was different from that given on the death certificate. The oral contraceptive practices of this enlarged group of infarction and control patients aged 40–44 years are shown in Table 2. The more reliable relative risk estimate derived from this study of a larger group of women is now very similar to that estimated for women below 40 years of age. When the mortality from myocardial infarction in women who use oral contraceptives and those who do not is estimated on the basis of the data given in Table 2 (enlarged group), the yearly death rates are 32 and 12 per 100,000, respectively. In absolute terms, therefore, the attributable mortality is still considerably greater in the older group of women (aged 40–44 years), there being a yearly excess of 20 deaths per 100,000 users of oral contraceptives.

In an investigation of fatal cases it was clearly not possible to get detailed information concerning other risk factors, but the data in Table 3 suggest that the association between myocardial infarction and oral contraceptives could not be explained by an association between these preparations and diabetes or hypertension (defined in this study as previous medical treatment for these conditions). No information was available concerning cigarette smoking habits or cholesterol levels.

The possible sources of bias which may have influenced these findings have

TABLE 2. *Oral contraceptive practice of myocardial infarction (MI) and control patients in the enlarged group of women aged 40–44 years*

Oral contraceptive practice	MI patients	Controls
Current users	18 (17.0%)	7 (6.9%)
Not current users	88 (83.0%)	95 (93.1%)

Relative risk estimate = 2.8 (X_1^2 = 4.35, $p < 0.05$)
(95% confidence limit: 1.2–7.2)

TABLE 3. *Estimated relative risk of death from MI in patients aged 40–44 currently using oral contraceptives after standardization for possible confounding variables*

Variable standardized	Relative risk estimate	X^2	Significance level
None	2.8	3.9	$p < 0.05$
Hypertension	2.7	3.8	$p < 0.05$
Diabetes	2.8	3.8	$p < 0.05$
Both variables simultaneously	2.7	3.8	$p < 0.05$

been considered in detail in the publication concerned. I would, however, like to mention briefly one particularly important aspect under this heading. The control population should be representative of the general population of women of childbearing age with regard to their oral contraceptive practice. Comparison with a national survey carried out in the United Kingdom suggests that current oral contraceptive use in the control population in all age groups appears to be greater than might have been expected (10), and this, if true, would have tended to reduce the association found between myocardial infarction and oral contraceptive use. One possible explanation might be an "overmatching" phenomenon, which could have occurred if the general practitioners had tended to fall into two distinct categories, i.e., those regularly prescribing oral contraceptives and those prescribing them either infrequently or not at all. An association between myocardial infarction and oral contraceptive use would then have led the investigator, when following up deaths from infarction, to practices where the prescribing of these drugs was more frequent; hence the control population selected from these practices would have tended to include more users than the general population of the same age group.

These data provide strong evidence for an increased risk of death from myocardial infarction in women using oral contraceptives. The observation that dead patients in this study appeared to have been using oral contraceptives for a longer duration than control patients, together with the fact that the use of oral contraceptives had increased almost threefold since 1966, may help to explain the more striking effect apparent in 1973. The implications of these data are discussed later.

A STUDY OF NONFATAL MYOCARDIAL INFARCTION

Procedure

Data were also obtained concerning nonfatal myocardial infarction by investigating women under age 45 years who were discharged from the major hospitals in three hospital regions in England and Wales during the years 1968–1972 (11–13). In the great majority of cases, information concerning oral contraceptive practice and other risk factors was obtained during an interview in the patients' homes. When this could not be arranged, a postal questionnaire was completed or the required information was obtained from the general practitioner. Three control patients were selected to match each patient with infarction with respect to age, marital status, and hospital and year of admission. They were selected at random from lists of patients admitted with a wide range of acute medical and surgical conditions, and for certain elective surgical procedures; they were investigated in the same manner as the infarction patients. Blood samples were collected from as many as possible of the infarction patients and the controls.

Results

The proportion of patients who used oral contraceptives during the month before admission to hospital was substantially higher in the infarction than the control group (Table 4). The relative risk of developing myocardial infarction, compared with that in women who had never used oral contraceptives, is estimated from these figures to be 4.3:1 for women who had used them during the month before admission and 1.1:1 for women who had stopped using them more than a month previously. Even when allowing for the effect of all the other risk factors measured, a statistically significant increased risk remained (Table 5). Diabetes was not considered in this analysis because only four patients were known to have the disease and none was using oral contraceptives.

This type of analysis cannot establish the quantitative effect of each combination of risk factors. To do so would require very large numbers of infarction patients and controls. However, the data in Table 6, derived from the study of survivors of infarction, show the proportions of patients known to have had various risk factors, those who had only one risk factor being subgrouped according to the nature of the factor in question. Information on the presence of one or more factors was not obtained for a few patients, and lipid analyses were

TABLE 4. *Oral contraceptive practice among myocardial infarction patients and controls*

Oral contraceptive practice	No. and (%) of MI patients	No. and (%) of controls
Never used	44 (61.1)	150 (78.9)
Used during month before admission	20 (27.8)	16 (8.4)[a]
Used only more than 1 month before admission	8 (11.1)	24 (12.6)
Used any time before admission	28 (38.9)	40 (21.0)[b]
Total	72 (100)	190 (100)

[a] Comparison between proportions of patients using oral contraceptives during the month before admission: $X_1^2 = 13.3$, $p < 0.001$.

[b] Comparison between proportions of patients using oral contraceptives at any time before admission: $X_1^2 = 7.5$, $p < 0.01$.

TABLE 5. *Estimated relative risk of MI in patients currently using oral contraceptives after standardization for possible confounding variables*

Variable standardized	Relative risk estimate	X^2	Significance level
None	4.3	13.3	$p < 0.001$
Cigarette smoking	3.2	6.6	$p < 0.01$
Pre-eclamptic toxemia or hypertension	3.8	10.1	$p < 0.001$
Type II hyperlipoproteinemia	3.6	8.3	$p < 0.01$
All of above variables simultaneously	3.1	5.5	$p < 0.05$

Data are based on the study of survivors of myocardial infarction.

TABLE 6. *Risk factors in myocardial infarction patients and controls*

Risk factor	No. and (%) of MI patients	No. and (%) of controls
No risk factor	14 (18.9)	128 (64.0)
One risk factor		
Current oral contraceptive use	4 (5.4)	9 (4.5)
Type II hyperlipoproteinemia	4 (5.4)	1 (0.5)
Diabetes	1 (1.4)	0
Cigarette smoking (15 or more daily)	12 (16.2)	33 (16.5)
Hypertension or pre-eclamptic toxemia	5 (6.8)	19 (9.5)
Two risk factors	20 (27.0)	9 (4.5)
Three or more risk factors	14 (18.9)	1 (0.5)
Total	74 (100)	200 (100)

carried out on only 70% of the patients with infarction, so the number who were exposed to one risk factor or to none at all is likely to have been smaller than appears from the table. It should also be recalled that hypertension and diabetes were recorded only when the patient had been treated for these conditions before the infarction occurred. The risk estimates derived from the data in Table 6 nevertheless strongly suggest that the combined effect of the factors is synergistic. In comparison with patients not known to have any risk factors, the relative risk increased from 4:1 in women with one factor to 20:1 in women with two factors and 128:1 in women with three or more factors. Of particular importance with regard to the present discussion, however, is the fact that none of the risk factors, except type II hyperlipoproteinemia, appeared to exert a strong effect when present on its own. Only four of the infarction patients studied had experienced an acute myocardial infarction while using oral contraceptives in the absence of other risk factors.

CLINICAL APPLICATIONS OF THESE STUDIES

I should like to consider briefly the relevance of these findings in drawing up a balance sheet of advantages and disadvantages of oral contraceptives. Such attempts have been made previously [e.g., by Potts and Swyer (14)], but the calculations involved many complicated assumptions, did not consider the different age groups separately, and were made at a time when myocardial infarction was not recognized as a complication of oral contraceptive use. The conclusions at that time were that the mortality associated with the use of oral contraceptives or intrauterine contraceptive devices were of the same order of magnitude as the mortality due to unplanned pregnancies occurring when less efficient contraceptive methods were used.

Ideally, any such balance sheet should be as simple as possible. In Table 7 I compare the annual mortality from thromboembolic events attributable to oral contraceptives among users of these preparations with the mortality resulting from the complications of unwanted pregnancies that might be expected among users of a less effective method of contraception (the diaphragm).

In these calculations I used data derived from the studies I mentioned, and the age breakdown was so chosen that comparable statistics from the different studies could be employed. It should be recalled that the data relating to pulmonary and cerebral thromboembolism were collected at a time when the majority of oral contraceptive preparations contained 100 μg estrogen, and those data relating to myocardial infarction were collected when the 50-μg preparations were most widely used. I have assumed oral contraceptives to be totally effective as a method of contraception (which is, of course, not true) and have also assumed a 10% failure rate among users of the diaphragm (Vessey, 1975, *personal communication*), which is a fairly pessimistic assessment. There is an excess of 1.3 deaths per 100,000 in the younger age group of women using oral contraceptives and an excess of 6.6 per 100,000 in women age 35–44 years. The excessive number of deaths attributable to oral contraceptives would have been even greater had

TABLE 7. *Mortality rates in women aged 20–44 using two contraception methods*

Measurement	Aged 20–34 years	Aged 35–44 years
Annual mortality attributable to oral contraceptives per 100,000 users of these preparations[a] from		
Myocardial infarction	1.1	8.1
Pulmonary and cerebral thromboembolism	1.3	3.4
Total	2.4	11.5
Annual mortality from all risks of pregnancy, delivery, and puerperium,[b] resulting from unwanted pregnancies per 100,000 users of the diaphragm[a]	1.1	4.9

[a] This assumes a 10% failure rate among women using the diaphragm as a method of contraception and no failures among users of oral contraceptives.

[b] I.C.D., 8th revision, Rubrics 630–678.

the 40–44 age group been considered, but data for pulmonary and cerebral thromboembolism are not available for this age breakdown.

These simple computations do not take into account a number of other aspects that may be relevant. Surgery for gallbladder disease (common among users of oral contraceptives) may be associated with a significant mortality rate, as may also cerebral hemorrhage and some of the less commonly suggested adverse reactions. However, thromboembolic complications at present probably account for the greatest number of fatal adverse reactions to oral contraceptives, and only these have been quantified with any accuracy. Furthermore, widespread recourse to legal abortion of unwanted pregnancies among users of the diaphragm would appreciably reduce the number of deaths in these women. These observations and the fact that fewer than 10% of women using the diaphragm are likely to become pregnant per year suggest that the estimate of excess deaths in oral contraceptive users is a conservative one.

I have not included statistics of morbidity associated with oral contraceptives or other methods of contraception—not because I consider nonfatal illness unimportant but because the difficulties of quantification are even greater here than with regard to mortality. Certain beneficial effects of oral contraceptives would need to be included in such a consideration too, e.g., the protective effect of oral contraceptives against benign breast disease. I also did not consider the mortality in women using other methods of contraception, e.g., intrauterine devices, which are themselves associated with potentially lethal unwanted effects that have not yet been accurately quantified.

These observations and the fact that oral contraceptives appear to increase the risk of myocardial infarction chiefly in the presence of other risk factors lead me to conclude that alternative methods of contraception should be recommended to women already at increased risk of ischemic heart disease. This may apply particularly to the older woman requiring a method of contraception.

REFERENCES

1. Maleki, M. and Lange, R. L. (1973): *Am. Heart J.,* 85:749.
2. Mann, J. I. (1975): Epidemiology of heart disease in young women. D. M. Thesis, University of Oxford.
3. Oliver, M. F. (1974): *Br. Med. J.,* 4:253.
4. Inman, W. H. W., and Vessey, M. P. (1968): *Br. Med. J.,* 2:193.
5. Fischer, A. J., and Mosbech, J. (1970): *Ugeskr. Laeger,* 132:2480.
6. Vessey, M. P., and Doll, R. (1969): *Br. Med. J.,* 2:651.
7. Inman, W. H. W., et al. (1970): *Br. Med. J.,* 2:203.
8. Mann, J. I., and Inman, W. H. W. (1975): *Br. Med. J.,* 2:245.
9. World Health Organization (1971): *Criteria for Myocardial Infarction, Ischaemic Heart Disease Register.* W.H.O., Copenhagen.
10. Bone, M. (1973): *Family Planning Services in England & Wales.* H.M.S.O., London, and *personal communication.*
11. Mann, J. I., et al. (1975): *Br. Med. J.,* 2:241.
12. Mann, J. I., et al. (1975): *Br. Med. J.,* 3:631.
13. Mann, J. I., and Thorogood, M. (1975): *Br. Heart J.,* 37:790.
14. Potts, D. M., and Swyer, G. I. M. (1970): *Br. Med. Bull.,* 26:26.

Pharmacology of Steroid Contraceptive Drugs
edited by S. Garattini and H. W. Berendes.
Raven Press, New York © 1977.

Comments on Epidemiologic Studies Relating Myocardial Infarction and Oral Contraceptives

F. M. Sturtevant

Searle Laboratories, G. D. Searle & Co., Chicago, Illinois 60680

One of the prime concerns and responsibilities of the pharmaceutical manufacturer in this era of exploding knowledge of the actions of new drugs is the ascertainment and analysis of such information and its disbursement to the practicing physician. Such new information is traditionally included in the labeling of the drug and accompanies it in interstate commerce. The manufacturer is charged with the appropriateness of the labeling, which means the adequacy of the information for use: indications, effects, dosages, and the like, plus relevant warnings, contraindications, side effects, and precautions.

The Food and Drug Administration (FDA) has the responsibility for both initial approval and continued marketing of new drugs. This sanction is based in part on the adequacy of the labeling, the contents of which understandably change from time to time as new information becomes available.

The ultimate recipient of this information is the practicing physician. It is incumbent on him to be aware of current information concerning the drugs he prescribes. To this end, he utilizes not only the labeling provided by the manufacturer but also informational material disbursed by the FDA, as well as the traditional methods of medical communication, e.g., professional journals, meetings, conferences. From all of these sources the physician builds his knowledge of the drug for use in making prescribing decisions.

REACTIONS TO THE BRITISH REPORTS

The difficulties attendant to notifying practicing physicians of new information are aptly illustrated by the events following the appearance in May of 1975 of epidemiologic studies in Great Britain relating myocardial infarction (MI) and oral contraceptives. In typical retrospective case-controlled studies, Mann and co-workers (1–5) reported that prior use of "the pill" was higher in women with a diagnosis of myocardial infarction—whether discharged alive from the hospital or officially reported as dead—than was the prior use of the pill by designated "controls." The observational data were reported in terms of relative risk ratios comparing prior pill use by cases and controls. The ratios were notably higher in groups aged over 40. Based on sets of assumptions, these ratios were then employed to estimate incidence figures for the general population of reproductive-age women. These estimates of incidence in Great Britain and the misstatement of relative risk ratios in terms of projected attributable risk to the individual made immediate headlines across the United States.

The *Associated Press* reported, "Women taking birth control pills run a higher risk of heart attacks, especially if they have other heart risk factors . . ." (6). *Medical World News* wrote that "women who use oral contraceptives—especially those over 40—stand a considerably greater than normal chance of suffering myocardial infarctions and of dying from that type of heart attack" (7). These are misstatements of the British data.

In September 1975 the FDA sent a bulletin to every physician in this country reporting on the risk of myocardial infarction in users of oral contraceptives (8). The FDA's Advisory Committee on Obstetrics and Gynecology reportedly recommended that "patients over 40 be made thoroughly aware of the increased risk and be urged to utilize other forms of contraception" (8). In contrast, however, the Family Planning Association in Great Britain, where the data were gathered, said it was not ready to make such a recommendation, citing the high risk of complications in pregnancy for this age group (7). The U.S. Planned Parenthood Federation, on the other hand, urged its affiliates to offer women over 40 another method of contraception (9).

The FDA announced its intention "to revise the labeling for oral contraceptives to reflect this recommendation" of its Advisory Committee (8). On the other hand, their British equivalent, the Committee on Safety of Medicines, apparently has no plans to make similar recommendations (10).

Meanwhile, the National Institutes of Health, also an entity of the U.S. Department of Health, Education, and Welfare (but distinct from the FDA) has been seeking sources for a case–control study, in part "to determine the nature and extent of the relationship between the use of oral contraceptives and the risk of myocardial infarction" (11).

At this point, it should be pointed out that prior practice in the field of oral contraceptives restricted the manufacturers from altering the labeling of these drugs on a unilateral basis because all such labeling was uniform from one manufacturer to another. However, according to a recent announcement of FDA policy, this is now permitted. Thus we find in the 1976 edition of the *Physicians' Desk Reference* that two of the seven[1] American manufacturers of the pill recount the findings of Mann et al. and list myocardial infarction as a possible adverse reaction; the other five do not, even though some describe products with identical active ingredients.

NATURE OF THE MI REPORTS

What is the nature of the Mann et al. reports on myocardial infarction that resulted in such a furor and ultimate confusion in the lay and medical press?

---

[1] One manufacturer has since discontinued its sole product for other reasons.

Detailed criticism of these specific papers (12,13) and the misuse of results from other, similar, retrospective case–control studies have been made previously (14–16). However, a brief review of some of the points is worthwhile to underscore the uncertainties that currently exist concerning the Mann reports. The discussion primarily concerns the mortality study because diagnosis and vital statistics are more certain here than in morbidity studies.

Mann and Inman (2) examined all 726 death certificates in England and Wales for women under 50 years of age whose deaths in 1973 were ascribed to acute myocardial infarction and coded ICD 410. After various exclusions, 145 cases were selected for tabulation according to the results of interviews with the patients' physicians. The cases were classified as "current users" of the pill if they had used it during the month before death. "Nonusers" must have been defined as those who had used the pill more than a month before death; the last category was "never users." Only this definition allows one to duplicate the relative risks given in their report. Thus an error of recollection of 1 day in the history of pill use by the deceased, a year or more previously, could change the classification of a case from user to nonuser. For an unknown reason, the definition of nonuser appears to change in Mann's morbidity report (1). Relative risk was calculated by matched pairs in the morbidity report, but insufficient data were provided to permit confirmation of the calculations. However, one is able to calculate risk ratios by the cross-products method, and only by now defining nonusers as never-users can one duplicate the risk ratio of 4.5 given in the text.

In the mortality study, deceased patients were compared with living controls selected from the physicians' records, matched for 5-year age group and marital status, but not for presence or absence of known risk factors for myocardial infarction or for other factors that could have affected the decision to prescribe the pill in the first place. The potential import of the latter point was recently discussed by Preston (12). Thus a history of treatment for hypertension or diabetes was significantly more frequent for the cases than for the controls, and it is impossible for the reader to correct for this in the tabulation of pill use by the various age groupings.

In the age group 30–39, 21 of the 47 cases were classified as users. Assuming that the 76 controls selected were identical in all relevant aspects, approximately 11 users would have been expected. This difference in pill use results in a cross-products calculation of relative risk of 2.8. In the age group 40–44, 8 of the 52 cases were users, compared with the 2 expected, giving a relative risk of 4.6. Note that this difference of 6 subjects forms the basis for the warnings of fatal myocardial infarction in women over 40 who use the pill!

Relative risk in retrospective studies such as this, however, refers to a difference between a history of pill use by dead women with the disease and live women without the disease. It is necessary to make further assumptions and calculations in order to project estimates for incidence. Accordingly, the authors state: "The data derived from this study and information on the structure of the female population of England and Wales derived from the Registrar General's report make it possible to estimate the mortality from myocardial infarction in women who use oral contraceptives and in those who do not" (2). No details are provided, and it is only by trial and error that the reader can reconstruct the calculations involved.

The reconstruction proceeded as follows for the age group 30–39. *First,* the relative risk of 2.8 comparing prior pill use for deceased patients and living controls is assumed to be identical to the degree by which the incidence of myocardial infarction would be increased by pill use in the general population of British women of this age group. *Second,* the number of such women is given in the Registrar General's 1973 report (17) as 2.83 million. *Third,* the pill use by the general female population aged 30–39 is assumed to be the same as the pill use by Mann's controls aged 30–49, which amounts to 19/181 or 10.5%. (This inclusion of older controls has the effect of decreasing the percentage of pill use and increasing the final mortality estimates.) Taking 10.5% of the population yields 297,150 users, with the balance of 2,532,850 being nonusers. *Fourth,* the incidence of fatal myocardial infarction for 1973 is obtained from the 65 deaths listed by the Registrar General (17) divided by the population of 2.83 million, giving 2.3 cases per 100,000. *Lastly,* the nonuser incidence x, and the user incidence $2.8x$, are estimated by the following equation:

$$2.3 = \frac{2,533\, x\, + 297\, (2.8x)}{2,830}$$

This yields 1.9 per 100,000 for nonusers and 5.4 for users. Had controls been employed who were of the same age group, these incidence figures would be 1.6 and 4.6, respectively. The utilization of such incidence estimates requires the assumption that the calculations based on the year 1973 are pertinent for the present and future years, which ignores the demonstrable change in mortality rates with time.

If the same reconstruction is performed for the age group 40–44, this time with the proper controls, we obtain approximately the same estimated incidences published by Mann, viz., 11 per 100,000 for nonusers and 55 for users. It should be emphasized that this large figure for users aged 40–44 develops directly from a difference of only 8 subjects in the relative risk calculation, and from a control use by only 2 subjects in the reconstruction procedure. Simply put, there is a high probability that these projected incidences are wrong, even though they have been carried out to three significant figures and broadcast throughout the world.

ACCURACY OF PREDICTIONS

If one accepts Mann's predicted incidence figures *arguendo*, the total myocardial infarction mortality for users and nonusers alike can be estimated and then compared with the number actually reported by the Registrar General.

One estimates the pill users in the age groups 30–39 and 40–44 by reducing the 1970 census figures for these groups by the number unmarried (18) and by

TABLE 1. *Predicted vs. observed mortality in England and Wales, 1970*

Age (years)	Predicted deaths			Registrar general	% Difference
	Users	Nonusers	Total		
30–39	26	45	71	87	−18
40–44	41	163	204	167	+22

applying the percentage thereof who are pill users (19); one similarly computes the small contribution from unmarried users (18,19). The total number of deaths is then estimated by applying Mann's incidence figures; the comparison with the Registrar General's entries (20) are shown in Table 1. Note that these estimates are for the year 1970 in order to render more applicable the data of Bone (18) and Kay (19), which were employed.

The small absolute number of deaths predicted is noteworthy. The younger group's deaths are underestimated and those for the older group overestimated, probably as a result of the misleadingly high relative risk ratios assumed for the older women.

PREDICTING FOR THE UNITED STATES

Patterns of oral contraceptive use, medical practice, autopsy, diagnostic zeal, prejudice, recording of vital statistics, etc. surely are not identical in the United States and the United Kingdom. Further, it is easily demonstrated that year-to-year trends in the vital statistics for myocardial infarction are markedly different in the two countries, and that within the United States qualitative differences exist between blacks and whites.

If all of this is ignored, the predictions by Mann for England and Wales, based on the statistics derived from England and Wales, can be extrapolated to the United States. Obviously, this invites gross error; yet it was done by the FDA without qualification (8), and their statements have had wide distribution in this country.

In order to calculate predicted mortality rates for the United States, it is necessary to partition the 30–39 and 40–44 age populations in 1970 by race and marital status. These variables affect both pill use and death rates (21) for myocardial infarction. Attention must be restricted to 1970, as that is the year of the most recent National Fertility Survey (22).

The appropriate white and black populations were obtained from 1970 census figures (23), reduced to the number who were married (24), and multiplied by the proportion of pill users in the National Fertility Survey (22,25). The number of married users so derived, and the nonusers obtained by difference, were multiplied by Mann's incidence estimates to obtain the predicted mortality figures, which were then compared to the appropriate vital statistics (26) (Table 2).

The mortality rates for younger whites and particularly for the blacks of both

TABLE 2. *Predicted vs. observed mortality in the United States, 1970*

Age (years)	Predicted deaths			U.S. vital statistics	% Difference
	Users	Nonusers	Total		
White					
30–39	63	142	205	418	−51
40–44	336	464	800	808	− 1
Black					
30–39	5	12	17	192	−91
40–44	27	40	67	292	−77

age groups have been markedly underestimated. It is incorrect to conclude from the apparent agreement in one subgroup that this projection from the British data, risk ratio, and vital statistics is appropriate. It is also incorrect to conclude from the underestimates that the attributable risk for use of the pill is higher in the United States than in the United Kingdom. Rather, the total mortality rate for myocardial infarction in the 40- to 49-year-old woman is some two to three times higher in America, both before and after the advent of the pill. It is of interest, however, that the increasing female mortality rate for MI in Great Britain is 1.4 times greater than in the United States for the years 1956–1973. The corresponding increase for British males is 6.2 times greater than for females, whereas in the United States a slight decrease has occurred. These quantitative and qualitative differences in the vital statistics of the two countries, as well as the other differences enumerated earlier, preclude the extrapolation of British risk ratios, British vital statistics, British pill usage percentages, and derived British incidence projections to the United States female population.

THE MORBIDITY STUDY

Using techniques similar to those in the mortality study (2), Mann et al. published a second report relating hospital discharges with a diagnosis of MI to certain risk factors and prior pill use. Only *one* user of the pill had an MI in the absence of other listed risk factors.

Additional assumptions were employed to derive incidence estimates in this study. Using these estimates, we attempted to match the projections with the second National Morbidity Survey in Great Britain (27) and the Framingham Study in the United States (28). The findings were widely disparate, but are not recounted here because the reasons for the differences may be many. It is noteworthy that a recent news item (29) reports that Mann et al. have recalculated their statistics and now predict only half as much morbidity for women over 40 as they had previously.

DISCHARGE OF RESPONSIBILITIES

It should be emphasized that the papers of Mann and co-workers (1,2) did contain caveats concerning possible misapplication of their data. However, the FDA perceived the necessity of publicizing the British incidence estimates as though they were directly applicable to the United States; furthermore, they combined rates for morbidity and mortality as though subjects never appeared in both categories.

The recommendation of the FDA's Advisory Committee and of Planned Parenthood concerning women over 40 has placed the practicing physician between the Scylla of prescribing less effective contraception for an age group at high risk during pregnancy and the Charybdis of a malpractice allegation in the event an older patient on the pill displays signs or symptoms of myocardial ischemia. The patient is in no less a quandary, unless she has decided by now to be tolerant of the succession of frightening reports with which she is bombarded. One can only question whether such a misuse of epidemiologic data avoids doing an injustice or disservice to medicine and the public.

REFERENCES

1. Mann, J. I., Vessey, M. P., Thorogood, M., and Doll, R. (1975): Myocardial infarction in young women with special reference to oral contraceptive practice. *Br. Med. J.*, 2:241–245.
2. Mann, J. I., and Inman, W. H. W. (1975): Oral contraceptives and death from myocardial infarction. *Br. Med. J.*, 2:245–248.
3. Mann, J. I., Thorogood, M., Waters, W. E., and Powell, C. (1975): Oral contraceptives and myocardial infarction in young women: A further report. *Br. Med. J.*, 3:631–632.
4. Mann, J. I., and Thorogood, M. (1975): Coffee-drinking and myocardial infarction. *Lancet*, 2:1215.
5. Mann, J. I., and Thorogood, M. (1975): Serum lipids in young female survivors of myocardial infarction. *Br. Heart J.*, 37:790–794.
6. *Chicago Sun Times,* July 25, 1975.
7. *Medical World News,* August 25, 1975.
8. *FDA Drug Bulletin,* July–August 1975.
9. *Today's Health,* March 1976.
10. Smith, J. (1975): *J. Fam. Plann. Doctors* 3:14; cited by Guillebaud, J. (1975): Oral contraceptives in women over 34. *Br. Med. J.*, 4:457–458.
11. *NIH Guide supplement for Grants and Contracts,* Synopsis No. NICHD-75–22, July 25, 1975.
12. Preston, S. N. (1976): Myocardial infarction and the pill. *J. Reprod. Med.*, 16:1–4.
13. Sturtevant, F. M. (1976): Current misconceptions concerning retrospective studies on the pill. North American Fertility Conference, Acapulco, Jan. 25–Feb. 4.
14. Feinstein, A. R. (1973): Clinical biostatistics. XX. The epidemiologic trohoc, the ablative risk ratio, and 'retrospective' research. *Clin. Pharmacol. Ther.*, 14:291–307.
15. Goldzieher, J. W., and Dozier, T. S. (1975): Oral contraceptives and thromboembolism: A reassessment. *Am. J. Obstet. Gynecol.*, 123:878–914.
16. Hougie, C. (1973): Thromboembolism and oral contraceptives. *Am. Heart J.*, 85:538–545.
17. *The Registrar General's Statistical Review of England and Wales for the Year 1973,* Part I (A), Tables, Medical. H.M.S.O., London.
18. Bone, M. (1973): Family Planning Services in England and Wales. Off. Pop. Censuses and Surveys, Soc. Survey Div. H.M.S.O., London.
19. Kay, C. R. (1974): *Oral Contraceptives and Health.* Pitman, London.
20. *The Registrar General's Statistical Review of England and Wales for the Year 1970,* Part I (A), Tables, Medical. H.M.S.O., London.

21. National Office of Vital Statistics (1956): Mortality from selected causes by marital status, United States, 1949–1951. *Vital Statistics Special Reports,* 39, No. 7, pp. 301–429. G.P.O., Washington, D.C.
22. Westoff, C. F. (1972): The modernization of U.S. contraceptive practice. *Fam. Plann. Perspect.,* 4:9–12.
23. Population Estimates and Projections. In: *Current Population Reports,* Series P-25, No. 519, April 1974. Bureau of the Census. G.P.O., Washington, D.C.
24. Population Characteristics. In: *Current Population Reports,* Series P-20, No. 212, February 1971. Bureau of the Census. G.P.O., Washington, D.C.
25. Westoff, C. F. (1975): *Personal communication.*
26. *Vital Statistics of the United States 1970, Vol. II: Mortality,* Part A. Public Health Service, National Center for Health Statistics. G.P.O., Washington, D.C.
27. *Morbidity Statistics from General Practice, Second National Study 1970–71.* Off. Pop. Censuses and Surveys, Studies on Medical and Population Subjects, No. 26, 1974. H.M.S.O., London.
28. Kannel, W. B., and Gordon, T. (1968–1973): An epidemiological investigation of cardiovascular disease. D.H.E.W. Publication No. (N.I.H.) 74–618.
29. *Medical World News,* April 26, 1976.

Pharmacology of Steroid Contraceptive Drugs
edited by S. Garattini and H. W. Berendes.
Raven Press, New York © 1977.

Discussion

J. I. Mann

*Department of Social and Community Medicine, Oxford University,
Oxford, OX1 3QN, England*

Dr. Sturtevant has made a number of comments concerning our data, which are answered as follows:

1. The relative risk estimates in the mortality study were calculated by defining "nonusers" as "never-users" plus "ex-users." This was made clear in the pre-edited version of the text but I agree with Dr. Sturtevant that to determine this from the published version the reader would need to carry out two simple arithmetical calculations. The method by which relative risk was calculated in the morbidity study is made clear in the text. I accept entirely that it is a pity that the estimates in the two studies were not made in identical fashion; however, it is of interest to note, and Dr. Sturtevant does not point this out, that had this been done the risk estimate for the 30–39 age group (in the mortality study) would be 3.4 rather than 2.8.

2. It is suggested that "an error of recollection of one day in the history of pill use by the deceased, a year or more previously, could change the classification of a case from user to nonuser." In this study of fatal cases, drug histories were not based on "recollection" but on information obtained from records. Current use was defined as use during the month before death because of the precedent established in numerous earlier studies, but in fact all the current users in our studies were using oral contraceptives at the time of death and had been using them for at least *six* weeks. The ex-users in our study had all stopped using the preparations more than *eight* weeks before the event.

3. Dr. Sturtevant criticizes our failure to match cases and controls for presence or absence of known risk factors for myocardial infarction. This was done quite deliberately so we could examine for the effect of these factors in the analyses. Failure to have done so would have prevented us from obtaining any data concerning interaction of factors. The aim of the investigation was to study myocardial infarction as it presents in young women and not to examine only the relationship between myocardial infarction and oral contraceptives.

4. Dr. Sturtevant states that 21 of the 47 fatal cases aged 30–39 years were classified as users of oral contraceptives. This is not correct. This proportion relates to all women under the age of 40 years and not to the 30–39 age group. This is clearly indicated in Table 2 and the early part of the text. It is this incorrect assumption which results in Dr. Sturtevant's inability to reproduce exactly our calculations aimed to determine the approximate incidence of myocardial infarc-

tion in users and nonusers of oral contraceptives. The details according to which our calculations were made were given in more detail in the pre-edited version of our text, but it is of some interest that even using an incorrect assumption Dr. Sturtevant's calculations provide a very similar estimate of attributable mortality for the 30–39 age group. (Our estimate was 3.5 per 100,000 users per year and his estimate 3.0 per 100,000 users per year.)

5. It is difficult to comment on Dr. Sturtevant's attempts to determine the accuracy of predictions based on our data since he makes a number of assumptions which are not valid. First, it seems that he used data from the Royal College of General Practitioners' Study to determine the proportion of women in different age groups in the population who might be expected to be using the pill. He quotes Table 2.2 of this report as his source. This table gives a percentage distribution by age group of women known to be using oral contraceptives and bears no relationship whatsoever to the proportion of women in the population who might be expected to be users of these preparations. Furthermore, as the mortality rate from myocardial infarction in this age group does tend to fluctuate from year to year, it is surely not possible to predict what might happen during one year from data collected 3 years later. It seems to me to be quite remarkable that his data "predict" as well as they do!

6. Dr. Sturtevant comments that a news item reports that we have recalculated our data collected in the study of nonfatal myocardial infarction and now predict only half as much morbidity for women over 40 as that reported previously. This is quite incorrect. We studied a larger number of cases of fatal myocardial infarction in the older age group. These data, presented in this volume, enable a more reliable estimate of risk to be calculated. Indeed, the results of our morbidity study suggest that the estimate of an approximately threefold increase in risk which now emerges from the study of fatal cases is a conservative one. In the study of nonfatal cases, the risk of myocardial infarction was found to be 5.7 times greater in women aged 40–44 years who currently used oral contraceptives than in women who had never used these preparations.

7. Finally, Dr. Sturtevant refers to a criticism made by Preston. He argued that the association between oral contraceptives and myocardial infarction could be a spurious one, arising merely because physicians were more likely to prescribe the pill (a particularly effective method of contraception) for women with risk factors for ischemic heart disease. The strongest evidence against this argument comes from the Royal College of General Practitioners' Study and the Oxford University/Family Planning Association Study (to be published). In both these investigations, the control group (women using methods of contraception other than oral agents) were less healthy than users of oral contraceptives; and, despite this, appreciably more cases of ischemic heart disease were seen among the pill users than the controls. In these prospective studies the total number of cases was small, but these data do provide evidence that the risk estimates made in our investigations might have been much greater if the pill was widely prescribed for women already at high risk of developing ischemic heart disease.

Pharmacology of Steroid Contraceptive Drugs
edited by S. Garattini and H. W. Berendes.
Raven Press, New York © 1977.

Drug Interactions with Oral Contraceptives: An Overview

A. Breckenridge

*Department of Pharmacology & Therapeutics, University of Liverpool,
Liverpool L69 3BX, England*

The topic of drug interactions with oral contraceptives (OCs) is of importance for two main reasons. Firstly, there is an increasing number of reports that interactions may lead to a failure of contraceptive efficacy. The magnitude of this problem can only be surmised, and one relies on isolated case reports whose accuracy and veracity undoubtedly vary. Secondly, many women taking OC therapy also take other drugs, and it is possible, at least in theory, that the response of these other agents may be altered owing to changes in either their pharmacokinetics or pharmacodynamics.

It is important not to extrapolate data obtained from women taking one form of OC therapy to those taking another. This is true not only between combined (estrogen–progestogen) OC agents and progestogen-only contraceptives, but also between OCs of different estrogen and progestogenic potency and content. Available data suggest that drug interactions leading to failure of contraceptive potency of OC therapy frequently involves only the estrogen component. Another important caveat to be kept in mind is the variation in the magnitude of drug–drug interactions in different individuals. With respect to liver microsomal enzyme induction, it has been shown (1) that administration of the same dose of quinalbarbitone may lead to a fall in steady-state plasma warfarin concentrations, varying from 5% to 65% of control values, and similar differences may be operative with respect to enzyme induction involving OC therapy.

DRUG INTERACTIONS OF OTHER DRUGS WITH ORAL CONTRACEPTIVES

Antituberculous Drugs

The first clinical evidence that antituberculous therapy might interfere with the efficacy of OC agents came in 1971 from a series of 51 patients with tuberculosis studied by Reimers and Jezek (2). Those patients whose drug regimen included rifampicin showed an increased evidence of breakthrough bleeding equated with a diminished efficacy of the oral contraceptive. In 1974 in a larger series of 88 women taking rifampicin and OC therapy, not only did 68 notice breakthrough bleeding but 5 became pregnant. In contrast, of 26 women with tuberculosis who were taking OC therapy and streptomycin, only one noticed breakthrough bleeding (3).

A possible explanation for these findings is to be found in the observation that rifampicin increases the rate of hepatic breakdown of both ethinylestradiol and estradiol (4), as shown by Bolt and his colleagues using microsomal preparations of human liver obtained at laparotomy from patients previously given rifampicin. Further, rifampicin is known to increase the rate of metabolism of other drugs such as tolbutamide (5). Theoretically, another explanation for the failure of contraceptive therapy is that rifampicin may alter the output of the hypo-thalamic–pituitary axis, but studies have shown that its administration has no influence on serum growth hormone levels (5).

Anticonvulsant Therapy

If one group of microsomal enzyme-inducing agents can cause a failure of OC efficacy, a similar situation may well be relevant in epileptic patients on anticon-vulsant drugs. Many anticonvulsants (e.g., phenobarbitone, phenytoin, primi-done, and pheneturide) are known enzyme inducers (6). In 1972 a woman who had become pregnant while on phenytoin and sulthiame, as well as OC therapy, was reported (7). In a larger series of patients taking an OC and other drugs simultaneously, epileptics were found to have a high incidence of breakthrough bleeding; and four, taking either phenobarbitone or phenytoin (or both), became pregnant (8). Pregnancy in another three epileptics on drug therapy and taking oral contraceptives was documented by Janz and Schmidt (9).

In 1968 Conney and his colleagues (10) showed that the uterotropic effects of the estrogens stilbestrol and ethinylestradiol could be inhibited by simultaneous administration of phenobarbitone at higher doses (Fig. 1). Presumably the con-

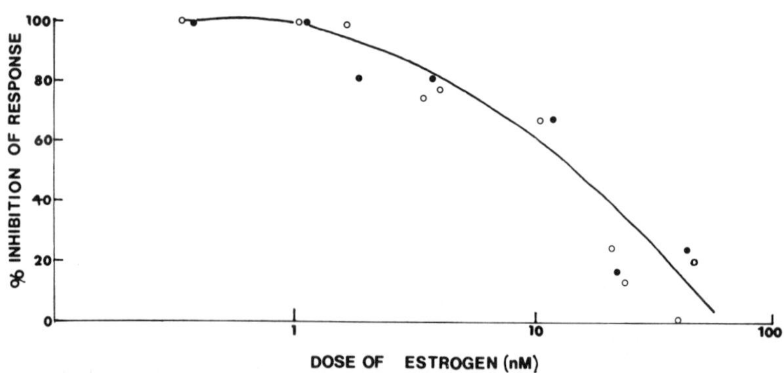

FIG. 1. Decrease in uterotropic potency of two estrogens—stilbestrol and ethinylestradiol (EE) —after various doses of phenobarbitone in rats. (Data from Levin et al., ref. 10.) Filled circles: stilbestrol, open circles: EE.

traceptive effect of these steroids would similarly be altered by barbiturate administration.

Analgesics and Tranquilizers

In the series of patients noted above (8) taking OCs and other agents and who became pregnant, 10 were taking amidopyrine, meprobamate, chlordiazepoxide, or phenacetin. There is good evidence that the first three of these drugs induce liver microsomal enzyme activity in man (11), thus perpetrating the failure of OC therapy. In a further investigation of women on amidopyrine and OC drugs, the same workers found that 11 of 24 women had significant breakthrough bleeding within 10–16 days of starting the analgesic. The basis of the interaction with phenacetin-containing compounds is uncertain, and its importance is unknown.

Antibiotics

Of possibly greater importance than any of the three drug interactions discussed above is that between antibiotics and OC therapy. The clinical data are sparse. Three women who became pregnant while taking ampicillin and OC therapy were reported (12); and in the large series of women already cited (8) who experienced OC failure while on other medication, two were taking either sulphamethoxypyridazine or chloramphenicol.

It is known that antibiotics (e.g., ampicillin and neomycin) in therapeutic doses, decrease both plasma and urine estriol levels during pregnancy within 2–3 days of their administration (13,14). The following explanation has been suggested (15) for this phenomenon. During pregnancy estriol produced in the fetoplacental unit is excreted in bile as a conjugate (probably a glucuronide), which is broken down in the gut by bacterial enzymic biotransformation. The estrogenic metabolite is reabsorbed from the gut, possibly undergoing conjugation again within the gut wall, completing the enterohepatic circulation cycle that is well known for estrogens. In the presence of antibiotics within the gut, with the consequent alteration of gut flora, this enterohepatic circulation may be disturbed, resulting in increased fecal excretion of estrogens. The estrogenic component of many OC agents may suffer a metabolic fate similar to that of natural estrogens, and a similar interaction with antibiotics may result, producing decreased plasma concentrations and increased fecal levels. This may be of relevance only in women taking low-estrogen-containing OC agents, and there may be other sources of interindividual variation as well.

INTERACTIONS OF OC AGENTS WITH OTHER DRUGS

Compared with the alteration of contraceptive efficacy produced by administration of other drugs, problems posed by this type of interaction are of considerably less importance and magnitude. Two studies (16,17) examined the effect of OC administration on the elimination of two drugs oxidized in the liver: antipyrine and phenylbutazone. In the first of these studies, O'Malley and his colleagues (16) showed that the plasma half-life of antipyrine was significantly ($p < 0.001$) shorter in 36 control subjects (10.8 ± 2.4 hr) than in 26 subjects taking OCs (14.1 ± 3.1 hr). In a similar study but using 8 subjects as their own controls (17), there was no significant change in the plasma antipyrine half-life (10.5 ± 1.2 hr versus 13.6 ± 1.3 hr) when subjects were given OC agents. Neither group of workers showed that OCs caused a change in the plasma half-life of phenylbutazone.

Solomon and colleagues (18) examined the effect of OC therapy on the disposition and effect of the oral anticoagulant bishydroxycoumarin. There was no change in its plasma half-life, although the anticoagulant effect of a single dose was decreased when OCs were given for 20 days. This is due to the known ability of OC therapy to increase the synthesis rate of clotting factors in the liver. This property appears to be most important in the case of combined oral contraceptives, as progestogen-only OC therapy has not been shown to alter clotting factor synthesis consistently.

Interactions between OC therapy and tricyclic antidepressants and anticonvulsants have been noted, but most of these reports consist of isolated cases, and the basis and importance of the putative interaction is in some doubt.

Administration of oral contraceptives can alter blood pressure and growth hormone levels, resulting in hypertension or exacerbation of diabetes mellitus. Thus in the hypertensive and the diabetic the wisdom of OC therapy must be questioned, and the treatment of one drug side effect by the administration of another drug appears to run counter to one of the basic principles of therapeutics.

CONCLUSIONS

Administration of a variety of drugs has been shown to alter the efficacy of simultaneously prescribed oral contraceptive agents manifested by either unwanted pregnancy or breakthrough bleeding. The magnitude of the problem is largely undetermined. The other facet of drug–drug interactions with OCs (i.e., their ability to alter the response to other agents) is of less importance.

REFERENCES

1. Breckenridge, A., Orme, M. L'E., Davies, L., Thorgeirsson, S. S., and Davies, D. S. (1973): Dose dependent enzyme induction. *Clin. Pharmacol. Ther.*, 14:514–520.
2. Reimers, D., and Jezek, A. (1971): The simultaneous use of rifampicin and other antitubercular agents with oral contraceptives. *Prax. Pneumonol.*, 25:255–265.
3. Reimers, D., Nocke-Finch, L., and Brever, H. (1974): In: *Proceedings of 22nd International Tuberculosis Conference.*
4. Bolt, H. M., Kappus, H., and Bolt, M. (1975): Effect of rifampicin treatment on the metabolism of oestradiol and 17α oestradiol by human liver microsomes. *Eur. J. Clin. Pharmacol.*, 8:301–307.
5. Syvalahti, E. K. C., Pihlajamaki, K. K., and Isalo, E. J. (1974): Rifampicin and drug metabolism. *Lancet*, 2:232–233.
6. Kutt, H. (1974): Interactions with antiepileptic form drugs involving multiple mechanisms. In:

Drug Interactions, edited by P. L. Morselli, S. Garratini, and S. N. Cohen, pp. 211–222. Raven Press, New York.

7. Nenyon, I. E. (1972): Unplanned pregnancy in an epileptic. *Br. Med. J.,* 1:686–687.

8. Von Hempel, E., Bohm, W., Carol, W., and Klinger, C. (1973): Medicinal enzyme induction and hormonal contraception. *Zeitblad. Gynakol.,* 95:1451–1455.

9. Janz, D., and Schmidt, D. (1974): Antiepileptic drugs and failure of oral contraceptives. *Lancet,* 1:1113.

10. Levin, W., Welch, R. M., and Conney, A. H. (1968): Decreased uterotropic potency of oral contraceptives in rats pretreated with phenobarbital. *Endocrinology,* 83:149–156.

11. Breckenridge, A. (1974): Clinical implications of enzyme induction. In: *Enzyme Induction,* edited by D. V. Parke, pp. 273–301. Plenum Press, New York.

12. Dossetor, J. (1975): Drug interactions with oral contraceptives. *Br. Med. J.,* 4:467–468.

13. Pulkinnen, M. O., and William, K. (1971): Reduced maternal plasma and urinary estriol during ampicillin treatment. *Am. J. Obstet. Gynecol.,* 109:893–895.

14. Pulkinnen, M. O., and Willman, K. (1973): Reduction of maternal oestrogen excretion by neomycin. *Am. J. Obstet. Gynecol.,* 115:1153–1154.

15. Tikkanen, M. J., Adlercreutz, H., and Pulkinnen, M. O. (1973): Effects of antibiotics on oestrogen metabolism. *Br. Med. J.,* 2:369.

16. O'Malley, K., Stevenson, I., and Crook, J. (1972): Impairment of human drug metabolism by oral contraceptive steroids. *Clin. Pharmacol. Ther.,* 13:552–557.

17. Carter, D. E., Goldman, J. M., Bressler, R., Huxtable, R. J., Christian, C. D., and Heine, M. W. (1974): Effect of oral contraceptives on drug metabolism. *Clin Pharmacol. Ther.,* 15:22–31.

18. Schrogie, J. J., Solomon, H. M., and Zieve, P. (1967): Effect of oral contraceptives on vitamin K-dependent clotting activity. *Clin. Pharmacol. Ther.,* 8:670–675.

Pharmacology of Steroid Contraceptive Drugs
edited by S. Garattini and H. W. Berendes.
Raven Press, New York © 1977.

Effect of Contraceptive Drugs on Liver Mono-oxygenases in Several Animal Species

A. Jori, M. Salmona, L. Cantoni, and G. Guiso

Istituto di Ricerche Farmacologiche "Mario Negri," 20157 Milan, Italy

Steroids and particularly synthetic steroid contraceptive drugs (SCDs) have been reported to affect the activity of the liver mono-oxygenase systems responsible for metabolism of endogenous and exogenous compounds. The interest in SCDs stems from the fact that these drugs are given to women for long periods of time during which it may become necessary to administer other medications for various therapeutic reasons, or the women may be exposed to chemicals by absorbing pollutants or food additives. These hypothetical interactions are not yet well documented in women. Impaired metabolic capacity for antipyrine (22) and meperidine (6) was reported, but more recently contradictory results have also been published (27). It has been suggested that any effect on drug metabolism in women taking contraceptives must be more theoretical than real (3). However, knowledge of the possible interactions of SCDs with the metabolism of other compounds has experimental interest in that it helps us to understand the meaning of results obtained when contraceptives are combined with other drugs in experimental models aimed at clarifying their mechanisms of action.

The results reported by different authors on the effect of SCDs on drug metabolism in experimental animals cover all possible effects: blockade, no change, and induction (2,7–9,16,24,26,30). Differences in animal species, strain, sex, type of steroid, and experimental design may, among other factors, account for the discrepancies in these results—hence the need for systematic re-evaluation of the problem.

Previous data from our laboratories indicated that SCDs increase the activity of liver microsomal enzymes in rats and mice (4,14,15,25). Now we report the results of a comparative investigation of the effect of several widely used contraceptive drugs in mature female rats, mice, and guinea pigs. In an attempt to reproduce the conditions required for human clinical use, estrogens and progestogens were combined in various fixed ratios at doses that produced an experimentally controlled antiovulatory effect; they were administered chronically by the oral route for periods covering at least one but generally more than one estrous cycle. The specific aim was to study the effect of such treatments on the *in vitro* activity of the liver mono-oxygenase enzymes.

MATERIAL AND METHODS

Animals

Adult female animals were used (Charles River rats weighing 220 ± 10 g, CD_1 mice weighing 25 ± 3 g, and PIR bright v/z guinea pigs weighing 350 ± 50 g). Animals were kept at a temperature of 20°C, with relative humidity 60% and a controlled light cycle of 12 hr (6:30 A.M. to 6:30 P.M.). Food and water were given *ad libitum.*

Treatments

The following progestogens were combined with mestranol in fixed ratios: norethynodrel (66.6:1), norethisterone (20:1), lynestrenol (16.6:1). The drugs were dissolved in corn oil and given orally for a period of 4 days consecutively (acute treatment) to cover one estrous cycle in rats and mice, or 30 days (chronic treatment) to cover approximately seven cycles in mice and rats and two cycles in guinea pigs. Controls received a corresponding amount of corn oil. The estrous cycle was cytologically determined by vaginal smears. Animals were killed by decapitation at various times after the last administration, as reported in the tables.

Enzymatic Activity

The following enzymatic reactions, catalyzed by microsomal mono-oxygenase systems, were studied: N-demethylase, O-demethylase, aromatic hydroxylase, and epoxide synthetase. The substrates used were aminopyrine, pNO_2 anisole, aniline, and styrene. The first three enzyme activities were measured on the 9,000 g supernatant fraction of a liver homogenate (18). The metabolites formed (4-aminopyrine, pNO_2-phenol, and pNH_2-phenol) were determined according to Gilbert and Goldberg (11). Epoxide synthetase activity was measured on microsome pellets obtained from various tissues according to Kato and Takayanaghi (17) using the method described by Belvedere et al. (1). Styrene epoxide hydratase activity was also measured in these liver microsomal preparations. Liver microsomes for determination of proteins according to Lowry et al. (19) and of cytochrome P-450 according to Omura and Sato (23) were prepared by Ca^{++} precipitation as described by Cinti et al. (5).

Contraceptive Test

Two female animals were caged with one fertile male for different periods depending on the animal species and the duration of treatment, as previously reported (4). The contraceptive activity was measured by bioassay, examining the uterine horns for the number of implantation sites.

RESULTS

Effect of SCDs on Liver Microsomal Enzyme Activity in Rats and Mice

Table 1 presents data concerning the efficacy of the SCD combinations in terms of their contraceptive effect in the same animal species and in the same experimental conditions in our studies of enzyme activity. This is useful for meaningful comparison of their activity on the mono-oxygenase systems. Rats need a fairly high dose of the three combinations for protection; mice require a similar dose of lynestrenol and norethisterone combinations but smaller doses of norethynodrel; the guinea pig is more sensitive, and smaller doses are sufficient. Prolonged treatment does not enhance the contraceptive activity of SCDs in rats and mice.

The highest doses of SCDs used block the estrus cycle in the diestrous phase; therefore for comparison with controls it was necessary to establish whether liver microsomal enzyme activity varied during the three cycle phases. Experiments in untreated animals killed during proestrus, estrus, and diestrus established that at least in mice and rats liver microsomal enzyme activity is not cycle-dependent. No differences in the microsomal enzyme activity were observed in the various estrous phases. Therefore in subsequent experiments no attempt was made to check the phases of estrus during which the animals were killed.

Table 2 shows the effect of SCDs on liver microsomal enzyme activity in rats treated daily for 30 consecutive days and killed 18 hr after the last treatment. An increase is always present after doses which are high in comparison to the ones utilized in women, although they are lower than the minimal doses with contraceptive effect in this animal species.

Table 3 shows the dose-effect relationship for the lynestrenol-mestranol combination on microsomal enzyme activity in rats. This effect increases with the dose of progestogen, from 1 to 5 mg/kg, but an appreciable effect is already present after 1 mg/kg, which protects only 33% of the animals from pregnancy. In Table 4 the effect of these treatments on liver epoxide synthetase and epoxide hydratase

TABLE 1. *Effective doses of steroid combinations for contraception*

| Treatment | Rat | | Mouse | | Guinea pig |
	4 Days	30 Days	4 Days	30 Days	30 days
Lynestrenol	2.2	2	1.8	1.65	0.82
+ mestranol	0.13	0.12	0.11	0.099	0.049
Norethynodrel	3	4.2	0.4	0.4	0.36
+ mestranol	0.045	0.063	0.006	0.006	0.0054
Norethisterone	2.2	1.8	0.85	1	0.38
+ mestranol	0.11	0.09	0.042	0.05	0.019

Figures indicate a graphically calculated ED_{90} (mg/kg p.o.): the dose of steroid combination which reduces the control level of implantations by 90%.

Rats and mice were killed 8 days and guinea pigs 25 days after the last treatment.

TABLE 2. *Effect of chronic treatment with SCDs on liver microsomal enzyme activity in rats*

| Treatment | | Enzyme activity (nmoles/g/hr $\pm$ SE) | | |
| | Dosage | | | |
Agent	(mg/kg/day $\times$ 30 Days	Aminopyrine	Aniline	pNO$_2$ anisole
Controls	—	230 $\pm$ 25	667 $\pm$ 68	615 $\pm$ 46
Lynestrenol + mestranol	1.25 0.075	379 $\pm$ 29[a]	829 $\pm$ 57[b]	803 $\pm$ 34[a]
Norethisterone + mestranol	2 0.1	435 $\pm$ 36[a]	1,233 $\pm$ 36[a]	794 $\pm$ 38[a]
Norethynodrel + mestranol	2 0.03	324 $\pm$ 20[a]	1,081 $\pm$ 49[a]	738 $\pm$ 27[a]

Each figure represents the average of at least six animals.

Rats were killed 18 hr after the last treatment. Enzyme activity is represented by the metabolites formed (4-NH$_2$-antipyrine, pNH$_2$-phenol, and pNO$_2$-phenol) from the 9,000 g supernatant fraction of liver homogenates.

[a] $p < 0.01$ versus the controls.
[b] $p < 0.05$ versus the controls.

TABLE 3. *Effect of different doses of lynestrenol + mestranol treatment on liver microsomal enzyme activity in rats*

Treatment		Enzyme activity (nmoles/g/hr $\pm$ SE)		
Agent	Dosage (mg/kg/day $\times$ 30 days)	Aminopyrine	Aniline	pNO$_2$ anisole
Controls	—	230 ± 25	667 ± 68	615 ± 46
Lynestrenol + mestranol	1.25 0.075	379 ± 29^a	829 ± 57^b	803 ± 34^a
Lynestrenol + mestranol	2.5 0.15	485 ± 33^a	977 ± 35^a	876 ± 34^a
Lynestrenol + mestranol	5 0.30	530 ± 24^a	$1,100 \pm 41^a$	892 ± 28^a

Each figure represents the average of at least six animals.

Rats were killed 18 hr after the last treatment. Enzyme activity is represented by the metabolites formed (4-NH$_2$-antipyrine, pNH$_2$-phenol, and pNO$_2$-phenol) from the 9,000 g supernatant fraction of liver homogenates.

[a] $p < 0.01$ versus the controls.
[b] $p < 0.05$ versus the controls.

TABLE 4. *Effect of chronic SCD treatment on liver microsomal epoxide synthetase and epoxide hydratase activity in rats*

Treatment		Enzyme activity (nmoles/mg protein/min $\pm$ SE)	
Agent	Dosage (mg/kg/day $\times$ 30 days)	Epoxide synthetase	Epoxide hydratase
Controls	—	1.36 ± 0.24	3.49 ± 0.79
Lynestrenol + mestranol	5 0.3	2.16 ± 0.13[a]	5.51 ± 0.74
Norethisterone + mestranol	4 0.2	2.13 ± 0.08[a]	5.99 ± 0.28[a]
Norethynodrel + mestranol	4 0.06	1.81 ± 0.16	6.25 ± 0.32[a]

Each figure represents the average of at least four animals. Rats were killed 18 hr after the last treatment.

Epoxide synthetase and epoxide hydratase enzyme activities are represented by the amount of phenethylenglycol formed from the substrates styrene and styrene epoxide by the microsomal fraction of liver homogenates.

[a] $p < 0.01$ versus the controls.

is reported. The three combinations, in contrast to the first enzyme activities tested (Table 2) behave differently. Lynestrenol plus mestranol according to previously reported data (25) increase the synthetase; norethisterone increases both enzymes; and norethynodrel only the hydratase. Thus in the first case an accumulation of epoxide may be obtained as synthesis increases, but not during the following step; no substantial effect is observed after norethisterone, as both enzyme activities are increased; and the third treatment produces shorter destruction of the epoxide formed. These differences are particularly interesting in view of the possible carcinogenicity of the epoxides; intermediates with high reactivity formed during metabolism of exogenous compounds such as polycyclic hydrocarbons (29).

The epoxide synthetase is also present in extrahepatic tissues of female rats where the hydratase is not found or is at least less active (25). In heart, spleen, and lung only the epoxide synthetase is detectable, and this may permit the epoxides to persist longer. It was therefore considered important to investigate the effects of SCDs on epoxide synthetase in a large number of tissues (Table 5). None of the combinations tested affect epoxide synthetase in the above-mentioned tissues. Moreover, a decrease in epoxide synthetase in kidney seems to be mediated by norethisterone and norethynodrel. In this tissue, where we also detected epoxide hydratase, the SCDs have no effect on this enzyme.

All the data reported so far apply to chronic treatment. When rats were acutely treated with contraceptives for a period covering only one estrous cycle (4 days), lynestrenol and norethynodrel combinations did not increase the activity of the microsomal enzymes, and norethisterone + mestranol treatment was active only

TABLE 5. *Effect of chronic SCD treatment on microsomal epoxide synthetase activity in various rat tissues*

| Tissue | Epoxide synthetase activity (nmoles/mg protein/min ± SE) | | | |
	Control	Norethynodrel-mestranol	Norethisterone-mestranol	Lynestrenol-mestranol
Heart	0.26 ± 0.09	0.20 ± 0.02	0.20 ± 0.02	0.21 ± 0.02
Lung	0.34 ± 0.13	0.21 ± 0.02	0.26 ± 0.03	0.28 ± 0.02
Kidney	0.34 ± 0.04	0.13 ± 0.02[a]	0.18 ± 0.03[a]	0.24 ± 0.03
Spleen	0.55 ± 0.10	0.38 ± 0.13	0.46 ± 0.09	0.44 ± 0.07
Uterus	0.54 ± 0.07	0.44 ± 0.10	0.43 ± 0.02	0.37 ± 0.10

Doses of SCD are as listed in Table 4.
Determinations were on the tissues of the rats used for the experiments in Table 4. For details see Table 4.
[a] $p < 0.01$ versus controls.

at a very large dose (4 mg + 0.2 mg, respectively). In mice the effect of contraceptive treatment on liver microsomal enzyme activity becomes evident after a few administrations (Table 6). The activity of the microsomal enzymes increases after very high doses as well as after the minimum antifertility dose of all combinations, except for norethynodrel + mestranol, which had no effect after either acute or chronic administration.

The time course of this effect shows that the activity of the microsomal enzymes is increased as early as 2 hr after the last treatment. The effect reaches a peak near 18 hr and is still present, although to a lesser extent, 40 hr after the end of SCD treatment (Table 7).

Whether the effect of contraceptive combinations was dependent on the estrogen or progestogen compound or on both steroids was also investigated. Table 8 shows that in mice and rats mestranol at the highest doses used does not alter the enzyme activity, whereas lynestrenol alone is responsible for the stimulation usually induced by the combined treatment.

Effect of SCDs on Liver Protein and Cytochrome P-450 Levels in Rats and Mice

Table 9 indicates that the lynestrenol + mestranol combination does not cause enlargement of the liver or increase the microsomal protein concentration or cytochrome P-450 content in rats. In mice the liver weight increased only after very high doses; an increase in P-450 is detectable after treatment with lynestrenol 5 mg/kg but is clearly demonstrable only after a 20 mg/kg dose.

Therefore, particularly in rats, the drug metabolism induction picture differs from that produced by the two classic inducing agents, phenobarbital and 3-methylcholanthrene (3-MC). Phenobarbital and lynestrenol-mestranol treatments induce the metabolism of substrates of type 1 (aminopyrine) and type 2 (aniline),

TABLE 6. *Effect of acute SCD treatment on liver microsomal enzyme activity in mice*

| Treatment | | Enzyme activity (nmoles/g/hr $\pm$ SE) | | |
Agent	Dosage (mg/kg/day p.o. $\times$ 4 days)	Aminopyrine	Aniline	pNO$_2$-anisole
Controls		392 ± 21	626 ± 22	821 ± 16
Lynestrenol + mestranol	5 0.3	707 ± 27^a	$1{,}034 \pm 112^a$	$1{,}337 \pm 34^a$
Lynestrenol + mestranol	1.25 0.075	609 ± 18^a	885 ± 67^a	$1{,}181 \pm 4^a$
Norethisterone + mestranol	4 0.2	686 ± 34^a	828 ± 33^a	$1{,}069 \pm 58^a$
Norethisterone + mestranol	1 0.05	473 ± 21^b	709 ± 21^b	922 ± 20^b
Norethynodrel + mestranol	4 0.06	335 ± 9	511 ± 23	721 ± 42
Norethynodrel + mestranol	0.5 0.0075^c	285 ± 8	574 ± 23	670 ± 48

Each figure is the average of five determinations. The animals were killed 18 hr after the fourth administration.

Experimental conditions are described in Table 2.

[a] $p < 0.01$ versus controls.

[b] $p < 0.05$ versus controls.

[c] Daily for 30 days.

TABLE 7. *Time course of the effect of acute treatment with lynestrenol + mestranol on liver microsomal enzyme activity in mice*

| Interval between treatment and killing (hr) | Enzyme activity (nmoles/g/hr $\pm$ SE)^a | | |
	Aminopyrine	Aniline	pNO$_2$-anisole
Controls	257 ± 17	442 ± 11	590 ± 40
Lynestrenol + mestranol			
2	524 ± 18	618 ± 27	941 ± 27
4	488 ± 46	700 ± 49	898 ± 52
8	649 ± 28	812 ± 49	1068 ± 65
18	707 ± 27	1034 ± 112	1337 ± 34
30	523 ± 24	740 ± 40	1084 ± 83
40	355 ± 20	572 ± 10	757 ± 38

Lynestrenol (5 mg/kg) and mestranol (0.3 mg/kg) were given daily for 4 days. Mice were killed at various times after the last administration.

[a] In all cases, $p < 0.01$ versus controls.

TABLE 8. *Effect of mestranol and lynestrenol on microsomal enzyme activity in rats and mice*

Treatment			Enzyme activity (nmoles/g/hr $\pm$ SE)		
Agent	Dosage (mg/kg p.o.)	No. of days	Aminopyrine	Aniline	pNO$_2$-anisole
Rat					
Controls			243 $\pm$ 11	790 $\pm$ 62	501 $\pm$ 40
Mestranol	0.3	30	282 $\pm$ 20	837 $\pm$ 48	691 $\pm$ 51[a]
Lynestrenol	5	30	345 $\pm$ 23[a]	1,135 $\pm$ 126[a]	819 $\pm$ 36[a]
Mouse					
Controls			208 $\pm$ 20	710 $\pm$ 34	695 $\pm$ 41
Mestranol	0.3	4	190 $\pm$ 27	674 $\pm$ 89	540 $\pm$ 46
Lynestrenol	5	4	593 $\pm$ 18[a]	916 $\pm$ 69[b]	1,303 $\pm$ 86[a]

Each figure represents the average of at least six animals.
Animals were killed 18 hr after the last treatment.
Experimental conditions were as described for Table 2.
[a] $p < 0.01$ versus controls.
[b] $p < 0.05$ versus controls.

TABLE 9. *Effect of lynestrenol + mestranol on various liver parameters in mice and rats*

Treatment			Liver weight (g/100 g b.w.)	Microsomal protein (mg/g)	Cytochrome P-450 (nmoles/mg protein)
Agent	Dosage (mg/kg/day)	No. of days			
Rat					
Controls			4.8 $\pm$ 0.02	19 $\pm$ 0.6	0.410 $\pm$ 0.03
Lynestrenol + mestranol	1.25 0.075	30	4.4 $\pm$ 0.17	22 $\pm$ 1.4	0.424 $\pm$ 0.04
Lynestrenol + mestranol	5 0.3	30	4.8 $\pm$ 0.19	24 $\pm$ 2.7	0.484 $\pm$ 0.04
Mouse					
Controls			5.5 $\pm$ 0.14	16 $\pm$ 0.5	0.610 $\pm$ 0.06
Lynestrenol + mestranol	5 0.3	4	5.9 $\pm$ 0.24	15 $\pm$ 0.4	0.780 $\pm$ 0.05[a]
Lynestrenol + mestranol	20 1.2	4	7.3 $\pm$ 0.5[b]	12 $\pm$ 0.6	1.350 $\pm$ 0.08[b]

Animals were killed 18 hr after the last treatment.
Results are the mean $\pm$ SE.
[a] $p < 0.05$ versus controls.
[b] $p < 0.01$ versus controls.

and increase epoxide synthetase activity; however, differently from phenobarbital with the steroids, this effect appears at a dose which does not increase cytochrome P-450. The differences from 3-MC are much more evident: 3-MC stimulates synthesis of a new heme cytochrome, P-448; selectively increases the metabolism of substrates of type 2 (20); and does not modify epoxide synthetase activity (21).

These results are not surprising: A similar picture showing increased microsomal enzyme activity but no effect on the cytochrome P-450 content was also reported for other steroids (12,28). Deeper analysis of the literature also clarifies some discrepancies concerning the activity of the steroids on drug metabolism.

Steroids are reported to induce and block microsomal enzyme activity or not to affect it at all (7,8,14,16,24,26,30); probably, as we suggested above, the opposite results obtained depend on the experimental conditions and/or animal species and sex, on the duration of treatment, and on the steroids employed. In fact Hamrick et al. (12), comparing the effect of various steroids in intact female and male rats, showed that repeated treatment with these compounds increases the microsomal enzyme activity only in females and is inactive in males. In animal species in which drug metabolism is not sex-dependent (e.g., hamsters and mice), steroids increase the activity of microsomal enzymes in males too (10,13,24).

Effect of SCDs on Liver Microsomal Enzyme Activity in Guinea Pigs

The effect of SCDs on the guinea pig mono-oxygenase system presents quite a different picture from that found in mice and rats. Although guinea pigs are extremely sensitive to the contraceptive effect of these treatments (Table 1), they do not respond with an increase in liver microsomal enzyme activity following chronic administration of SCDs, either at the minimum antifertility doses or at very high doses similar to those used for rats (Table 10). Similar results have been obtained for the effect on the other enzymes tested, epoxide synthetase and epoxide hydratase (Table 11). It should be added that liver microsomal enzymes can be increased by classic inducers such as phenobarbital and 3-MC.

TABLE 10. *Effect of combined treatment with contraceptive drugs on liver microsomal enzyme activity in guinea pigs*

Treatment (mg/kg daily)			Enzyme activity (nmoles/g/hr ± SE)		
Agent	Dosage (mg/kg/day)	No. of days	Aminopyrine	Aniline	pNO$_2$ anisole
Controls			302 ± 28	767 ± 37	1,592 ± 132
Lynestrenol +mestranol	0.3 p.o. 0.018 p.o.	32	374 ± 47	843 ± 35	1,704 ± 67
Lynestrenol + mestranol	5 p.o. 0.3 p.o.	32	304 ± 19	565 ± 14	1,599 ± 17
Norethisterone + mestranol	4 p.o. 0.2 p.o.	32	331 ± 18	812 ± 49	1,511 ± 82
Phenobarbital	80 i.p.	2	985 ± 153[a]	1,195 ± 76[a]	2,836 ± 281[a]
Eucalyptol	500 s.c.	3	769 ± 44[a]	847 ± 43	2,188 ± 104[a]

The activity was measured on the 9,000 *g* supernatant fraction of liver homogenate. Experimental conditions were as described in Table 2.

[a] $p < 0.01$ versus controls.

TABLE 11. *Effect of chronic SCD treatment on liver microsomal epoxide synthetase and epoxide hydratase in guinea pigs*

Treatment		Enzyme activity (nmoles/ mg protein/min ± SE)	
Agent	Dosage (mg/kg/day × 30 days)	Epoxide synthetase	Epoxide hydratase
Controls	—	3.09 ± 0.35	8.57 ± 0.66
Lynestrenol + mestranol	1.25 0.075	3.04 ± 0.38	7.79 ± 0.44
Lynestrenol + mestranol	5 0.3	2.98 ± 0.29	6.80 ± 0.56
Norethisterone + mestranol	0.5 0.025	2.90 ± 0.50	7.55 ± 0.91
Norethisterone + mestranol	4 0.2	2.29 ± 0.14	7.14 ± 1.04
Norethynodrel + mestranol	1 0.015	2.87 ± 0.21	7.47 ± 0.82
Norethynodrel + mestranol	4 0.06	3.40 ± 0.40	6.18 ± 1.18

For details see Table 4.

CONCLUSIONS

The most obvious finding in this investigation is that the effect of SCDs on liver microsomal enzymes is species-dependent. SCDs do not affect microsomal enzyme activity in guinea pigs, but they clearly increase it in mice and rats. However, within the same animal species, the various steroids behave differently. For instance, the combination norethisterone + mestranol increases aniline hydroxylase, N-demethylase, and O-demethylase activity in rats but does not affect epoxide synthetase. The same steroid combination is practically inactive on liver microsomal enzymes of mice.

In conclusion, SCDs may interfere with the metabolism of other drugs but only in given conditions. Our data emphasize the difficulties of extrapolating the effect of contraceptive steroids on drug metabolism from one animal species to another, even in similar experimental conditions. It is also hazardous to state that steroid contraceptives are inducers of drug metabolism in any particular animal species, as each steroid combination can elicit its own spectrum of activity.

REFERENCES

1. Belvedere, G., Pachecka, J., Cantoni, L., Mussini, E., and Salmona, M. (1976): A specific gas chromatographic method for the determination of microsomal styrene monooxygenase and styrene epoxide hydratase activities. *J. Chromatogr.*, 118:387–393.
2. Blackham, A., and Spencer, P. S. J. (1969): The effects of oestrogens and progestins on the response of mice to barbiturates. *Br. J. Pharmacol.*, 37:129–139.

3. Breckenridge, A. (1976): Drug interactions with oral contraceptives: An overview. *This volume.*
4. Briatico, G., Guiso, G., Jori, A., and Ravazzani, C. (1976): Effect of contraceptive agents on drug metabolism in various animal species. *Br. J. Pharmacol.,* 58:173–181.
5. Cinti, D. L., Moldeus, P., and Schenkman, J. B. (1972): Kinetic parameters of drug-metabolizing enzymes in Ca^{2+}-sedimented microsomes from rat liver. *Biochem. Pharmacol.,* 21:3249–3256.
6. Crawford, J. S., and Rudofsky, S. (1966): Some alterations in the pattern of drug metabolism associated with pregnancy, oral contraceptives, and the newly-born. *Br. J. Anaesth.,* 38:446–454.
7. Freudenthal, R. I., and Amerson, E. (1974): Effect of synthetic estrogens and estrogen-progestin combinations on the hepatic microsomal enzyme system. *Biochem. Pharmacol.,* 23:2651–2656.
8. Freudenthal, R. I., Amerson, E., Martin, J., and Wall, M. E. (1974): The effect of norethynodrel, norethindrone and ethynodiol diacetate on hepatic microsomal drug metabolism. *Pharmacol. Res. Commun.,* 6:457–469.
9. Garg, R. C., and Ahmad, A. (1974): Effect of some oral contraceptives on the response of mice to pentobarbitone. *Pharmacol. Res. Commun.,* 6:47–54.
10. Gerald, M. C., and Feller, D. R. (1970): Evidence for spironolactone as a possible inducer of liver microsomal enzymes in mice. *Biochem. Pharmacol.,* 19:2529–2532.
11. Gilbert, D., and Goldberg, L. (1965): Liver response tests. 3. Liver enlargement and stimulation of microsomal processing enzyme activity. *Food Cosmet. Toxicol.,* 3:417–432.
12. Hamrick, M. E., Zampaglione, N. G., Stripp, B., and Gillette, J. R. (1973): Investigation of the effects of methyltestosterone, cortisone and spironolactone on the hepatic microsomal mixed function oxidase system in male and female rats. *Biochem. Pharmacol.,* 22:293–310.
13. Jones, A. L., and Emans, J. B. (1969): The effects of progesterone administration on hepatic endoplasmic reticulum: An electron microscopic and biochemical study. In: *Metabolic Effects of Gonadal Hormones and Contraceptive Steroids,* edited by H. A. Salhanick, D. M. Kipnis, and R. L. Vande Wiele, pp. 68–85. Plenum Press, New York.
14. Jori, A., Bianchetti, A., and Prestini, P. E. (1969): Effect of contraceptive agents on drug metabolism. *Eur. J. Pharmacol.,* 7:196–200.
15. Jori, A., Guiso, G., and Ravazzani, C. (1976): Variations of the enzyme inducing effects of contraceptive agents in different animal species. *J. Pharm. Pharmacol.,* 28:714–716.
16. Juchau, M. R., and Fouts, J. R. (1966): Effects of norethynodrel and progesterone on hepatic microsomal drug-metabolizing enzyme systems. *Biochem. Pharmacol.,* 15:891–898.
17. Kato, R., and Takayanaghi, M. (1966): Differences among the action of phenobarbital, methyl-cholanthrene and male sex hormone on microsomal drug-metabolizing enzyme systems of rat liver. *Jap. J. Pharmacol.,* 16:380–390.
18. Kato, R., and Takanaka, A. (1967): Effect of starvation on the "in vivo" metabolism and effect of drugs in female and male rats. *Jap. J. Pharmacol.,* 17:208–217.
19. Lowry, O. H., Rosebrough, N. J., Farr, A. L., and Randall, R. J. (1951): Protein measurement with the folin phenol reagent. *J. Biol. Chem.,* 193:265–275.
20. Mannering, G. J., Sladek, N. E., Parli, C. J., and Shoeman, D. W. (1969): Formation of a new P-450 hemoprotein after treatment of rats with polycyclic hydrocarbons. In: *Microsomes and Drug Oxidations,* edited by J. R. Gillette, A. H. Conney, G. J. Cosmides, R. W. Estabrook, J. R. Fouts, and G. J. Mannering, pp. 303–330. Academic Press, New York.
21. Oesch, F., Jerina, D. M., and Daly, J. (1971): A radiometric assay for hepatic epoxide hydrase activity with [7–^{3}H] styrene oxide. *Biochim. Biophys. Acta,* 227:685–691.
22. O'Malley, K., Stevenson, I. H., and Crooks, J. (1972): Impairment of human drug metabolism by oral contraceptive steroids. *Clin. Pharmacol. Ther.,* 13:552–557.
23. Omura, T., and Sato, R. (1964): The carbon monoxide-binding pigment of liver microsomes. *J. Biol. Chem.,* 239:2370–2378.
24. Rumke, Chr. L., and Noordhoek, J. (1969): The influence of lynestrenol on the rate of metabolism of phenobarbital, phenytoin and hexobarbital in mice. *Eur. J. Pharmacol.,* 6:163–168.
25. Salmona, M., Pachecka, J., Cantoni, L., Belvedere, G., Mussini, E., and Garattini, S. (1976): Studies on microsomal styrene monooxygenase and styrene epoxide hydratase activities in rats. *Xenobiotica (in press).*
26. Soyka, L. F., and Deckert, F. W. (1974): Further studies on the inhibition of drug metabolism by pregnanolone and related steroids. *Biochem. Pharmacol.,* 23:1629–1639.
27. Stambaugh, J. E., and Wainer, I. W. (1975): Drug interactions. I. Meperidine and combination oral contraceptives. *J. Clin. Pharmacol.,* 15:46–51.
28. Stripp, B., Hamrick, M. E., Zampaglione, N. G., and Gillette, J. R. (1971): The effect of

spironolactone on drug metabolism by hepatic microsomes. *J. Pharmacol. Exp. Ther.,* 176: 766–771.

29. Swaisland, A. J., Grover, P. L., and Sims, P. (1974): Reactions of polycyclic hydrocarbon epoxides with RNA and polyribonucleotides. *Chem. Biol. Interact.,* 9:317–326.
30. Tuttenberg, K. H., Huthwohl, B., Kahl, R., and Kahl, G. F. (1974): Effects of synthetic progestogens on drug metabolism in rat liver microsomes. *Biochem. Pharmacol.,* 23:2037–2043.

Pharmacology of Steroid Contraceptive Drugs
edited by S. Garattini and H. W. Berendes.
Raven Press, New York © 1977.

Hormonal Control of Cytochrome P-450-Dependent Ethylmorphine N-Demethylase Activity of the Mouse

Terry R. Brown, C. Wayne Bardin, and Frank E. Greene

Departments of Pharmacology and Medicine, The Milton S. Hershey Medical Center, The Pennsylvania State University, Hershey, Pennsylvania 17033

The effects of sex steroids on drug metabolism in the rat have been studied extensively (2,14,19–21). Since males of this species metabolize a number of substrates much faster than females, the effects of androgens were examined in detail. Several investigators indicated that these steroids play a key role in determining the sex difference and that estrogens are less important. Although synthetic and natural progestins can also influence the metabolism of drugs by the liver, a physiologic role for this action has not been established.

In contrast to these observations in the rat, most studies in mice indicate little or no sex difference in the rate of drug metabolism. In a few experiments when differences were observed, females metabolized certain substrates faster than males (1,7–9,31,32,39–41). In view of the lack of uniformity concerning the possible effect of sex steroids in the mouse, we thought it pertinent to investigate hepatic drug metabolism not only in males and females but in animals treated with androgens, estrogens, and progestins. The mouse was chosen for study since certain hepatic cytochrome P-450-linked mono-oxygenases appear to be under genetic control, with regard to constitutive levels and in their response to enzyme inducers (29,42). These differences appeared to offer a means of probing the mechanism by which steroid hormones regulate the activity of hepatic microsomal enzymes. In the present study, ethylmorphine demethylase activity and cytochrome P-450 content were used as endpoints of hormone action. Ethylmorphine was selected because it is a typical type I substrate which is known to exhibit a sex difference in its rate of metabolism in some rodents (7,9).

SEX AND STRAIN DIFFERENCES

The inbred strains of mice studied were BALB/cJ, DBA/2J, C57BL/10J, and C3H/HeJ. These strains were selected because they exhibited known differences in sex steroid sensitivity and drug metabolism. BALB/cJ mice are in the "high class" for androgen inducibility of kidney β-glucuronidase activity, whereas DBA/2J and C57BL/10J mice are in the "low class" (37). The response of kidney β-glucuronidase activity of C3H/HeJ mice to androgen administration is uniquely different from the other strains tested (37). There are also differences between DBA/2J and C3H/HeJ mice for induction of hepatic arylhydrocarbon hydroxylase activity (29) and for the basal and induced level of hepatic coumarin hydroxylase activity (42).

Two noninbred strains of mice were also studied. The CRL:CD-1(Swiss) mice were included since a sex difference in hepatic microsomal drug metabolism has been reported for this strain (41). The HMC mice were examined because the tfm mutation is carried in these animals (24,33). Mice which carry this gene (tfm/y) have a defect of the androgen receptor and as a consequence are insensitive to testosterone and other androgens (4). By contrast, normal males (+/y) and females (+/+) have normal responses to these steroids.

The results of these studies are summarized in Table 1. No evidence of a sex difference in ethylmorphine N-demethylase activity could be demonstrated in C3H/HeJ, C57BL/10J, or HMC mice. Although a sex difference in the DBA/2J strain was seen in some experiments, the difference was small and not always statistically significant. The specific activity of ethylmorphine N-demethylation in female mice was not affected in any of these four strains by the administration of 1, 2, or 5 mg testosterone per day for 6 days. Since these strains differ widely in their inducibility of kidney β-glucuronidase (37) and hepatic microsomal aryl hydrocarbon hydroxylase (29), it is apparent that factors which determine the inducibility of these enzymes by androgens and polycyclic hydrocarbons, respectively, are not the same as those controlling the effects of androgens on ethylmorphine N-demethylase. The apparent absence of a sex difference in the rate of ethylmorphine metabolism of these four strains suggested a relatively minor role for sex hormones in the regulation of the hepatic microsomal drug-metabolizing enzyme system. Therefore subsequent experiments utilized HMC mice, in which the genetic defect causing androgen insensitivity has been identified, and the two strains discussed below.

In contrast to the strains described above, male BALB/cJ mice metabolized

TABLE 1. *Sex differences in ethylmorphine metabolism*

Strain	Sex difference	Testosterone responsiveness[a]
CRL:CD-1	Yes (♀ > ♂)	No
BALB/cJ	Yes (♂ > ♀)	Yes
DBA/2J	No	No
C3H/HeJ	No	No
C57BL/10J	No	No
HMC	No	No[b]

[a] Response was defined as an alteration of the specific activity of ethylmorphine N-demethylation following the treatment of intact female mice with testosterone (5 mg/day, 6 days).

[b] Response measured in androgen-insensitive (tfm/y) mice rather than female mice.

ethylmorphine faster than females. In this strain, this aspect of drug metabolism was similar to that in rats (19). On the other hand, CRL:CD-1 male mice metabolized this substrate at a slower rate than did females. The latter results from CRL:CD-1 mice are in agreement with results reported by other investigators (41). Additional studies, except those using HMC mice, were confined to gonadectomized BALB/cJ and CRL:CD-1 mice.

In the studies summarized below, three effects of sex steroids on the liver were evaluated: (a) a generalized growth-promoting action manifested by increases in liver wet weight and microsomal protein content; (b) changes in the specific activity of ethylmorphine N-demethylase activity, expressed in terms of microsomal protein; and (c) the total activity of N-demethylase activity, which takes into account changes in liver weight and microsomal protein content. The latter way of expressing the results is especially useful in those instances where there was an increase in the microsomal protein content without equivalent changes in the specific activity of the N-demethylase system, and it provides information relevant to possible *in vivo* effects on the metabolism of drugs and other foreign compounds.

EFFECTS OF ANDROGENS

The effects of testosterone (Ts) and dihydrotestosterone (DHT) on liver weight and microsomal protein content appear to be independent of sex and strain (Fig. 1, top). This effect of androgen was most evident in the hepatic microsomal protein content.

In contrast to the general action of androgens on hepatic weight and protein, these steroids had a different effect on ethylmorphine N-demethylase activity of BALB/cJ and CRL:CD-1 mice (Fig. 1, bottom). Androgen treatment increased the specific activity of ethylmorphine N-demethylation by approximately 100% in male and 50% in female BALB/cJ mice. Even greater increases in the rate of ethylmorphine metabolism were observed in terms of total activity per liver, since, as noted previously, androgens also increase the hepatic microsomal protein content and liver weight. Androgen administration caused no significant changes in the rate of ethylmorphine demethylation by hepatic microsomes from male or female CRL:CD-1 mice. The total capacity of the liver (per gram of liver or total liver activity) to metabolize ethylmorphine remained unchanged following treatment of CRL:CD-1 mice with either Ts or DHT, since the slight decrease in specific activity was offset by an increase in microsomal protein and liver weight.

Cytochrome P-450 content was significantly increased in BALB/cJ mice by Ts and DHT treatment. However, the ethylmorphine N-demethylase activity of androgen-treated males increased to a much greater extent than the cytochrome P-450 content. In contrast, parallel increases in demethylase activity and cytochrome P-450 content were observed in androgen-treated female BALB/cJ mice. Furthermore, neither Ts nor DHT altered cytochrome P-450 levels in hepatic

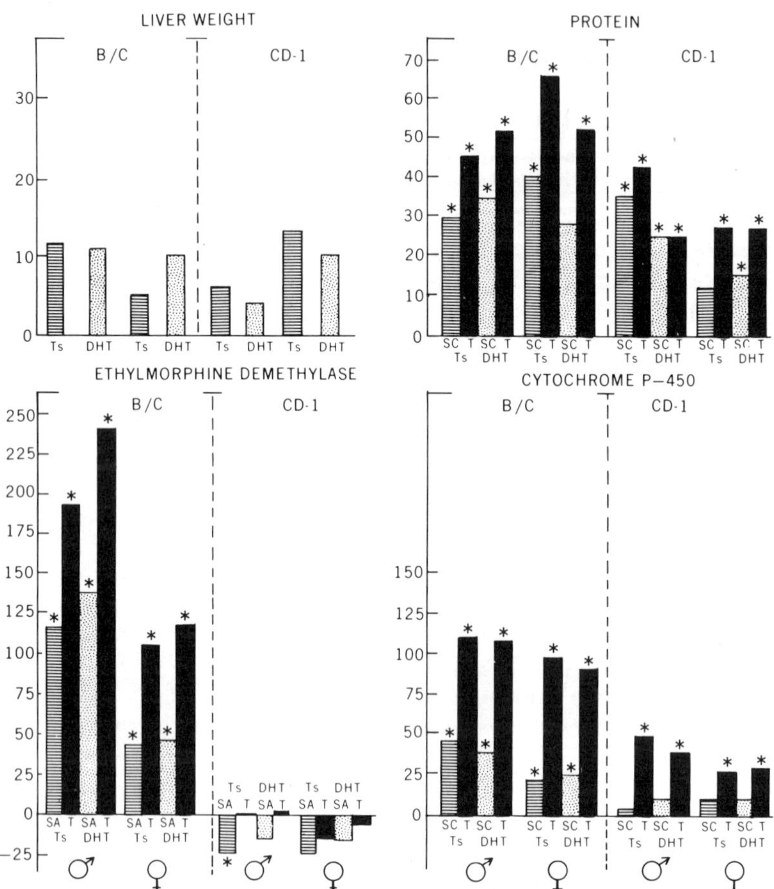

FIG. 1. Effects of androgens on the liver of gonadectomized BALB/cJ (B/C) and CRL:CD-1 (CD-1) mice. Animals were gonadectomized 2 weeks prior to initiation of treatment. Male (♂) and female (♀) mice were administered testosterone (Ts) or 5α-dihydrotestosterone (DHT) (2 mg/day, 6 days, s.c.). All values represent the percent change from the gonadectomized control values (mean ± SE) for each parameter. Striped and dotted bars represent specific activity (SA) or specific content (SC). Solid bars represent total (T) activity or content. *$p < 0.05$ vs. control; $N = 6$.

microsomes from male and female CRL:CD-1 mice. However, the specific activity of ethylmorphine N-demethylase of males was significantly decreased by Ts, and a similar trrend was observed in other androgen-treated CRL:CD-1 mice. Our results thus suggest that there are three levels of response by the hepatic N-demethylase system to androgen administration: stimulation (male BALB/cJ), no effect (female BALB/cJ), and impairment (male and female CRL:CD-1). This is of particular interest when considering a model for hepatic androgen responsiveness.

EFFECTS OF ESTROGENS

Estradiol-17β (E$_2$) and diethylstilbestrol (DES) produced increases in liver weight and total microsomal protein content of male and female CRL:CD-1 mice (Fig. 2, top). In the BALB/cJ strain, however, neither E$_2$ nor DES affected liver weights, but small increases in microsomal protein were detected. Thus although

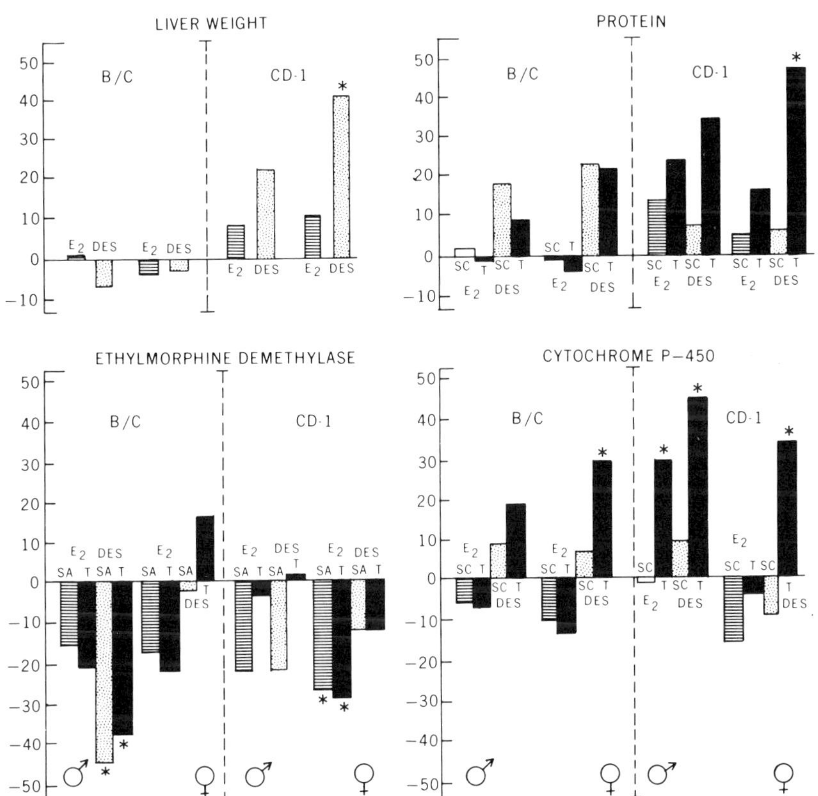

FIG. 2. Effects of estrogens on the liver of gonadectomized BALB/cJ (B/C) and CRL:CD-1 (CD-1) mice. Animals were gonadectomized 2 weeks prior to initiation of treatment. Male ($\male$) and female ($\female$) mice were administered estradiol-17β (E$_2$) or diethylstilbestrol (DES) (2 μg/day, 6 days, s.c.). All values represent the percent change from the gonadectomized control values (mean $\pm$ SE) for each parameter. Striped and dotted bars represent specific activity (SA) or specific content (SC). Solid bars represent total (T) activity or content. *$p < 0.05$ vs. control; $N = 6$.

estrogens and androgens affect microsomal protein content and liver wet weight, there appear to be subtle strain differences in their relative effects on these two parameters.

It seemed possible that estrogens could play an active role in the control of N-demethylation in the CRL:CD-1 strain, since the rate was faster in females than in males. However, as shown in Fig. 2 (bottom), the specific activity of N-demethylase was decreased in both strains. These decreases were offset by increases in liver weights and total microsomal protein in the CRL:CD-1 strain, resulting in little net change in the total N-demethylase activity in the estrogen-treated males. The net effect of estrogens on the total N-demethylase activity in the BALB/cJ strain tended to be greater, since the increases in total protein content were not enough to offset the decreases in the specific activity of N-demethylase in this strain.

The effects of estrogens on cytochrome P-450 content of both strains appeared to be due primarily to an effect on total microsomal protein content of the livers, since the specific content was not significantly affected by estrogen treatment. Comparisons of the effects of estrogens on cytochrome P-450 content and N-demethylase activity show that the changes are equivalent in female mice of both strains, but in males the changes in N-demethylase activity were greater than changes in cytochrome P-450 content. These results suggest that a functional impairment of cytochrome P-450 may have developed in males as a result of estrogen treatment. In females, however, it seems likely that estrogens are not affecting N-demethylase activity directly but are producing this apparent effect through changes in membrane composition that affect the calculation of specific activity.

It is difficult to relate the observations of these studies with the limited number of published studies on the effects of estrogen administration on *in vivo* estimates of drug metabolism. For example, Westfall et al. (41) reported that DES decreased the duration of pentobarbital anesthesia in intact Swiss mice, whereas Gessner et al. (13) found that DES prolonged the duration of hexobarbital- and chlorzoxazone-induced sleep in intact Swiss mice. Our results predict that the pharmacologic response of certain drugs might be increased somewhat in DES-treated castrated BALB/cJ mice and ovariectomized CRL:CD-1 mice treated with E_2. Only in these groups was the total metabolism of ethylmorphine, expressed per liver, significantly different from control.

EFFECTS OF PROGESTINS

Administration of progesterone (P), medroxyprogesterone acetate (MPA), and cyproterone acetate (CPA) resulted in a generalized increase in hepatic microsomal protein content in both BALB/cJ and CRL:CD-1 mice (Fig. 3, top). Each of these steroids produced an increase in the specific activity of demethylation in BALB/cJ animals, but only CPA was effective in CRL:CD-1 mice. In BALB/cJ mice the relative potency, in order of increasing activity, was MPA,

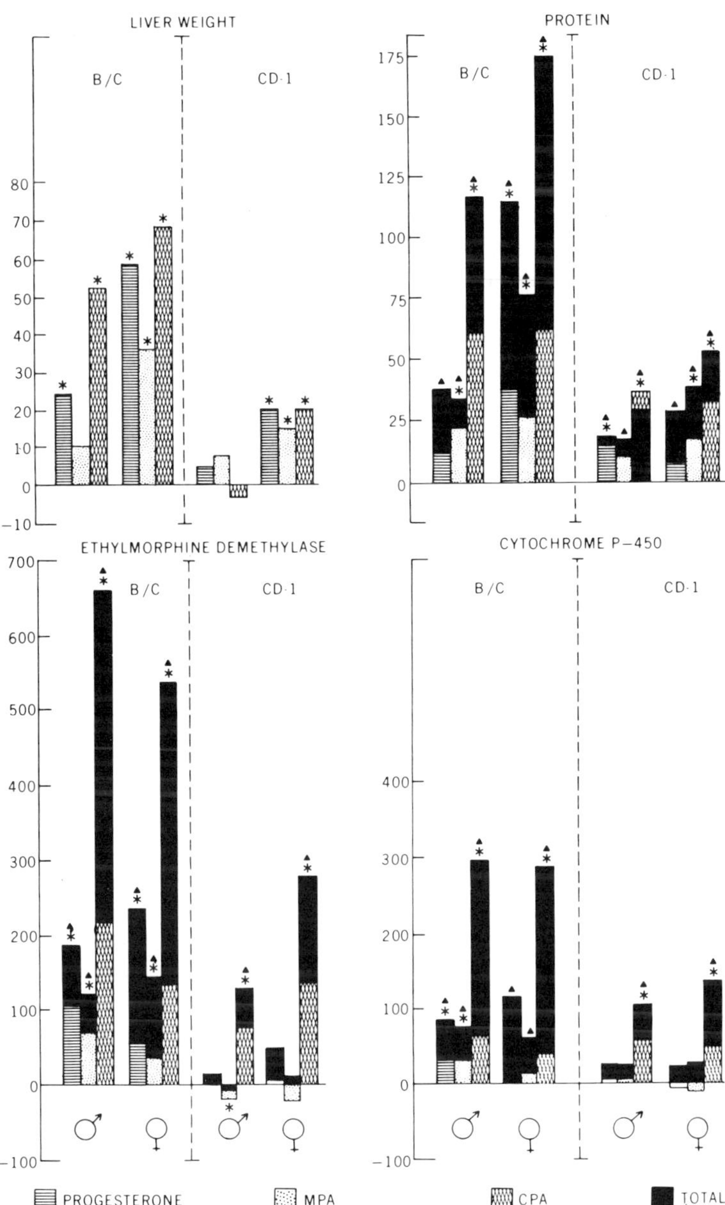

FIG. 3. Effects of progestins on the liver of gonadectomized BALB/cJ (B/C) and CRL:(CD-1) (CD-1) mice. Animals were gonadectomized 2 weeks prior to initiation of treatment. Male (♂) and female (♀) mice were administered progesterone (P), medroxyprogesterone acetate (MPA), or cyproterone acetate (CPA) (5.0 mg/day, 6 days, s.c.). All values represent the percent change from the gonadectomized control values (mean ± SE) for each parameter. The striped, dotted, and cross-hatched portions of each bar represent specific activity or specific content (*$p < 0.05$ vs. control). The solid portion of each bar represents the total activity or content (▲ $p < 0.05$ vs. control); $N = 6$.

P, and CPA. The effects of these progestins on mouse liver did not correlate with their progestational activity since both MPA and CPA have much greater gestagenic activity than progesterone. Similarly, the activity of these steroids could not be attributed to their androgenic activity since the most androgenic progestin, MPA, was the least effective in stimulating ethylmorphine N-demethylase activity.

In fact, MPA decreased demethylase specific activity in CRL:CD-1 mice, whereas P had no effect. Since all three progestins increased microsomal protein content, the net effect was to increase the total activity of N-demethylation of the CPA-treated mice whereas the activity of the MPA- and P-treated mice remained at control levels. Although CPA increased the total demethylase activity in CRL:CD-1 mice two- to fourfold, the activity was increased seven- to eightfold in BALB/cJ mice.

The actions of progestins on the cytochrome P-450 content were also strain-specific and, in addition, displayed a dependence on sex in BALB/cJ mice. All three progestins significantly increased the P-450 content of microsomes of male BALB/cJ mice, but only CPA did so in females. However, the total microsomal cytochrome P-450 content was significantly increased in livers from male and female BALB/cJ mice by each of the progestins. In contrast, only CPA significantly increased cytochrome P-450 content (per milligram of protein or per liver) in male and female CRL:CD-1 mice. Although the direction of change for demethylase activity and cytochrome P-450 content are similar following progestin treatment, the magnitude of the observed increases are greater for demethylase activity than cytochrome P-450 content.

In conclusion, progestins exhibit two effects on mouse liver. First, they increase liver weight and microsomal protein. These effects were observed in all groups and are therefore independent of sex and strain. Second, progestins stimulated N-demethylase activity and increased P-450 content. The latter effects were strain-, sex-, and steroid-specific. Although it is not possible to assign either of these effects to androgenic or progestational actions, it may be significant that both male and female BALB/cJ mice responded to MPA and P, whereas CRL:CD-1 mice did not.

Although there have been several studies in which the effects of P, MPA, and CPA on the hepatic metabolism of foreign compounds have been investigated, these results are often conflicting and are difficult to relate to the present study; this is because most were done with intact rats, thus allowing expression of antihormone activity of the progestins to be manifested. P, for example, has been reported to increase the metabolism of chlorpromazine (27) and certain anticholinesterase compounds (10), whereas the metabolism of hexobarbital and zoxazolamine were decreased (18). P given 2 hr prior to sacrifice inhibited the metabolism of hexobarbital by 9,000 g supernatant from rat livers (18), indicating that P or its metabolites can also inhibit drug metabolism directly. MPA (10 mg/kg, 30 days) has been shown to increase the *in vitro* metabolism of *p*-

nitroanisole, aminopyrine, and aniline by 9,000 g supernatant prepared from livers of female rats (17). CPA increased the metabolism of aniline by hepatic microsomes from male and female rats, and of hexobarbital metabolism in female rats but not in males (38).

EVIDENCE THAT ANDROGENS AND PROGESTINS STIMULATE HEPATIC DRUG METABOLISM BY INDEPENDENT MECHANISMS

Androgens, as well as other steroids and drugs, increase liver weight and microsomal protein content. The general nature of this response suggests that it is independent of the androgen receptor. To test this possibility, the effects of testosterone on androgen-insensitive HMC (tfm/y) mice were examined. Since the action of progestins on mouse kidney (28) and submaxillary gland (6) were mediated via the androgen receptor, the effect of these steroids on livers of tfm/y mice were also examined.

Effects of Androgens and Progestins on Livers of Androgen-Insensitive (tfm/y) Mice

The effects of testosterone on the livers of tfm/y mice are shown in Table 2. As expected, there was no increase in N-demethylase activity or cytochrome P-450 content. By contrast, there was a small increase in hepatic weight and a larger increase in microsomal protein content. These observations are consistent with the hypothesis that some effects of androgens on liver are not mediated through the androgen receptor.

The effects of progestins on the livers of tfm/y mice are shown in Table 3. Both progesterone and cyproterone acetate stimulated several of the endpoints examined. These observations support the conclusion that effects of progestins are independent of their androgenic activity.

TABLE 2. *Effect of testosterone on tfm/y mice[a]*

Measurement	Control[b]	+ Testosterone 2.0 mg/day[c]	+ Testosterone 5.0 mg/day[c]
Liver weight (g)	1.20	113	108
Microsomal protein (mg/g)	19.1	110	137[d]
Ethylmorphine N-demethylase (nm/mg/10 min)	174	100	99
Cytochrome P-450 (nm/mg)	0.86	94	95

[a] All treatments were for 6 days, s.c.
[b] Expressed as the mean value for five animals.
[c] Expressed as percent of the control value.
[d] Different from control, $p < 0.05$.

TABLE 3. *Effect of progestins on tfm/y mice[a]*

Measurement	Control[b]	Medroxy progesterone acetate[c]	Progesterone[c]	Cyproterone acetate[c]
Liver weight (g)	1.45	100	115	117
Microsomal protein (mg/g)	19.0	89	132[d]	137[d]
Ethylmorphine N-demethylase (nm/mg/10 min)	193	120	269[d]	244[d]
Cytochrome P-450 (nm/mg)	0.72	86	123	156[d]

[a] All treatments 5.0 mg steroid/day, 6 days, s.c.
[b] Expressed as the mean value for five animals.
[c] Expressed as percent of the control value.
[d] Different from control, $p < 0.05$.

Effects of the Antiandrogen Flutamide (SCH 13521) on Testosterone-Induced Changes in Livers of BALB/cJ Mice

Flutamide is a new, nonsteroidal antiandrogen devoid of hormonal activity (30). This compound, or more likely a metabolite, exerts its effects by inhibiting androgen uptake and retention by the androgen receptors of the target tissues (22,25,34,39). It seemed reasonable, therefore, that it could also block androgen receptor-mediated events in the liver as well. The effect of flutamide on the androgen-induced increase of N-demethylase activity and P-450 content are shown in Fig. 4. As expected, testosterone given alone produced significant increases in ethylmorphine N-demethylase activity and cytochrome P-450 content of hepatic microsomes. Flutamide blocked the testosterone-induced increases

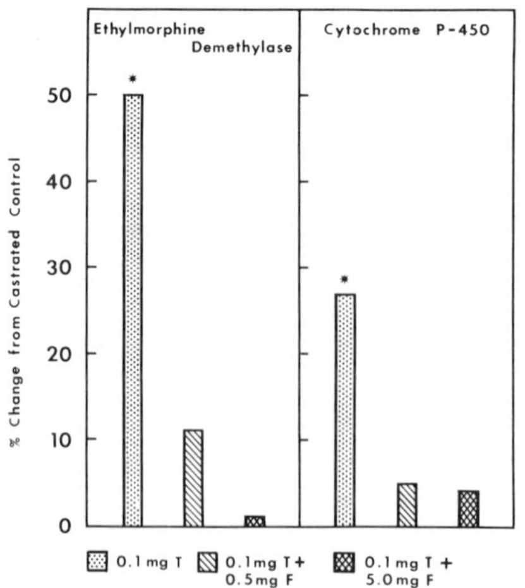

FIG. 4. Effect of flutamide on testosterone stimulation of hepatic ethylmorphine N-demethylase activity and cytochrome P-450 content in castrated male BALB/cJ mice. Mice were castrated 2 weeks before initiation of treatment. Animals were administered testosterone (T) (0.1 mg/day) alone and concurrently with flutamide (F; 0.5 mg or 5.0 mg/day, 6 days, s.c.) Values represent the percent change from the castrated control values *$p < 0.05$ vs. castrated control; $N = 5$.

in both N-demethylase activity and cytochrome P-450 content (3). Although the mechanism of the flutamide blockade of testosterone actions in the liver has not been established, it is tempting to speculate that the mechanism is identical to its action in the male reproductive tract, i.e., blockade of an androgen receptor.

PROPOSED MECHANISM OF SEX STEROID ACTION ON THE LIVER

Our studies indicate that there are at least two ways in which sex steroids can affect drug-metabolizing enzyme systems of the liver. First, steroids may act via an apparently nonspecific mechanism characterized by liver growth and an increase in the net microsomal protein content, a property not only of androgens, estrogens, and progestins but also of such drugs as phenobarbital. An increase in liver weight and microsomal protein content was a common feature of steroid action in BALB/cJ, CRL:CD-1, and tfm/y mice. Secondly, sex steroids may exert specific effects on enzyme activity that are not only an inherent property of a particular steroid but also may be specific for the sex and strain of mice involved. In the present studies, the nonspecific effects always accompanied the specific effect, but the inverse was not true.

To explain in part the mechanism by which sex steroids produce these two kinds of effect on mouse liver, a model was developed that relates the effects of steroids on liver growth to a pleiotypic effect (16) and the effect on N-demethylase activity to a specific receptor mechanism. In a variety of mammalian cell types, a constant set of metabolically unrelated biochemical reactions responds coordinately when changes in the environment affect cellular growth. Because of the multiplicity and diversity of the reactions involved, the entire regulatory program is referred to as the "pleiotypic response" (16) (Fig. 5). When growth-promoting substances are withdrawn, the changes taking place are called the negative pleiotypic response, and when growth is stimulated reference is made to the positive

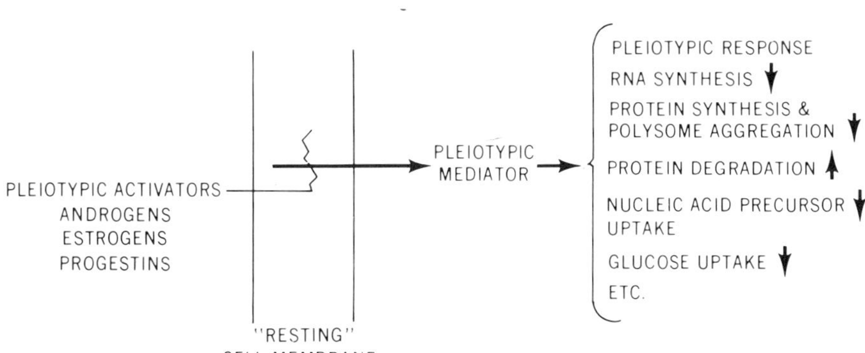

FIG. 5. Proposed mechanism for pleiotypic control of mouse liver by sex steroids. See text for discussion.

pleiotypic response. It has been hypothesized that under resting conditions in a variety of cells a pleiotypic mediator is formed which dampens cellular activity (16). Under appropriate stimulation (e.g., by steroids or drugs) apparently involving specific membrane interactions, the concentration or activity of the mediator decreases, allowing the cell to prepare for active growth. This action would account for the increases in liver weight and total microsomal protein content observed following the administration of androgens, estrogens, and progestins. The cellular response to a given hormone may be both pleiotypic and specific. This dual action probably accounts for differences in the spectra of activity produced by different steroids.

The specific activity of ethylmorphine N-demethylase (expressed per milligram of microsomal protein) was used as the endpoint for determining the specific effects of steroids on the hepatic microsomal drug-metabolizing enzyme system. Changes in cytochrome P-450 content could not account for the induction of demethylase activity in most instances. For example, although cytochrome P-450 content increased in testosterone-treated BALB/cJ mice, the increase was not equivalent to the increase in demethylase activity. Changes in the efficiency of the demethylase system are most likely associated with cytochrome P-450 rather than other components of the membrane, since spectral studies (12,36), reconstitution of the microsomal drug-metabolizing system (23), and purification of the reductase and cytochrome P-450 fractions (15) suggest that specificity resides in the P-450 fraction.

As a result of the present study of steroid effects on mouse liver, the specific mechanism can be described only from observations of various endpoints rather than at the molecular level. The model is based on the measurement of hepatic microsomal ethylmorphine N-demethylase activity relative to functional changes in the terminal oxidase of the system, cytochrome P-450.

Studies utilizing BALB/cJ and CRL:CD-1 strains, as well as the tfm/y mouse and flutamide, suggest that a specific mechanism is responsible for the stimulation of ethylmorphine demethylase activity in BALB/cJ mice, a mechanism which is not operable in CRL:CD-1 or tfm/y mice (Fig. 6). Activation of this mechanism by androgens results in the accumulation of a "demethylase-specific" form of cytochrome P-450 (P-450$_{DS}$). This could occur basically in two ways: (a) synthesis of a new demethylase-specific form of cytochrome P-450; or (b) configurational or allosteric alteration of the microsomal membrane resulting in a more enzymatically efficient association of electron-transport components for demethylation. The first mechanism would require activation of an androgen-specific genome with specific macromolecular synthesis leading to increases in a specific form of cytochrome P-450. The second could result from a more direct effect on the microsomal membrane without activation of the genetic machinery of the hepatocyte. As shown in Fig. 6, either of these actions could be mediated via an intracellular androgen receptor.

Failure of the CRL:CD-1 and tfm/y mice to respond to androgens could be explained by either the absence of an androgen receptor or a chromatin acceptor

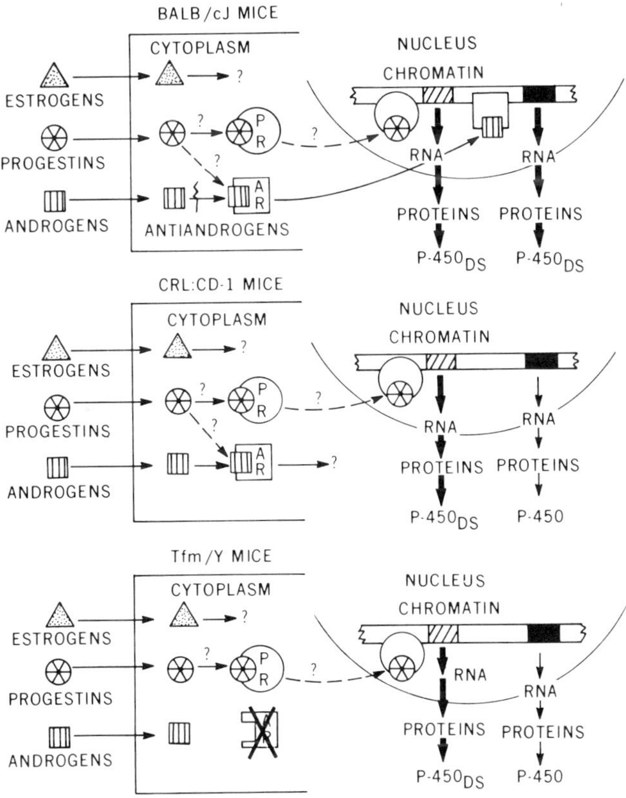

FIG. 6. Proposed model of a receptor mechanism for hormone actions in the mouse liver. See text for discussion.

site for the androgen-receptor complex. The former possibility is more likely in tfm/y mice, since other organs from these mice lack an androgen receptor, whereas the latter possibility is more likely in CRL:CD-1 mice since other tissues of CRL:CD-1 mice possess an androgen receptor. In addition to differences in receptor and acceptor sites in responsive and nonresponsive mice, these sites may be under additional genetic control mechanisms which determine their availability or concentration in hepatocytes of certain strains.

Several lines of evidence favor the concept of an intracellular receptor protein(s) being responsible for androgen action in the liver. First, androgen-insensitive pseudohermaphroditic (tfm) rats do not respond to androgen treatment with increased demethylase activity as do normal male rats (5). Subsequently tfm rats have been shown to lack a specific cytoplasmic androgen-binding protein found in the livers of normal male rats (26,35). Secondly, the androgen receptor found in kidneys of normal mice is absent in tfm/y mice (4). This androgen receptor presumably functions in the androgen induction of mouse kidney β-glucuronidase activity, which is highly inducible in BALB/cJ mice, much less inducible in CRL:CD-1 mice, and noninducible in tfm/y mice. This suggests that the androgen receptor is absent in tissues of tfm/y mice. We showed that androgen administration to tfm/y mice does not result in an increase in the specific activity of N-demethylase. Three possibilities then exist for the less inducible CRL:CD-1 strain: (a) the receptor is present in very low concentration; (b) the receptor is defective in some way so that androgens are not bound; or (c) receptor steroid binding is normal, but the chromatin acceptor site is absent or defective.

Although estrogen receptors have been identified in hepatic cytosol (11), estrogens appear to be capable of evoking only the pleiotypic cellular response without a specific effect on demethylase activity. Since this action does not appear to require a receptor mechanism, the estrogen receptor does not seem to play a role in the parameters we measured.

A mechanism to explain the actions of progestins on the liver is considerably more difficult to envision. A hypothetical progestin receptor is included in the model (Fig. 6) for the purpose of discussion, although a progesterone receptor for liver has not been identified. A satisfactory model of a progestin receptor-mediated increase in demethylase-specific cytochrome P-450 would have to take into account the observations that the ability of progestins to increase the level of this cytochrome appears not to be related to androgenic or progestational activity as measured in extrahepatic tissues. Although progestins lack some of the strain-dependent specificity exhibited by androgens, they still manifest some specificity with regard to their effects on demethylase activity and cytochrome P-450 content of specific strains, as well as an apparent inherent specificity related to chemical structure. However, as noted previously, there is no evidence at present to support a receptor-mediated mechanism of progestin action. Moreover, indirect evidence such as that presented in favor of an androgen receptor is difficult to obtain for progestins, since there does not appear to be an animal model comparable to the tfm rat or tfm/y mouse for progestin insensitivity, and because antiprogestin compounds tend to have intrinsic hormone actions of their own.

SUMMARY

Hepatic demethylase activity is sensitive to androgens, progestins, and to a lesser extent estrogens. The effects of androgens are specific among different mouse strains and therefore may be genetically controlled. Some degree of specificity also exists for progestin actions but not for estrogens. In the case of progestins, there appears to be some overlap with androgens, such that their mechanisms of action may be related. However, the ability of progestins to stimulate N-demethylase in androgen-insensitive mice clearly indicates that differences in the modes of action for androgens and progestins do exist.

A model has been proposed to explain the actions of sex steroids on the mouse liver based on a "pleiotypic" (or general) effect on the liver and a specific effect related to a "receptor-dependent" mechanism for androgens which affects demethylase activity. Future experiments using androgen-"responsive" and androgen-"nonresponsive" mouse strains may further elucidate the genetic control of androgen action on the mouse liver as well as the relationship of androgen and progestin mechanisms of stimulation of drug-metabolizing enzymes. Use of the techniques available for purification of cytochrome P-450 from hepatic microsomes and reconstitution of the drug-metabolizing enzyme system may aid in identifying the site of androgen-specific effects on the demethylase system. In addition, studies of the molecular events of steroid action in the liver and the identification of specific macromolecules involved in this action will lead to further delineation of hepatic steroid responsiveness.

ACKNOWLEDGMENTS

We thank the Schering Corporation (Bloomfield, N.J.) and Schering AG (Berlin, Germany) for kindly providing the flutamide and cyproterone acetate, respectively; and the Upjohn Co. (Kalamazoo, Mich.) for the gift of medroxyprogesterone acetate. This research was supported by NIH Contract No. NO1–HD-2-2730.

REFERENCES

1. Backus, B., and Cohn, V. H. (1966): Genetic differences in metabolism of hexobarbital in mice. *Fed. Proc.,* 25:531 (abstract).
2. Booth, J., and Gillette, J. R. (1962): The effect of anabolic steroids on drug metabolism by microsomal enzymes in rat liver. *J. Pharmacol. Exp. Ther.,* 137:374–379.
3. Brown, T. R., Greene, F. E., and Bardin, C. W. (1976): Androgen receptor dependent and independent activities of testosterone on hepatic microsomal drug metabolism. *Endocrinology,* 99:1353–1362.
4. Bullock, L. P., and Bardin, C. W. (1974): Androgen receptors in mouse kidney: A study of male, female and androgen-insensitive (tfm/y) mice. *Endocrinology,* 94:746–756.
5. Bullock, L. P., Bardin, C. W., Gram, T. E., Schroeder, D. H., and Gillette, J. R. (1971): Hepatic ethylmorphine demethylase and Δ^4-steroid reductase in the androgen-insensitive pseudohermaphroditic rat. *Endocrinology,* 88:1521–1523.
6. Bullock, L. P., Barthe, P. L., Mowszowicz, I., Orth, D. N., and Bardin, C. W. (1975): The effect of progestins on submaxillary gland epidermal growth factor: Demonstration of androgenic, synandrogenic and antiandrogenic actions. *Endocrinology,* 97:189–195.
7. Castro, J. A., and Gillette, J. R. (1967): Species and sex differences in the kinetic constants for the N-demethylation of ethylmorphine by liver microsomes. *Biochem. Biophys. Res. Commun.,* 28:426–430.
8. Catz, C. S., and Jaffe, S. Y. (1967): Strain and age variations in hexobarbital response. *J. Pharmacol. Exp. Ther.,* 115:152–156.
9. Davies, D. S., Gigon, P. L., and Gillette, J. R. (1968): Sex differences in the kinetic constants for the N-demethylation of ethylmorphine by rat liver microsomes. *Biochem. Pharmacol.,* 17: 1865–1872.
10. Dubois, K. P., and Kinoshita, F. (1965): Modification of the anticholinesterase action of O,O-diethyl-O(4-methylthio-m-tolyl)phosphorothioate (DMP) by drugs affecting hepatic microsomal enzymes. *Arch. Int. Pharmacodyn.,* 156:418–431.
11. Eisenfeld, A. J., Aten, R., Weinberger, M., Haselbacher, G., Halpern, K., and Krakoff, L. (1976): Estrogen receptor in the mammalian liver. *Science,* 191:862–864.
12. El Defrawy El Masry, S., and Mannering, G. J. (1974): Sex-dependent differences in drug

metabolism in the rat. II. Qualitative changes produced by castration and the administration of steroid hormones and phenobarbital. *Drug Metab. Dispos.,* 2:279–284.

13. Gessner, T., Acara, M., Baker, J. A., and Edelman, L. L. (1967): Effects of sex hormones on the duration of drug action in mice. *J. Pharm. Sci.,* 56:405–407.

14. Gram, T. E., and Gillette, J. R. (1969): The role of sex hormones in the metabolism of drugs and other foreign compounds by hepatic microsomal enzymes. In: *Metabolic Effects of Gonadal Hormones and Contraceptive Steroids,* edited by H. A. Salhanick, D. M. Kipnis, and R. L. Van de Wiele. Plenum Press, New York.

15. Haugen, D. A., van der Hoeven, T. A., and Coon, M. J. (1975): Purified liver microsomal cytochrome P-450: Separation and characterization of multiple forms. *J. Biol. Chem.,* 250: 3567–3570.

16. Hershko, A., Mamont, P., Shields, R., and Tomkins, G. M. (1971): Pleiotypic response. *Nature [New Biol.],* 232:206–211.

17. Jori, A., Bianchetti, A., and Prestini, P. E. (1969): Effect of contraceptive agents on drug metabolism. *Eur. J. Pharmacol.,* 7:196–200.

18. Juchau, M. R., and Fouts, J. R. (1966): Effects of norethynodrel and progesterone on hepatic microsomal drug-metabolizing enzyme systems. *Biochem. Pharmacol.,* 15:891–898.

19. Kato, R. (1974): Sex-related differences in drug metabolism. *Drug Metab. Rev.,* 3:1–32.

20. Kato, R., and Gillette, J. R. (1965): Sex differences in the effects of abnormal physiological states on the metabolism of drugs by rat liver microsomes. *J. Pharmacol. Exp. Ther.,* 150:285–291.

21. Kato, R., and Onoda, K. (1970): Studies on the regulation of the activity of drug oxidation in rat liver microsomes by androgen and estrogen. *Biochem. Pharmacol.,* 19:1649–1660.

22. Liao, S., Howell, D. K., and Chang, T-M. (1974): Action of a non-steroidal antiandrogen, flutamide, on the receptor binding and nuclear retention of 5α-dihydrotestosterone in rat ventral prostate. *Endocrinology,* 94:1205–1209.

23. Lu, A. Y. H., and Levin, W. (1974): The resolution and reconstitution of the liver microsomal hydroxylation system. *Biochim. Biophys. Acta,* 344:205–240.

24. Lyon, M. F., and Hawkes, S. G. (1970): X-linked gene for testicular feminization in the mouse. *Nature (Lond.),* 227:1217–1219.

25. Mainwaring, W. I. P., Mangan, F. R., Feherty, P. A., and Freifeld, M. (1974): An investigation into the anti-androgenic properties of the nonsteroidal compound, Sch 13521 (4'-nitro-3'-trifluoro-methylisobutyrylanilide). *Mol. Cell. Endocrinol.,* 1:113–128.

26. Milin, B., and Roy, A. K. (1973): Androgen "receptor" in rat liver: Cytosol "receptor" deficiency in pseudohermaphrodite rats. *Nature [New Biol.],* 242:248–250.

27. Miya, T. S., Adams, E. H., and Saunders, R. (1966): Effects of estradiol and progesterone on the metabolism of chlorpromazine. 113th Annual Meeting, American Pharmaceutical Association, Dallas, Texas, p. 66 (abstract).

28. Mowszowicz, I., Bieber, D. E., Chung, K. W., Bullock, L. P., and Bardin, C. W. (1974): Synandrogenic and antiandrogenic effect of progestins: Comparisons with non-progestational antiandrogens. *Endocrinology,* 95:1589–1599.

29. Nebert, D. W., Robinson, J. R., Niwa, A., Kumaki, K., and Poland, A. P. (1975): Genetic expression of aryl hydrocarbon hydroxylase activity in the mouse. *J. Cell Physiol.,* 85:393–414.

30. Neri, R., Florance, K., Koziol, P., and van Cleave, S. (1972): A biological profile of a non-steroidal antiandrogen, Sch 13521 (4'-nitro-3'-trifluoromethylisobutyranilide). *Endocrinology,* 91:427–437.

31. Noordhoek, J. (1972): The effect of castration and testosterone on some components of the microsomal drug metabolizing enzyme system in mice. *FEBS Lett.,* 24:255–259.

32. Noordhoek, J., and Rumke, C. L. (1969): Sex differences in the rate of drug metabolism in mice. *Arch. Int. Pharmacodyn.,* 182:401.

33. Ohno, S., and Lyon, M. F. (1970): X-linked testicular feminization in the mouse as a non-inducible regulatory mutation of the Jacob-Monod type. *Clin. Genet.,* 1:121–127.

34. Peets, E. A., Henson, M. F., and Neri, R. (1974): On the mechanism of the antiandrogenic action of flutamide (α,α,α-trifluoro-2-methyl-4'-nitro-m-propionotoluidide) in the rat. *Endocrinology,* 94:532–540.

35. Roy, A. K., Milin, B. S., and McMinn, D. M. (1974): Androgen receptor in rat liver: Hormonal and developmental regulation of the cytoplasmic receptor and its correlation with the androgen-dependent synthesis of $\alpha_{2\mu}$-globulin. *Biochim. Biophys. Acta,* 354:213–232.

36. Stripp, B., Greene, F. E., and Gillette, J. R. (1971): Extinction coefficient for cytochrome P-450 in hepatic microsomes from male and female rats. *Pharmacology,* 6:56–64.

37. Swank, R. T., Paigen, K., and Ganschow, R. E. (1973): Genetic control of glucuronidase induction in mice. *J. Mol. Biol.,* 81:225–243.
38. Talcott, R. E. and Stohs, S. J. (1973): The effect of cyproterone acetate pretreatment on the in vitro metabolism of aniline, hexobarbital, and ^{3}H-digitoxigenin. *J. Pharmacol. Exp. Ther.,* 184: 419–423.
39. Vesell, E. S. (1968): Factors altering the responsiveness of mice to hexobarbital. *Pharmacology,* 1:81–97.
40. Vesell, E. S. (1968): Genetic and environmental factors affecting hexobarbital metabolism in mice. *Ann. NY Acad. Sci.,* 151:900–912.
41. Westfall, B. A., Boulos, B. M., Shields, J. L., and Garb, S. (1964): Sex differences in pentobarbital sensitivity in mice. *Proc. Soc. Exp. Biol. Med.,* 115:509–513.
42. Wood, A. W., and Conney, A. H. (1974): Genetic variation in coumarin hydroxylase activity in the mouse (Mus musculus). *Science,* 185:612–614.

Pharmacology of Steroid Contraceptive Drugs
edited by S. Garattini and H. W. Berendes.
Raven Press, New York © 1977.

Increased Metabolism of Estrogens during Rifampicin Treatment

Herbert Remmer, Hermann-Maximilian Bolt, Mechthild Bolt, and Hermann Kappus

Institute of Toxicology, University of Tübingen, D-7400 Tübingen, West Germany

Reimers and Ježek (12) reported in 1971 that women experienced an increased incidence of breakthrough bleeding and spotting when using oral contraceptives during antituberculosis therapy. A further study revealed that of 88 rifampicin-treated women taking oral contraceptives 5 became pregnant (9). The reason for this unexpected side effect of rifampicin was not clear. The authors speculated that rifampicin either interferes with the hormonal action of estrogens or gestagens or with their conversion in the liver. The latter mechanism seemed to be not very likely, because any real evidence for an interaction of rifampicin with the metabolism of drugs or hormones was lacking at the time the first observations were published.

Several results obtained when our group studied quite different problems shed light on this strange phenomenon. When testing the amount of enzymes involved in drug metabolism, and the hydroxylation rate of a model compound in liver biopsy samples from patients with different kinds of hepatic diseases, we found that these parameters were decreased only in a few cases with serious pathological alterations of the liver due to heavy cholestasis, considerable cell necrosis, or cirrhosis (15). For comparison we determined the activity of two other enzymes involved in drug metabolism but also located in the membranes of the endoplasmic reticulum (Fig. 1).

We had to limit the investigation, since not more than 20 mg of liver tissue could be provided by the clinician—who had performed the liver biopsy for diagnostic purposes and had sent the major portion to the pathologist for histological examinations. After developing suitable micromethods we were able to carry out five tests (Fig. 1) in addition to measurement of the protein content. In a first unselected trial we collected 33 liver biopsy samples from patients with normal parameters of drug metabolism in spite of the presence of indications for existing liver disease.

We classified the patients from whom we received the tissue into three groups. The first group was comprised of all those who took no drugs; and the second and third groups received common drugs for therapeutic purposes. The second group presented no signs of increased drug metabolism in their livers. However,

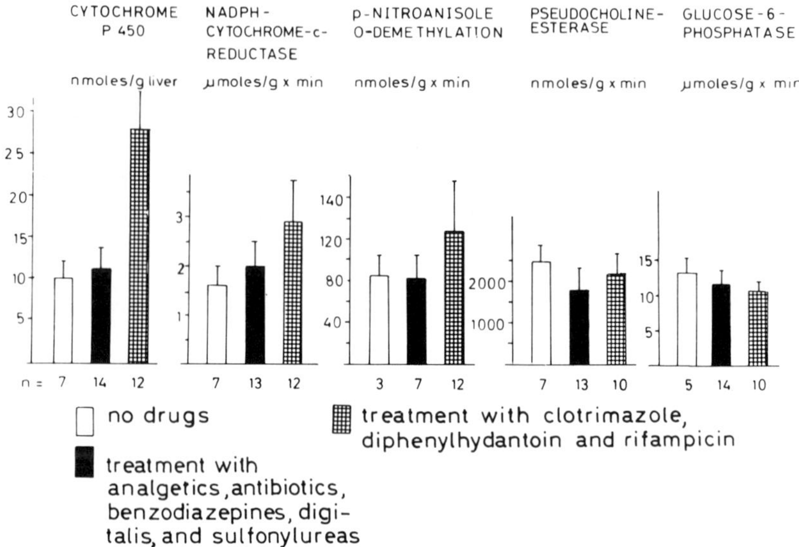

FIG. 1. Amount of cytochrome P-450 and activities of microsomal enzymes measured in the homogenate of liver biopsy samples.

the *in vitro* tests with biopsy samples from the third group indicated a typical induction of drug-metabolizing enzymes.

The high number (12 patients) with a more than twofold rise of cytochrome P-450 in their liver, but a minor increase of the activities concerning the accompanying reductase and oxidase, should not mislead us. In reality, the induction of drug-metabolizing enzymes in human liver during therapy is an unusual event. Incidentally, von Oldershausen, a liver specialist, has been interested in the extent to which antituberculosis agents prescribed for a long period of time, cause injury to the liver. He found very few cases, but we discovered that during antituberculosis therapy a considerable increase of cytochrome P-450 in the liver occurred almost regularly (13). After comparing patients treated with different schedules, it became apparent that all those receiving rifampicin belonged to this group. However, we were puzzled by the fact that the reductase, which provides reducing equivalents for the activation of molecular oxygen on the heme iron of cytochrome P-450, and the hydroxylation rate did not increase comparably. The results were not consistent with the values we observed in the liver of an epileptic treated with phenytoin and phenobarbital and two patients receiving an antimycotic drug, clotrimazol. In these three cases all parameters of drug metabolism increased, as we expected from animal experiments.

The livers of two patients treated exclusively with rifampicin reacted in a similar manner. A 2- or 2.5-fold increase of cytochrome P-450, but a much smaller and incompatible rise of reductase and the hydroxylation rate of *p*-nitroanisole, have been observed. *In vitro* results are meaningless if they cannot be confirmed *in vivo*. Therefore we tested the oxidation rate of monomethyl-aminoantipyrine in these two patients by determining the amount of the oxidative demethylated metabolite aminoantipyrine in the urine, collected over a 6-hr period after one injection of novaminsulfonum (15 mg/kg i.v.), a highly water-soluble drug closely related to aminopyrine. We observed no increase in the first patient and only 30% higher excretion of this metabolite in the other; we realized again that we were dealing with an unusual type of induction, one that is not accompanied by a comparably elevated drug hydroxylation.

In order to exclude any factor which might interfere with drug metabolism in the patient's liver (e.g., other drugs or nutritional compounds), we performed a trial, asking members of our institute to join as volunteers. In this study we also tried to assess the reliability of the *in vivo* test for drug oxidation, performing the determination twice before, once during, and three times after a 6-day treatment with rifampicin, 0.6 g daily (14).

The results were surprisingly much more reproducible than we had expected, taking into account all influences which may alter hydroxylation in the liver and excretion of the metabolite in the urine. Values in one individual did not vary more than 5%. Even the interindividual results did not differ by more than 10%.

During the treatment with rifampicin we observed no real change except in one subject who reacted with a 70% increase of the amount found as metabolite in the urine. However, 2–3 days after ending the intake of rifampicin metabolism was significantly enhanced, with an average increase of 60%. Probably a high concentration of rifampicin in the liver inhibits the hydroxylation rate, but this seems to be outbalanced by the inducing action of rifampicin. Inhibition of drug metabolism during induction is a well-known phenomenon, first observed during administration of phenobarbital. Two to three weeks after the impact of rifampicin on the liver, the amount of the hydroxylated metabolite in urine was normal, indicating that the small increase of the metabolic rate has disappeared.

Of course such a small rise in the oxidation of a compound should hardly interfere with the therapeutic effect. Only for drugs with a very low therapeutic index, which are hydroxylated to ineffective compounds, could a 50% rise of the metabolic rate lower the pharmacological action. Normally, however, differences like these do not alter the therapeutic effect because a sufficient margin of safety must be allowed when a therapeutic dose is recommended. Besides, individual pharmacodynamic or pharmacokinetic differences considerably exceed any small increase of drug metabolism like this.

The small, insignificant increase of drug oxidation is the reason we first refused to accept the concept that rifampicin reduces the effectiveness of contraceptive agents by activating their metabolism. This opinion seemed to be concordant with the fact that the number of women becoming pregnant while taking oral con-traceptives is practically insignificant, although probably millions use drugs si-multaneously with contraceptive compounds. Mention should be made of an-tiepileptics and higher doses of hypnotics, which are known to increase drug metabolism in the dosage range prescribed: Only 13 pregnancies among epileptic women taking contraceptive formulations regularly had been reported up to the end of 1974 (7).

The low incidence of failure due to inducers of the phenobarbital type contrasts with the high percentage of pregnancies during rifampicin treatment, 5 of 88 women using oral contraceptives. A crucial experiment clarified the divergency (3). Several patients who underwent surgical treatment because of gallbladder disease gave their consent for receiving 0.6 g rifampicin per day 6 days before the operation. A small piece of liver (not more than 0.5 g) was removed and microsomes prepared. They were incubated with estradiol (E) or ethynylestradiol (EE). Both substrates were tritiated either in position 2, 4, 6, and 7 or only at C6 and C7. We calculated the hydroxylation rate from the amount of tritium lost in the water of the incubation medium. The amount of ^3H removed from C6 and C7 was never higher than 5% of the total loss during incubation with the compound labeled in all four positions, indicating that C6 hydroxylation of estrogens by microsomal enzymes obviously plays no significant role as a metabolic step. Approximately 95% of the tritium is displaced from C2 and C4. Steric considerations speak against any reaction at C4. An exchange of T for H is very unlikely. However, it is well known that women excrete methylated 2-hydroxyethynylestradiol in urine (1). Furthermore, the enzymic system used contains a mono-oxygenase which converts ethynylestradiol and estradiol to the 2-hydroxy metabolites in rats (4). This reaction explains the loss of tritium.

Hydroxylation was achieved only if NADPH or an enzymic system was present which regenerates NADPH from NADP. The reaction could be almost completely inhibited by carbon monoxide and reduced by some compounds known for their inhibiting action on the cytochrome P-450-containing mono-oxygenase. These additional tests presented evidence that the 2-hydroxylase of estrogens is a cytochrome P-450-dependent enzyme.

The hydroxylation rate of EE is twice as high as that of E, showing that EE is a better substrate for this enzyme (Table 1). Most important and completely unexpected was the three- to sevenfold increase of the hydroxylation rate of both substrates with liver microsomes from patients pretreated with rifampicin.

It is now feasible that such a marked rise in the hydroxylation rate of ethynylestradiol prevents an effective level of this contraceptive agent from being reached in the organism, by oxidizing the compound too rapidly. Aromatic hydroxylation at the C2 position of estradiol is an important but not the main metabolic step

TABLE 1. *C2 hydroxylation of estradiol and ethynylestradiol by liver microsomes from untreated and rifampicin-treated patients[a]*

Patients	Estradiol	Ethynylestradiol
Controls (*N*-12)	120 ± 58	237 ± 104
Rifampicin-treated (*N*-4)	610 ± 180	$1,140 \pm 380$

Values in pmoles/mg protein × minutes.
[a] Rifampicin: 0.6 g/day for 6 days.

in the conversion of natural estrogens to ineffective compounds (Fig. 2). According to Fishman, 33% of estradiol uses this step in the human liver, whereas 55% is hydroxylated at 16α (6). However, derivatives of the natural hormone having an alkyl group in the α-position of C17, which prevents or strongly inhibits the hydroxylation at C17, are compelled to find another hydroxylating enzyme. Thus it is very likely that 2-hydroxylation of ethynylestradiol is the major route of metabolism *in vivo* as far as C17-alkylated compounds are concerned. The catechol formed is further transformed by the action of the COMT enzyme to 2- or 3-methyl ethers of 2-hydroxy ethynylestradiol (1). Of course, at each conversion level the parent compound or the metabolites may be conjugated either with glucuronic acid or sulfate. Any average fivefold increase of the hydroxylation rate at C2 of ethynylestradiol in patients treated with rifampicin should arise the overall metabolism of this contraceptive agent at least two- to threefold.

The disappearance rate of labeled ethynylestradiol (50 μg per subject) was demonstrated from plasma of patients before and after treatment with rifampicin. Two elimination phases could be distinguished; both were accelerated (2). During the second, slower phase the drug disappeared from plasma two to three times faster when the patients had been pretreated with rifampicin. Correspondingly

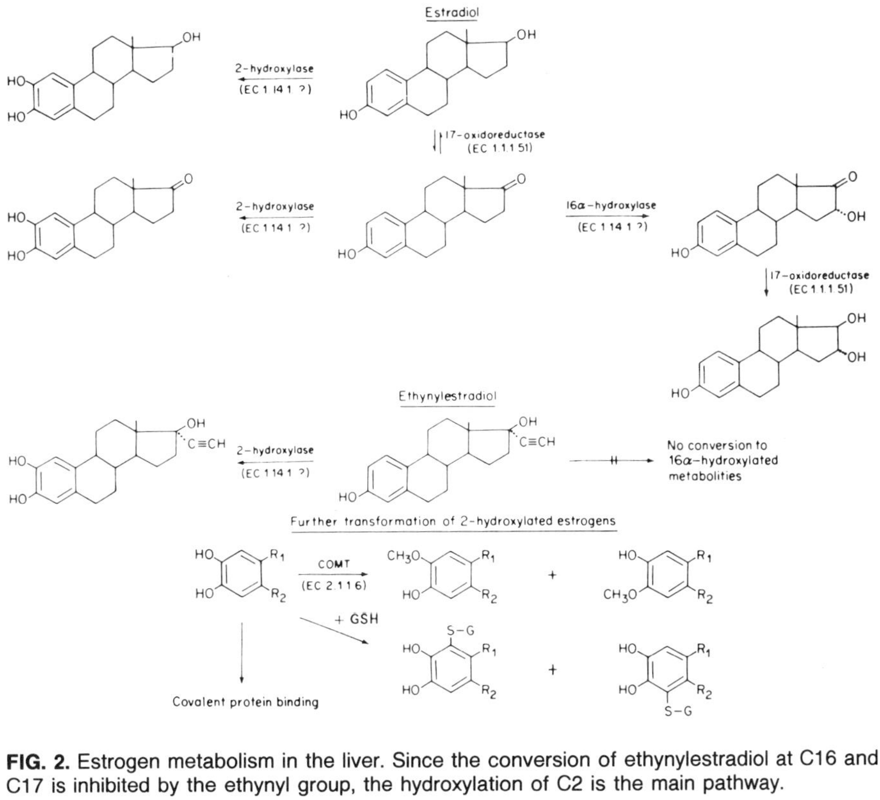

FIG. 2. Estrogen metabolism in the liver. Since the conversion of ethynylestradiol at C16 and C17 is inhibited by the ethynyl group, the hydroxylation of C2 is the main pathway.

lower were the plasma levels of ethynylestradiol in these subjects. A first-pass effect with diminished systemic bioavailability contributes to the rapid decline of EE, which behaves similarly to estradiol, which is more rapidly metabolized in the liver than EE and is therefore ineffective orally in a normal dosage range. Obviously the concentrations EE reaches in the plasma of patients treated with rifampicin are too low to sustain the contraceptive action. It is very likely that reducing the dose of the estrogenic component in the contraceptive formulation lowered the side effects but diminished the margin of safety. A decreased estrogenic dose leads to levels which become ineffective if further reduced considerably by an inducing agent.

When we observed rifampicin's powerful capacity to enhance the hydroxylation rate at position C2, we tried to confirm these results in animal experiments but were unsuccessful. All species we tested (mice, rats, and guinea pigs) failed to show that rifampicin induces cytochrome P-450 (10). In accordance with these results, drug hydroxylation also did not increase. Similar results have been obtained in experiments with rabbits. Only rats (not guinea pigs and mice) responded with a 50% rise of C2 hydroxylation after several days of pretreatment with rifampicin 25 mg/kg.

We interpret our divergent observations by assuming that the species man seems to be unique in that a considerable portion of cytochrome P-450 in the liver belongs to a form which is inducible by rifampicin and hydroxylates aromatic steroids at C2 preferentially. The other species tested seem not to possess this particular cytochrome P-450.

If the dose of rifampicin is increased, this compound is also able to stimulate drug hydroxylation in man (Table 2). This indicates either that other forms of cytochrome P-450 are induced concomitantly but to a much lesser extent, or that the rifampicin-inducible form may also have an affinity to drugs but a much smaller one, so that only a huge increase of this unknown cytochrome P-450 can cause a higher rate of drug oxidation.

That the rifampicin-induced cytochrome P-450 should be viewed as an excep-

TABLE 2. *Increase of drug metabolism in patients receiving Rifampicin*

| | | | | Ethynylestradiol | |
| | *In vivo* Aminopyrine hexobarbital | *In vitro* Hydroxylation rate | Cytochrome | | *In vivo* Elimination |
Rifampicin dose	tolbutamide (%)	(type I) (%)	P-450 (%)	*In vitro* C2 hydroxylation	rate
0.45	0	—	—	—	—
0.6	20–70	0–100	100–300	300–700	50–250
1.2	100–200	—	—	—	—

Adapted from Zilly et al. (1975): *Eur. J. Clin. Pharmacol.* 9:219–227.
There is no increase of cytochrome P-450 and the hydroxylation rate after pretreatment (1–6 days) with rifampicin (10–50 mg/kg) in mice, rats, and guinea pigs—except a 50% enhanced C2 hydroxylation of ethynylestradiol and estradiol, but only in rats.

tional form—probably more specific for steroid hydroxylation—can also be deduced from the fact that antiepileptic agents act contrary to rifampicin in that they increase steroid hydroxylation in women only weakly (as indicated by epidemiological investigations) but induce drug metabolism considerably. This agrees with rat experiments in which we found that high doses of phenobarbital never increased the C2 hydroxylation of estrogens more than 50–100% but induced drug metabolism much more effectively (4). It is unlikely that induction as high as in rats might be achieved in man, but even a doubling of the estrogen hydroxylation rate should fall in the variation range of drug metabolism and can be responsible for the ineffectiveness of contraceptive drugs only if exceptional circumstances prevail. A reduced dose might explain the first reports of failure of oral contraceptives in epileptic women in 1973.

It should be mentioned that rifampicin treatment decreases the digitoxin level in patients receiving this glycoside chronically. Its half-life in plasma decreased from 8.2 to 4.5 days (11). However, typical inducers of drug hydroxylations (e.g., phenobarbital) have also been reported to decrease the effectiveness of digitoxin in man.

Similarly, the therapeutically effective doses of anticoagulants—e.g., acenocoumarol (8) and glucocorticoids (5)—must be increased if patients receive rifampicin. Correspondingly, a 50–100% increase of cortisol production in man occurs if patients are treated with rifampicin. It may be that 6β-hydroxylation is stimulated considerably in all cases of rifampicin therapy, but the same is true if patients receive drugs known for their inducing action. It remains to be elucidated if the interactions of rifampicin with the metabolism of digitoxin, anticoagulants, and glucocorticoids occur because rifampicin increases drug hydroxylation in an unspecific manner or if the increased digitoxin and cortisol elimination rate may be related to the more specific inducing action of rifampicin on estrogens in which another form of cytochrome P-450 seems to be involved, possessing a higher affinity to steroids.

SUMMARY

Reimers and Ježek reported in 1971 that women experienced an increased incidence of breakthrough bleeding and spotting when taking oral contraceptives during antituberculosis therapy. Further study revealed that of 88 rifampicin-treated women taking oral contraceptives 5 became pregnant.

Concurrently investigators in our department found that among more than 50 liver examinations there were 15 with a considerably increased amount of cytochrome P-450 (50–250%). Only two of these patients had *not* received rifampicin. Surprisingly, the substrate hydroxylation (aminopyrine and *p*-nitroanisol) as well as the activity of the cytochrome-c-reductase were enhanced only slightly or not at all. *In vivo* studies with volunteers produced similar results. An unimportant increase of the drug hydroxylation rate (20–70%) cannot be the reason for the considerable loss of contraceptive activity during rifampicin therapy.

However, microsomes of liver samples removed during abdominal surgery from patients who received 0.6 g rifampicin daily before the operation were compared for their capacity to hydroxylate estradiol or ethynylestradiol at position 2 of the aromatic ring with the activity of liver microsomes from 12 untreated patients. We found a fivefold increased hydroxylation rate of estradiol and ethynylestradiol, explaining the lack of contraceptive activity. A first-pass effect with a diminished systemic availability may contribute to the rapid disappearance of ethynylestradiol, behaving similarly to estradiol, which is orally inactive.

The 2-hydroxy hydroxylation of aromatic steroids seems to be achieved by a special rifampicin-inducible type of cytochrome P-450 present in considerable amounts only in human but not in animal liver, which seems not to be involved in drug hydroxylation.

ACKNOWLEDGMENT

We are indebted to Professor von Oldershausen, Medizinische Klinik, Universität Tübingen, for his essential and encouraging support.

REFERENCES

1. Abdel-Aziz, M. T., and Williams, K. I. H. (1970): Metabolism of radioactive 17α-ethinylestradiol by women. *Steroids,* 15:695–710.
2. Bolt, H. M.: *Unpublished observations.*
3. Bolt, H. M., Kappus, H., and Bolt, M. (1975): Effect of rifampicin treatment on the metabolism of oestradiol and 17α-ethinyloestradiol by human liver microsomes. *Eur. J. Clin. Pharmacol.,* 8:301–307.
4. Bolt, H. M., Kappus, H., and Remmer, H. (1973): Studies on the metabolism of ethinylestradiol in vitro and in vivo: The significance of 2-hydroxylation and the formation of polar products. *Xenobiotica,* 3:773–785.
5. Edwards, O. M., Courtenay-Evans, R. J., Galley, J. M., Hunter, J., and Tait, A. D. (1974): Changes in cortisol metabolism following rifampicin therapy. *Lancet,* 2:549–551.
6. Fishman, J. (1976): Entry and Metabolism of Estrogens in the Brain. Symposium on the Pharmacology of Steroid Contraceptive Drugs, Milan.
7. Janz, D., and Schmidt, D. (1975): Antiepileptika und die Sicherheit oraler Kontrazeptiva. *Bibl. Psychiatr.,* 151:82.
8. Michot, F., Bürgi, M., and Büttner, J. (1970): Rimactan (Rifampicin) und Antikoagulantientherapie. *Schweiz. Med. Wochenschr.,* 100:583–584.
9. Nocke-Finck, L., Breuer, H., and Reimers, D. (1973): Wirkung von Rifampicin auf den Menstruationszyklus und die Östrogenausscheidung bei Einnahme oraler Kontrazeptiva. *Dtsch. Med. Wochenschr.,* 98:1521–1523.
10. Otani, G., Stohrer, F., Bolt, H. M., Kappus, H., and Remmer, H.: Unpublished observations.
11. Peters, U., Hausamen, T-U., and Grosse-Brockhoff, F. (1974): Einfluß von Tuberkulostatika auf die Pharmakokinetik des Digitoxins. *Dtsch. Med. Wochenschr.,* 99:2381–2386.
12. Reimers, D., and Ježek, A. (1971): Rifampicin und andere Antituberkulotika bei gleichzeitiger oraler Kontrazeption. *Prax. Pneumol,* 25:255–262.
13. Remmer, H., Schoene, B., and Fleischmann, R. A. (1973): Induction of the unspecific microsomal hydroxylase in the human liver. *Drug Metab. Dispos.,* 1:224–230.
14. Remmer, H., Schoene, B., and Reid, W.: Unpublished observations.
15. Schoene, B., Fleischmann, R. A., Remmer, H., and von Oldershausen, H. F. (1972): Determination of drug metabolizing enzymes in needle biopsies of human liver. *Eur. J. Clin. Pharmacol.,* 4:65–73.

Pharmacology of Steroid Contraceptive Drugs
edited by S. Garattini and H. W. Berendes.
Raven Press, New York © 1977.

Progestin Simulation and Alteration of Androgen Action in Rodent Tissues

Leslie P. Bullock, Yen Chiu Lin, Samson Jacob, and
C. Wayne Bardin

*Departments of Medicine, Pharmacology, and Comparative Medicine, The Milton S.
Hershey Medical Center, The Pennsylvania State University,
Hershey, Pennsylvania 17033*

The widespread use of progestins, alone and in combination with other agents, for fertility control in men and women has stimulated interest in the biological effects of these streoids. They are known to stimulate responses other than those associated with their gestagenic actions. Androgenic effects of progestins have been described for embryonic, immature, and adult animals and man. It should be noted, however, that the sensitivity and type of response varies with species, steroid, and endpoint tested. The variation in species response is well illustrated by the virilization of external genitalia that occurs in guinea pigs but not rats following cyproterone acetate treatment (23,35). Differences in streoid potency are evident in the minimal effects of progesterone and its C_{21} derivatives on male rat reproductive tract while progestins related to 19-nortestosterone stimulate these tissues (16,24,31,41). By contrast, progesterone and 19-nortestosterone derivatives masculinize the external genitalia of the female rat and hamster fetus (37,39,42). Structure-function differences exist even within classes of progestins as medroxyprogesterone acetate (MPA) is equipotent to testosterone propionate in the rat fetus (37,39) whereas the structurally similar megestrol acetate is inactive (13).

Progestins that are not androgenic may alter androgen action. For example, cyproterone acetate inhibits androgen response (35), an activity shared by other gestagens (14,15,32). Progestins may also enhance androgen action, as recently described by several investigators (11,30,34,36). As with the androgenic effects of progestins, the antiandrogenic and synandrogenic actions vary with the progestin and endpoint studied.

This chapter summarizes recent *in vivo* and *in vitro* studies on the androgenic, synandrogenic, and antiandrogenic actions of several C_{21} progestins in mice and rats. In contrast to many of the previous experiments on reproductive tissues, these studies focus primarily on responses in nonreproductive organs.

BIOLOGIC ACTIONS OF PROGESTINS

Androgenic Action of Progestins in the Mouse

KIDNEY

Androgens increased organ weight and stimulated RNA and general protein synthesis in mouse kidney (20,29,44). They also induced an increase in the specific activity of several proteins, including β-glucuronidase, alcohol dehydrogenase, arginase (40), and 3-ketosteroid reductase (33). The progestin MPA also stimulated kidney weight and produced a significant dose-dependent increase in all four enzymes (34; L. P. Bullock, *unpublished observation*). When other C_{21} progestins were tested for their ability to increase β-glucuronidase activity, megestrol acetate was less active and progesterone and progesterone caproate had no effect. Although cyproterone acetate was usually inactive, in three of nine studies it produced a slight increase in enzyme activity which was not dose-dependent (34). The variable response of mouse kidney to several progestins with similar structures remains to be explained.

Since one of the early effects of testosterone on mouse kidney was an increase in RNA polymerase I and II activities (26), we thought it pertinent to compare this response to androgen with that to MPA. RNA polymerase I and II activities were therefore measured in whole nuclei at various times following steroid administration (Table 1). Testosterone and MPA produced an early rise in the activity of both enzymes, which declined and then increased again without further steroid treatment. Although both steroids produced a biphasic response, further

TABLE 1. *Comparative effects of MPA and testosterone on RNA polymerase I and II activities of mouse kidney*

Treatment time (hr)	MPA[a]		Testosterone	
	RNA polymerase		RNA polymerase	
	I	II	I	II
0	100[b]	100	100	100
0.25	103	117	120	160
0.5	142	133	120	142
1	171	156	135	158
2	160	153	150	110
4	165	185	115	80
12	55	87	150	140
20	353	111	180	122
24	135	99	—	—
28	286	90	155	105

[a] Mice were given MPA (10 mg) or testosterone (1 mg) subcutaneously, and RNA polymerase activities were measured in renal nuclei as previously described (26).
[b] The changes in the RNA polymerase activities are expressed as percent of controls.

experiments are required to determine if the absolute time pattern of response to both steroids is similar.

SUBMAXILLARY GLAND

Androgens also increased the weight and the RNA and protein synthesis in mouse submaxillary gland (12,27). Epidermal growth factor (6) is one of several specific proteins that increase in specific activity in response to testosterone treatment. Administration of MPA simulated the androgen-induced response of this protein. Megestrol acetate and progesterone also produced an increase in epidermal growth factor, but the responses were small and only the megestrol acetate response appeared to be dose-dependent. As in the kidney, in some experiments a small variable response to cyproterone acetate was detected (9).

OTHER TISSUES

The androgenic effects of progestins on mouse preputial gland and prostate seminal vesicles have been studied less extensively. Of the agents evaluated, only MPA stimulated preputial gland weight (34). This steroid also increased both weight and epithelial cell activity in seminal vesicles of castrated, immature mice (10).

Androgens have been shown to stimulate mouse hepatic ethylmorphine N-demethylase as well as total microsomal protein. The progestins cyproterone acetate, MPA, and progesterone also elicit similar responses. However, the fact that these progestins stimulate a similar response in androgen-insensitive tfm/y mice suggests that these actions of progestins should not be classified as androgenic but are apparently mediated by a separate mechanism. Interestingly, MPA, more potent than progesterone in stimulating the uterus, was less effective in stimulating ethylmorphine N-demethylase activity. This suggests that these hepatic actions of progestins are also not related to their progestational function. These observations are discussed in more detail by Brown et al. elsewhere in this volume.

Androgenic Action of Progestins in the Rat

Preputial glands in the rat responded to both androgens and progestins with an increase in RNA, DNA, and protein synthesis (25,38). In addition, specific enzyme synthesis was stimulated as evidenced by the increase in β-glucuronidase activity. Progesterone and androgens also influence hepatic drug-metabolizing enzymes in rats (3,8,17). However, it is not known if these responses are mediated by similar mechanisms.

Action of Progestins in Androgen-Insensitive Animals

Male mice and rats with the tfm mutation have an inherited end-organ insensitivity to androgens. In these animals large doses of androgens did not produce the increases in organ weight or specific protein activity observed in normal animals (4,6). In tfm/y mice, MPA, as well as progesterone and cyproterone acetate, were ineffective in stimulating androgenic responses (9,34). In androgen-insensitive tfm rats, neither testosterone nor progesterone produced a preputial gland response (weight or β-glucuronidase activity) similar to that observed in normal animals (38). The insensitivity of tfm mice and rats to androgens and progestins suggests that in some organs the actions of these steroids are mediated via a common mechanism.

Combined Actions of Testosterone and Progestins

The actions of testosterone plus cyproterone acetate, MPA, megestrol acetate, progesterone caproate, or progesterone were compared in several tissues of male and female mice (34). The basic protocol consisted of groups of mice treated daily for 6 days with 0.1 mg testosterone alone or in combination with 0.1–10 mg progestin.

KIDNEY

At low doses cyproterone acetate and megestrol acetate enhanced the action of testosterone on mouse kidney (Fig. 1). This unexpected response was seen consistently when the experiment was repeated. It was also evident when a 3-day study was performed with a similar ratio but greater doses of testosterone (1 mg) and cyproterone acetate (5 mg). This suggests that the ratio of androgen to progestin may be an important determinant of synandrogenic activity. Low doses of megestrol acetate also synergized with testosterone. As the progestin/androgen ratio was increased, cyproterone acetate and megestrol acetate exhibited inhibitory effects, whereas a synandrogenic action was seen with MPA and progesterone caproate. The synandrogenic response induced by testosterone plus MPA or megestrol acetate was greater than if the androgenic responses had only been additive.

The interaction of androgens and progestins on another renal androgen responsive enzyme, 3-ketoreductase, was also examined. Both MPA and progesterone caproate potentiated androgen action on this enzyme. Megestrol acetate had no effect, and cyproterone acetate was not examined. In addition, Ohno and Lyon (36) reported potentiation by cyproterone acetate of testosterone-stimulated renal alcohol dehydrogenase. The latter observations provide evidence that the synandrogenic action of progestins is not limited to the product of a single gene.

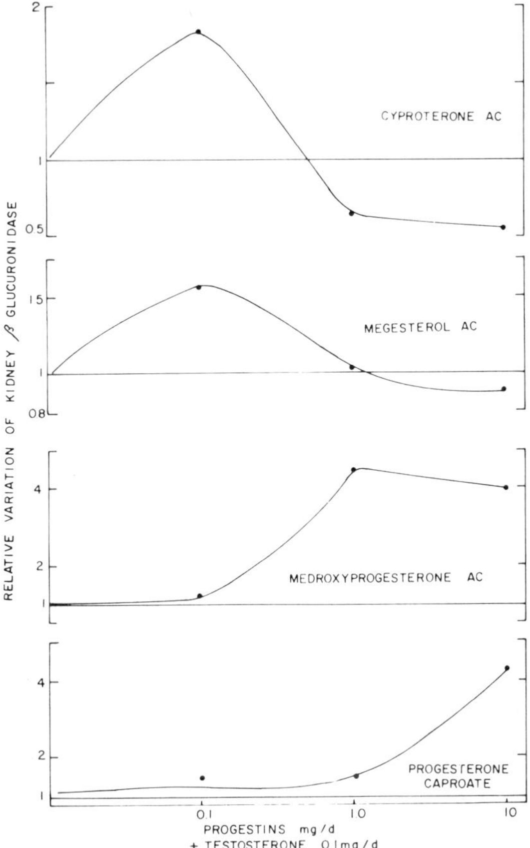

FIG. 1. Syn- and antiandrogenic effects of progestins on mouse kidney β-glucuronidase. For each steroid, the enzyme activity induced by 0.1 mg testosterone alone is taken as 1. The subsequent enzyme activity achieved when testosterone was combined with various doses of each progestin is shown relative to this normalized value. Groups of five female mice were treated daily for 6 days. (From Mowszowicz et al., ref. 34.)

Since some progestins were both syn- and antiandrogenic, it was of interest to see if androgen action could also be enhanced by low doses of nonprogestational antiandrogens. Two steroidal (cyproterone, BOMT) and one nonsteroidal (flutamide) compounds were studied. These three agents did not potentiate androgen-stimulated renal β-glucuronidase activity, and only flutamide had a significant inhibitory effect. This was despite the simultaneous demonstration of antiandrogenic activity on prostate-seminal vesicles by all three compounds. These studies suggest that the *in vivo* synandrogenic activity of progestins is associated with a progestational structure-function relationship whereas antiandrogenic activity is not (34).

SUBMAXILLARY GLANDS

In contrast to the synandrogenic response elicited by several progestins in mouse kidney, in submaxillary gland only progesterone caproate produced this effect. Cyproterone acetate was antiandrogenic even when administered at an equal ratio to testosterone. Progesterone and megestrol acetate were weakly antiandrogenic at the highest ratio used (9).

PREPUTIAL GLAND

The response of the preputial gland to combinations of testosterone and progestins was similar to that of submaxillary gland. Only progesterone caproate had a synandrogenic effect. Both cyproterone acetate and megestrol acetate acted as antiandrogens (34).

PROSTATE-SEMINAL VESICLES

Male accessory sex tissue is the usual target organ examined in studies of the antiandrogenic effects of high doses of cyproterone acetate. It was of interest to determine if a synandrogenic response could be elicited in this tissue when progestin/androgen ratios were used that were synandrogenic in other organs. When such an experiment was performed, cyproterone acetate inhibited testosterone stimulation of prostate-seminal vesicle weight despite a simultaneous synandrogenic action on renal β-glucuronidase activity. It is not known if this represents a qualitative difference in the mechanism of hormone action or a difference in endpoint responsiveness (34).

RAT PROSTATE

Progestins can also enhance androgen action on rat prostate. Carter et al. (11) found that cyproterone acetate increased the response of rat prostate DNA polymerase to three daily doses of testosterone if progestin was given 18 hr before animals were killed. If given earlier, cyproterone acetate acted as an antiandrogen. Cyproterone enhancement of testosterone-stimulated growth of rat prostate in organ culture was reported by Lasnitzki et al. (30).

From these studies it is evident that progestins are capable of altering androgen action on multiple endpoints in different tissues. However, the response elicited is tissue- and steroid-specific, as well as dependent on the progestin/androgen ratio used.

MECHANISM OF ANDROGENIC ACTION OF PROGESTINS

Although it is possible that the different actions of progestins involve separate molecular mechanisms, it would be satisfying to account for all of these actions by a common pathway. The fact that progestins with androgenic, synandrogenic, and antiandrogenic effects bind to androgen receptors (10,18,28) suggests that these actions may be mediated via this protein. The insensitivity of two species of tfm animals, lacking androgen receptors, to androgens and the androgenic effects of progestins supports this hypothesis.

To elucidate further the interactions of progestins and the androgen receptor, ^{3}H-medroxyprogesterone acetate (^{3}H-MPA) was synthesized (19), and a series of *in vivo* and *in vitro* studies were done using this ^{3}H-steroid (10). These studies are described below.

In Vivo Nuclear Uptake of ^{3}H-MPA

MOUSE

To determine if MPA, like testosterone, is concentrated by nuclei of androgen-responsive tissues, ^{3}H-MPA was administered intravenously to castrated, functionally hepatectomized mice. Low-capacity retention of unmetabolized ^{3}H-MPA was demonstrated in purified kidney, prostate-seminal vesicle, and submaxillary gland nuclei (Table 2). The role of the androgen receptor as a mediator of this nuclear retention was suggested by: (a) Inhibition of nuclear concentration of ^{3}H-MPA by excess dihydrotestosterone. (b) Suppression of nuclear uptake of ^{3}H-androgen by excess MPA. MPA blocked nuclear androgen accumulation irrespective of whether the predominant steroid was testosterone, as in kidney and submaxillary gland, or dihydrotestosterone, as in prostate-seminal vesicle. (c) The absence of nuclear concentration of ^{3}H-MPA in nuclei of tfm/y mice.

RAT

Since MPA was androgenic in the rat, studies similar to those described above were repeated in this species. Results suggest that, as in the mouse, MPA was

TABLE 2. *Nuclear concentration of ^{3}H-MPA in androgen target tissues of the mouse* [a]

Steroid administered	Route	No. of experiments	^{3}H-MPA (cpm/10^7 nuclei)		
			Kidney	Prostate-seminal vesicle	Submaxillary gland
^{3}H-MPA	i.v.	6	124	1,338	392
^{3}H-MPA	s.c.	3	46	710	91
^{3}H-MPA + MPA	s.c.	3	17	120	35

[a] ^{3}H-MPA (60 μCi) $\pm$ 50-fold excess unlabeled MPA was administered to castrated, functionally eviscerated male Balb/C mice 30 min before kill. Nuclear steroid (^{3}H-MPA) was extracted from purified nuclei by organic solvent and purified by thin-layer chromatography. Tissues from three mice were pooled for each experiment (10).

TABLE 3. *Nuclear concentration of ^{3}H-MPA in androgen target tissues of the rat*[a]

Steroid administered	No. of experiments	^{3}H-MPA (cpm/10[7] nuclei)	
		Prostate	Seminal vesicle
[3]H-MPA	6	401	749
[3]H-MPA + MPA	2	102	128

[a] Conditions were the same as in Table 1 except 150 μCi ^{3}H-MPA was administered intravenously (10).

specifically bound *in vivo* by the androgen receptor in prostate and seminal vesicles (Table 3).

In Vitro Binding of Progestins

[3]H-MPA was bound by macromolecules in mouse kidney cytosol which cosedimented with testosterone in the 8S region of surose gradients (Fig. 2) (5). Androgen, estrogen, and progestins abolished ^{3}H-MPA binding, whereas the glucocorticoid dexamethasone had no effect. This specificity was similar to that reported for ^{3}H-testosterone binding by the androgen receptor (7). In addition, unlabeled MPA inhibited 8S binding of ^{3}H-testosterone. ^{3}H-MPA and ^{3}H-testosterone binding was also compared in kidney cytosol from tfm/y mice and their normal littermates. Similar amounts of the two steroids were bound by 8S macromolecules in cytosol from males and females. By contrast, there was no evidence of 8S binding in kidney cytosol from tfm/y mice. These findings support the hypothesis, suggested by *in vivo* studies, that MPA is bound by the androgen receptor in mouse kidney. The ability of another progestin, cyproterone acetate,

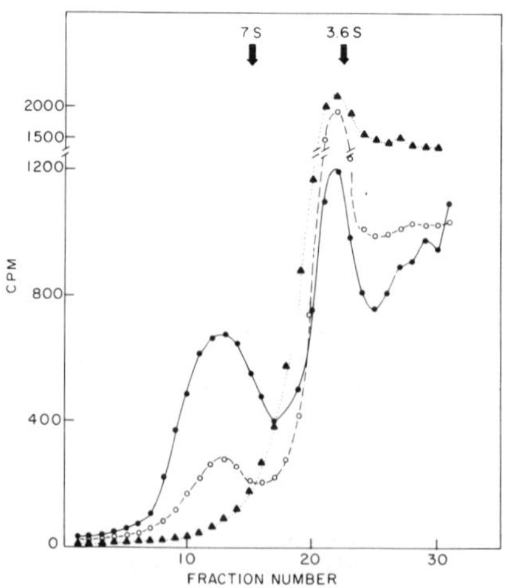

FIG. 2. ^{3}H-testosterone (●) and ^{3}H-MPA 2 nm (○) binding in kidney cytosol from normal mice. ^{3}H-testosterone plus MPA 200 nm (▲). No specific binding of either ^{3}H-steroid was demonstrated in kidney cytosol from androgen-insensitive (tfm/y) mice (not shown). (From Bardin et al., ref. 5.)

to bind to androgen receptors in mouse kidney (7,10) and other tissues (18,28) has been well documented.

Progestins are thus bound by androgen receptors in multiple tissues, and this interaction can account for their androgenic and antiandrogenic effects. The mechanism by which progestins synergize with testosterone, or how a tissue determines which of these actions is to be manifested, remains to be elucidated.

Nonreceptor-Mediated Effects of Progestins

Although our studies have dealt with the effects of progestins that are mediated through the androgen receptor of target organs, progestins may also affect androgen action in indirect ways. These have not been discussed specifically in this chapter, but they should be considered in assessing progestin alteration of androgen response. Progestins may reduce gonadotropin levels in rats (T. Worgul, *unpublished observation*) and man (2,43), which in intact animals may affect androgen action by reducing end-organ androgen concentration. Progestins may also decrease androgen effects by increasing androgen metabolic clearance rates (22). MPA treatment has been associated with an elevation of hepatic Δ^4-steroid reductase activity in rats and man (1,21,22). Within different tissues, steroid metabolism and various degrees of sensitivity may also modulate the final response.

SUMMARY

In addition to their action on uterus and vagina, progestins exert diverse metabolic effects on a variety of tissues. These actions include androgenic, synandrogenic, and antiandrogenic effects of androgen-responsive tissues of rats and mice. The androgenic and antiandrogenic effects of progestins have been demonstrated in multiple tissues. These actions appear to be mediated via the androgen receptor. A synandrogenic effect of progestins has also been detected in some tissues. However, there are few data to indicate how this response is mediated. Progestins may also affect androgen action indirectly through changes in steroid synthesis and metabolism. The overall biologic effect of a steroid may thus be determined by the sum of its actions on a variety of tissues.

ACKNOWLEDGMENTS

We wish to acknowledge the secretarial assistance of Marlene Brinser and Susan Keller. We also wish to thank the Upjohn, Hoffmann-LaRoche, Mead Johnson, Schering AG (Berlin, Germany), and Merrell-National companies for kindly providing the drugs used in this study. This study was supported by NIH Grant No. HDO5276 and NIH Contract No. NO1-2-2730.

REFERENCES

1. Altman, K., Gordon, G. G., Southren, A. L., Vittek, J., and Wilker, S. (1972): *Endocrinology,* 90:1252–1260.
2. Angeli, A., Boccuzzi, G., Bisbocci, D., Fonzo, D., Frajria, R., de Sanctis, C., and Ceresa, F. (1976): *J. Clin. Endocrinol. Metab.,* 42:551–560.
3. Bardin, C. W., Bullock, L. P., Schneider, G., Allison, J. E., and Stanley, A. J. (1970): *Science,* 167:1136–1137.
4. Bardin, C. W., Bullock, L. P., Sherins, R. J., Mowszowicz, I., and Blackburn, W. R. (1973): *Recent Prog. Horm. Res.,* 29:65–109.
5. Bardin, C. W., Janne, O., Bullock, L. P., and Jacob, S. T. (1975): Physicochemical and biological properties of androgen receptors. In: *Hormonal Regulation of Spermatogenesis,* edited by F. S. French, V. Hansson, E. M. Ritzen, and S. N. Nayfeh, pp. 237–255. Plenum Press, New York.
6. Barthe, P. L., Bullock, L. P., Mowszowicz, I., Bardin, C. W., and Orth, D. N. (1974): *Endocrinology,* 95:1019–1025.
7. Bullock, L. P., and Bardin, C. W. (1974): *Endocrinology,* 94: 746–756.
8. Bullock, L. P., Bardin, C. W., Gram, T. E., Schroeder, D. H., and Gillette, J. R. (1971): *Endocrinology,* 88:1521–1524.
9. Bullock, L. P., Barthe, P. L., Mowszowicz, I., Orth, D. N., and Bardin, C. W. (1975): *Endocrinology,* 97:189–195.
10. Bullock, L. P., Sherman, M. R., and Bardin, C. W. (1976): *Endocrinology (in press).*
11. Carter, M. F., Chung, L. W. K., and Coffey, D. S. (1972): The temporal requirements for androgens during the cell cycle of the prostate gland. In: *Urological Research,* edited by L. R. King and G. P. Murphy, pp. 27–38. Plenum Press, New York.
12. Charreau, E. H. (1969): *Acta Physiol. Lat. Am.,* 19:188–195.
13. David, A., Edwards, K., Fellowes, K. P., and Plummer, J. M. (1963): *J. Reprod. Fertil.,* 5: 331–346.
14. Dorfman, R. I. (1965): In: *Methods in Hormone Research, Vol. IV,* edited by R. I. Dorfman, pp. 77–93. Academic Press, New York.
15. Dorfman, R. I. (1970): *Br. J. Dermatol.,* 82:3–8.
16. Edgren, R. A., Jones, R. C., and Peterson, D. L. (1967); *Fertil. Steril.,* 18:238–256.
17. Fahim, M. S., and Hall, D. G. (1970); *Am. J. Obstet. Gynecol.,* 106:183–186.
18. Fang, S., Anderson, K. M., and Liao, S. (1969): *J. Biol. Chem.,* 244:6584–6595.
19. Feil, P. D., Miljkovic, M., and Bardin, C. W. (1976): *Endocrinology,* 98:1508–1515.
20. Frieden, E. H., and Ku, C. (1971): *Proc. Soc. Exp. Biol. Med.,* 137:1110–1144.
21. Gordon, G. G., Altman, K., Southren, A. L., and Olivo, J. (1971): *J. Clin. Endocrinol. Metab.,* 32:457–461.
22. Gordon, G. G., Southren, A. L., Tochimoto, S., Olivo, J., Altman, K., Rand, J., and Lemberger, L. (1970): *J. Clin. Endocrinol. Metab.,* 30:449–456.
23. Graf, K-J., Kleinecke, R-L., and Neumann, F. (1974): *J. Reprod. Fertil.,* 39:311–320.
24. Greene, R. R., Burrill, M. W., and Ivy, A. C. (1939): *Endocrinology,* 24:351–357.
25. Huggins, C., Parsons, F. M., and Jensen, E. V. (1955): *Endocrinology,* 57:25–32.
26. Janne, O., Bullock, L. P., Bardin, C. W., and Jacob, S. T. (1976): *Biochim. Biophys. Acta,* 418:330–343.
27. Junqueira, L. C., Fajer, A., Rabinovitch, M., and Frankenthal, L. (1949): *J. Cell. Comp. Physiol.,* 34:129–158.
28. King, R. J. B., and Mainwaring, W. I. P.: In: *Steroid-Cell Interactions,* edited by R. J. B. King and W. I. P. Mainwaring. University Park Press, Baltimore.
29. Kochakian, C. D. (1969): *Gen. Comp. Endocrinol.,* 13:146–150.
30. Lasnitzki, I., and Robel, P. (1969): Effects of cyproterone on the rat prostate gland grown in organ culture. In: *Advances in the Biosciences,* Vol. 3, edited by G. Raspe, pp. 175–184. Pergamon Press, Vieweg.
31. Lyster, S. C., Lund, G. H., Dulin, W. E., and Stafford, R. O. (1959): *Proc. Soc. Exp. Biol. Med.,* 100:540–543.
32. McKinney, G. R., and Braselton, J. P. (1970): *Steroids,* 15:405–411.
33. Mowszowicz, I., and Bardin, C. W. (1974): *Steroids,* 23:793–807.
34. Mowszowicz, I., Bieber, D. E., Chung, K. W., Bullock, L. P., and Bardin, C. W. (1974): *Endocrinology,* 95:1589–1599.

35. Neumann, F., von Berswordt-Wallrabe, R., Elger, W., Steinbeck, H., Hahn, J. D., and Kramer, M. (1970): *Recent Prog. Horm. Res.,* 26:337–410.
36. Ohno, S., and Lyon, M. F. (1970): *Clin. Genet.,* 1:121–127.
37. Revesz, C., Chappel, C. I., and Gaudry, R. (1960); *Endocrinology,* 66:140–144.
38. Sherins, R. J., and Bardin, C. W. (1971): *Endocrinology,* 89:835–841.
39. Suchowsky, G. K., and Junkmann, K. (1961): *Endocrinology,* 61:341–349.
40. Swank, R. T., Paigen, K., and Ganschow, R. E. (1973): *J. Mol. Biol.,* 81:225–243.
41. Tisell, L-E., and Salander, H. (1975): *Acta Endocrinol. (Kbh.),* 78:316–324.
42. Vomachka, A. J., Paup, D. C., Coniglio, L. P., McManus, M. J., and Clemens, L. G. (1974): *J. Reprod. Fertil.,* 37:269–276.
43. Warren, M. P., Mathews, J. H., Morishima, A., and Vande Wiele, R. (1975): *Am. J. Med. Sci.,* 269:375–381.
44. Yamanaka, H., Furuya, N., Shimazaki, J., and Shida, K. (1969): *Endocrinol. Jap.,* 16:29–34.

Subject Index